Handbook of Neurology

Handbook of Neurology

Charles Warlow

BA, MB, BChir, MD, FRCP (London), FRCP (Edinburgh)
Professor of Medical Neurology
Department of Clinical Neurosciences
University of Edinburgh

OXFORD

Blackwell Scientific Publications

LONDON EDINBURGH BOSTON

MELBOURNE PARIS BERLIN VIENNA

© 1991 by
Blackwell Scientific Publications
Editorial Offices:
Osney Mead, Oxford OX2 0EL
25 John Street, London WC1N 2BL
23 Ainslie Place, Edinburgh EH3 6AJ
3 Cambridge Center, Cambridge
  Massachusetts 02142, USA
54 University Street, Carlton
  Victoria 3053, Australia

Other Editorial Offices:
Arnette SA
2, rue Casimir-Delavigne
75006 Paris
France

Blackwell Wissenschaft
Meinekestrasse 4
D-1000 Berlin 15
Germany

Blackwell MZV
Feldgasse 13
A-1238 Wien
Austria

First published 1991

Set by Excel Typesetters, Hong Kong
Printed and bound in Great Britain
by Hartnolls Ltd, Bodmin, Cornwall

DISTRIBUTORS

  Marston Book Services Ltd
  PO Box 87
  Oxford OX2 0DT
  (*Orders*: Tel: 0865 791155
          Fax: 0865 791927
          Telex: 837515)

USA
  Mosby-Year Book, Inc.
  11830 Westline Industrial Drive
  St Louis, Missouri 63146
  (*Orders*: Tel: 800 633-6699)

Canada
  Mosby-Year Book, Inc.
  5240 Finch Avenue East
  Scarborough, Ontario
  (*Orders*: Tel: 416 298-1588)

Australia
  Blackwell Scientific Publications
  (Australia) Pty Ltd
  54 University Street
  Carlton, Victoria 3053
  (*Orders*: Tel: 03 347-0300)

British Library
Cataloguing in Publication Data

Warlow, Charles
  Handbook of neurology.
  1. Medicine, neurology
  I. Title
  616.8

  ISBN 0–632–01113–0

This book is dedicated to the Neurology Junior Staff who keep the show on the road; if they learn half as much from reading it as I did from writing it, I shall be well pleased

Contents

Acknowledgements

I would like to acknowledge my debt to the University of Edinburgh who allowed me a sabbatical period to get this book finished and to the neurologists in Auckland, New Zealand, who gave me a place to write it in which was far enough away to make it difficult for the time to be eroded.

I would also like to thank the friends, colleagues and teachers who commented on parts of the manuscript at various times during its gestation. When writing this handbook I did not believe that I could allow myself the luxury of too many 'ifs, buts and maybes' and I wanted to be sure that my more dogmatic recommendations were acceptable to those more expert in various fields of neurology than myself:

Dr John Bamford
Dr David Bates
Dr David Chadwick
Professor Alastair Compston
Dr Roger Cull
Dr Richard Greenhall
Dr Graeme Hankey
Professor Michael Harrison
Ms Shona Henderson
Dr David Hilton-Jones
Dr John Hodges
Dr Richard Knight
Professor Harold Lambert

Dr Andrew Lees
Professor Douglas Miller
Dr Pauline Monro
Professor John Newsom-Davis
Dr Michael O'Brien
Dr David Parkes
Dr Peter Sandercock
Dr Robin Sellar
Dr John Taylor
Dr David Thrush
Dr Chris Ward
Dr Bob Will

I am extremely grateful to the several secretaries who toiled with the manuscript over the years — June Gillam, Vanessa Langsbury, the late Joan Lennie, Jan Mackenzie, Jill Ratcliff and Helen Storey.

Finally, I would like to thank my family for their tolerance and for keeping out of the way for most of the time, particularly the children.

C.W.

Common abbreviations

AIDS	Acquired immune deficiency syndrome
BIH	Benign intracranial hypertension
BP	Blood pressure
CK	Creatine kinase
CNS	Central nervous system
CSF	Cerebrospinal fluid
CT	Computerized tomography
CXR	Chest X-ray
EEG	Electroencephalogram
EM	Electronmicroscopy
EMG	Electromyography
EP	Evoked potential
GCS	Glasgow coma score
ICP	Intracranial pressure
LP	Lumbar puncture
MRI	Magnetic resonance imaging
PICH	Primary intracerebral haemorrhage
SAH	Subarachnoid haemorrhage
SXR	Skull X-ray
TIA	Transient ischaemic attack

Introduction

Clinical neurology is to do with the diagnosis and care of patients with symptoms and disorders of the nervous system. This is far more than what consultant neurologists do with their day since, in the UK, each one covers a population of 150 000 to 600 000. And yet about 20% of all medical admissions to hospital are 'neurological' (e.g. stroke, epilepsy) and neurological symptoms, if not identifiable disorders, account for about 10% of contacts with general practitioners (e.g. headache, memory loss, dizziness, weakness). Indeed, it is obvious from the incidence (Table 1) and prevalence (Table 2) of various neurological conditions that neurologists cannot possibly see anything like all the patients presenting with neurological disease, as well as those who have no identifiable diagnosis but who are referred to them, and be responsible for more than a tiny fraction of their long-term management. Even to see each neurologically disabled patient once a year a consultant neurologist would have to see about 28 every working day. Therefore it is hardly surprising that most consultant neurologists in the UK must concentrate on the diagnosis of rare neurological disorders and common neurological disorders presenting in unusual ways, the management of the rare disorders themselves along with a small proportion of the common ones, trying to give advice on the management of all the rest, and teaching.

Since most neurological conditions are dealt with by non-neurologists (general practitioners, general physicians, geriatricians), medical students and others must learn the basic principles of making a neurological diagnosis, how to alleviate neurological disability and manage a few common disorders such as migraine, stroke, epilepsy and Parkinson's disease, and when to refer to a neurologist or neurosurgeon. This basic approach is important since many neurological disorders (and Tables 1 and 2 are far from exhaustive) are rare, so rare that general practitioners will not see more than one new case in their professional lifetime and yet some are treatable (e.g. polymyositis, myasthenia gravis). General practitioners will not even have a patient in their practice with some conditions and may therefore have insufficient experience to provide really good management (e.g. for motor neurone disease, Huntington's disease).

This handbook contains the sort of advice that a non-neurologist would expect to get from a neurologist and is meant to be consulted by specialists in other fields, neurologists in training, general practitioners and perhaps medical students. Even consultant neurologists might want to sneak a look at it if only to discover a mistake. It does not contain much in the way of

Table 1 The approximate incidence of some neurological disorders in the UK

	New patients per 100 000 population per annum	Number of new cases per consultant neurologist per annum[*]	Number of years between two new cases for each general practitioner[†]
Migraine (p. 137)	250	700	0.2
Stroke (p. 206)	200	560	0.25
Acute lumbar disc (p. 326)	150	420	0.33
Carpal tunnel syndrome (p. 372)	100	280	0.5
Non-febrile seizures (p. 66)	50	140	1
Transient ischaemic attack (p. 219)	35	98	1.4
Bell's palsy (p. 191)	25	70	2
Essential tremor (p. 294)	25	70	2
Parkinson's disease (p. 280)	20	56	2.5
Cerebral metastasis (p. 276)	15	42	3.3
Subarachnoid haemorrhage (p. 228)	15	42	3.3
Benign intracranial tumour (p. 266)	10	28	5
Bacterial meningitis (p. 491)	10	28	5
Malignant cerebral tumour (p. 266)	5	14	10
Giant cell arteritis (p. 450)	5	14	10
Trigeminal neuralgia (p. 145)	5	14	10
Multiple sclerosis (p. 341)	5	14	10
Guillain–Barré syndrome (p. 398)	2	6	25
Neuralgic amyotrophy (p. 368)	1.6	4	31
Motor neurone disease (p. 357)	1.5	4	33
Polymyositis (p. 434)	0.5	1	100
Syringomyelia (p. 334)	0.4	1	125
Myasthenia gravis (p. 407)	0.4	1	125
Huntington's disease (p. 298)	0.4	1	125
Herpes simplex encephalitis (p. 498)	0.2	<1	250
Tuberculosis of the nervous system (p. 512)	0.2	<1	250
Acute thoracic disc (p. 326)	0.1	<1	500
Creutzfeldt–Jakob disease (p. 531)	0.1	<1	500
Tetanus (p. 518)	0.06	<1	833
Subacute sclerosing panencephalitis (p. 525)	0.04	<1	1250
Cryptococcal meningitis (p. 533)	0.02	<1	2500

[*] Approximately 200 consultant neurologists in the UK, population 56 million.
[†] Approximate list size 2000.

Table 2 The approximate prevalence of some neurological disorders in the UK

	Patients per 100 000 population	Number of patients per neurologist[*]	Number of patients per general practitioner[†]
All physical neurological disability	2000	5600	40
Migraine (severe) (p. 137)	2000	5600	40
Stroke (p. 206)	800	2240	16
Active epilepsy (p. 66)	500	1400	10
Essential tremor (p. 294)	300	840	6
Parkinson's disease (p. 280)	150	420	3
Multiple sclerosis (p. 341)	100	280	2
Benign intracranial tumour (p. 266)	50	140	1
Nacrolepsy syndrome (p. 114)	50	140	1
Subarachnoid haemorrhage (p. 228)	50	140	1
Trigeminal neuralgia (p. 145)	40	112	<1
Cerebral metastasis (p. 276)	10	28	<1
Syringomyelia (p. 334)	7	20	<1
Huntington's disease (p. 298)	6	17	<1
Motor neurone disease (p. 357)	6	17	<1
Malignant cerebral tumour (p. 266)	5	14	<1
Myasthenia gravis (p. 407)	5	14	<1
Friedreich's ataxia (p. 336)	2	6	<1
Steele–Richardson–Olszewski syndrome (p. 290)	1.4	4	<1

[*] Approximately 200 consultant neurologists in the UK, population 56 million.
[†] Approximate list size 2000.

basic neurophysiology, neurochemistry, molecular biology or immunology because in the world of the jobbing neurologist these things which take up so much of the medical curriculum are not yet particularly helpful. Of far more use is a little neuroanatomy (much less than we were all taught and slightly more than we actually remember), an idea of what is likely, some clinical pharmacology, and the fruits of the experience of seeing a lot of patients. So, I hope this book will provide help with diagnosis, a tip or two on treatment when things are not going according to plan, and the reassurance that not even a specialist always knows what is going on.

1 Assessing the neurological patient

Symptoms and signs

Neurological disorders do not occur in isolation and should always be considered in their general medical and social context. There is no disease of the nervous system which fails to affect some other system, and many diseases of other systems have neurological consequences. For example, it is no good diagnosing a stroke without measuring the blood pressure, nor Parkinson's disease without considering the patient's occupation and lifestyle. Equally, diabetes cannot be properly managed without considering the neurological complications, and looking for the cause of respiratory failure is incomplete if neuromuscular weakness is forgotten.

Therefore, neurology is part of general medicine and making a neurological diagnosis is only one part of the evaluation of the whole patient, but it is that part which will be emphasized in this chapter.

There are four fundamental questions to be answered: 'Is there a neurological lesion?', 'Where is the lesion?', 'What is it?' and, 'What can be done about it?' The answer to the first two questions requires a little knowledge of neuroanatomy; the answer to the third some knowledge of pathology and general medicine along with experience of the sort of disorders which affect the nervous system under various conditions of age, sex, geography, etc.; and the answer to the last familiarity with the pharmacological, surgical, rehabilitative and other treatment options available. Whatever the lesion is, the actual neurological *deficit* depends more on *where* it is than *what* it is because destruction of a particular part of the nervous system produces much the same clinical deficit whatever the cause. On the other hand, the speed of onset of a deficit is a clue to its cause; strokes occur suddenly, a migrainous aura develops over some minutes, cerebral tumours cause progressive deterioration over weeks or longer, etc.

When tackling a diagnostic problem one must keep a clear head, concentrate on the history, be able to do a reasonable examination without finding things that are not there, and then have some idea whether investigation will delineate the site and nature of the lesion more accurately *and* affect the patient's management. Remember, the telephone is *the* most important neurological instrument, even more important than the tendon hammer. It can be used to complement the patient's history by using it to talk to relatives, friends and eyewitnesses who do not necessarily come to the doctor with the patient; it can be used to seek advice from neurologists and neurosurgeons in a distant specialist centre; and, unlike the tendon hammer, all doctors know how to use it.

Exactly how to elicit a history and perform a neurological examination will not be described here. The main concern is how to *interpret* the symptoms, signs and investigations.

Taking a neurological history cannot be learnt from books but at least a check list of possible neurological symptoms can be quickly run through after the history of the presenting complaint has been obtained, omitting those which have already been dealt with:

- headache and other pains around the head (face, orbits, neck, jaw, etc.)
- faintness, loss of consciousness, vertigo and other funny turns
- memory
- speech, reading, writing
- sleep, snoring
- mood
- vision, hearing, taste and smell
- swallowing
- facial weakness and numbness
- weakness, clumsiness, numbness, tingling and pain in the limbs
- walking, balance, falls
- bladder and bowels
- impotence in males
- back or neck pain

The *neurological examination* serves to confirm the diagnosis which has almost always been deduced after an adequate history; to exclude other diagnostic possibilities which may or may not have been suggested by the history; perhaps to refine more precisely where and what the lesion is; and to gather some semi-objective information about the state of the patient. It must be *directed* at the problem revealed by the history; it is impractical to examine obsessionally all parts of the nervous system in all patients.

Fortunately, making a neurological diagnosis usually requires only a proportion of the symptoms and signs actually present to be found; as in reading, it is not always necessary to see all the letters in a word to understand it.

One can be certain of some physical signs ('hard signs') and these should be relied on. Uncertain (or 'soft') signs can be noted but must *not* be used for making a diagnosis since they are as, or more, likely to be misleading as helpful. Signs may be 'soft' because they are only just emerging or have nearly disappeared, are variable with time, or the examiner is inexperienced. A neurologist is more likely than a non-specialist to deem a real but subtle sign 'hard', particularly if he has elicited it himself, and is more confident to say that there are no abnormal signs, so perhaps making the diagnosis more secure and further investigation less necessary. Signs which do not fit in with the diagnosis deduced from the history and other signs may be because they are 'soft' and really do not exist, or because they reflect a second disorder, or, more likely, because they are a residue of some previous neurological episode (e.g. an absent ankle jerk years after a prolapsed lumbar disc or polio).

At this stage, a brief description of the organization of the nervous system is needed, at least to the extent that it makes it possible to deduce the site of lesions; the *causes* of lesions in particular sites will mostly be dealt with in subsequent chapters.

The motor system

Voluntary willed movements are mediated by the upper motor neurone (pyramidal) system and by the bulbar and spinal motor nerves along with the muscles they supply (the lower motor neurone system). Lesions of the upper and lower motor neurone pathways cause two distinctive and different clinical pictures which help to localize the position of lesions affecting voluntary movement (Table 1.1). Voluntary movement itself is modulated by the extrapyramidal motor system, cerebellum, postural sensation and vision, which will all be considered later.

Table 1.1 The features of upper and lower motor neurone lesions

	Upper motor neurone lesion	Lower motor neurone lesion
Weakness	Yes: Pyramidal distribution Disproportionate loss of skill	Yes: Root distribution, peripheral nerve distribution, or global
Wasting	No, unless prolonged disuse	Yes, if chronic
Tone	Increased (spasticity)	Normal or reduced
Fasciculation	No	Yes, under some circumstances
Tendon reflexes	Increased (and clonus sometimes)	Depressed or absent
Plantar response	Up	Absent or down
Abdominal reflexes	Absent	Present

Note: One does not need a full house of clinical features to make a diagnosis any more than one needs to see everything about a cat to know it is a cat. A definite extensor plantar response is enough to indicate a lesion of the upper motor neurone just as a cat's head is enough to indicate that a cat is around somewhere; even a purr would be enough in the appropriate place, but not in the jungle!

The pyramidal, upper motor neurone or corticospinal and corticobulbar pathways (Fig. 1.1)

These start mainly in the cerebral motor cortex which is organized topographically in the posterior part of the frontal lobe; lesions in a particular place will affect the movement of a predictable part of the body (Fig. 1.2). These upper motor neurones descend through the internal capsule, cerebral peduncle and ventral part of the brainstem, cross to the other side in the medulla and continue in the lateral column of the spinal cord. They end by

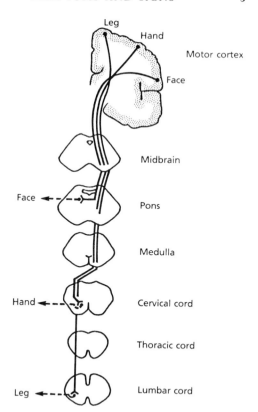

Fig. 1.1 The voluntary motor pathways. Dashed lines indicate lower motor neurones, solid lines indicate upper motor neurones.

synapsing on the cell bodies of the motor cranial nerves in the brainstem (i.e. the corticobulbar pathway), and on the cell bodies of the motor nerves in the anterior horns of the spinal cord (i.e. the corticospinal pathway).

Pyramidal lesions cause some combination of the following conditions:

Weakness

This may be complete in all muscle groups of a limb but, when incomplete, it tends to have a characteristic distribution; in the arms the extensors are weaker than the flexors and in the legs the flexors are weaker than the extensors (dorsiflexion of the foot is part of flexion and plantar flexion is part of extension of the lower limb). A motor cortex lesion will cause weakness of the contralateral part of the body corresponding to the site of the lesion (Fig. 1.2). A lesion large enough to affect the whole motor strip to cause weakness of all the contralateral body will almost always be accompanied by some disturbance of cerebral cognitive function (e.g. aphasia if in the dominant hemisphere). On the other hand, a lesion in the internal capsule, where the pyramidal tract is concentrated in a very small area, can also cause weakness of all the contralateral body (or sometimes just one limb) but there

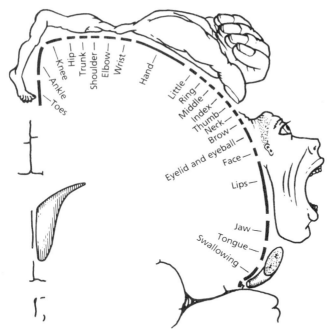

Fig. 1.2 Topographical organization of the motor cortex in the cerebral hemisphere. (After W. Penfield and T. Rasmussen (1950) *The Cerebral Cortex of Man*. Macmillan.)

is *no* cognitive deficit. A unilateral lesion below the pons spares the face and a lesion below the brainstem causes weakness of the same side of the body (arm and/or leg). In practice, spinal cord lesions are rarely small enough and unilateral enough to cause weakness of one arm and leg without at least some motor signs (e.g. extensor plantar response) if not symptoms on the other side as well.

Loss of skilled fine movements

This is usually out of proportion to any weakness which can be slight, or absent. Pyramidal lesions may cause profound clumsiness of the fingers for rapid coordinated movements even when power in the hand is normal.

Note: The non-dominant limb normally tends to be slightly clumsier than the dominant limb and sometimes even a little weaker as well.

Wasting

Wasting is absent, even when weakness is profound, although with prolonged disuse some mild wasting may develop.

Muscle tone

This is increased and is of the 'spastic' type in the sense that it preferentially affects the flexors and pronators in the arm, and the extensors and adductors in the leg (so producing the characteristic hemiplegic posture). It tends to be most obvious at the beginning of a passive movement (like opening a pen-knife) and wears off with repetition of the movement. On the other hand, in extrapyramidal rigidity there is increased tone equally in extensors and flexors which is present throughout the whole range of movement (so-called lead pipe rigidity) or is jerky (so-called cogwheel rigidity).

Reflexes

Tendon reflexes below the site of the lesion become brisk (e.g. brisk reflexes in both legs but not the arms indicate a thoracic spinal cord lesion), the plantar response becomes extensor, and the abdominal reflexes are lost if the lesion is above the T7 spinal segment.

A tendon reflex may also be brisk enough to be activated from a distance, e.g. striking the tendon of brachioradialis may produce not just a brisk supinator jerk but a finger jerk as well; eliciting the knee jerk may also produce adduction of both hips. Symmetrically brisk reflexes with no other pyramidal signs (i.e. the plantars are flexor, etc.) may be due to excessive sympathetic stimulation as a result of:

- anxiety
- hyperthyroidism or thyroxine abuse (p. 456)
- withdrawal of sedatives, alcohol, opiates
- drugs (e.g. salbutamol, amphetamines, lithium, etc.)

The notation for recording the tendon reflexes is:

0	absent tendon reflex
±	present only with reinforcement
+	just present without reinforcement
++	easily obtained
+++	brisk
++++	very brisk

Clonus has exactly the same significance as a very brisk tendon reflex so is not a particularly helpful sign.

The abdominal reflexes may be lost:
- in pyramidal lesions above T7
- in spinal cord/root lesions at T7–T12 segmental level
- in the elderly
- in the obese
- if the abdomen is tense
- after multiple pregnancies
- after abdominal surgery

A pout (or snout) reflex can be found in the normal elderly and may also indicate widespread cerebral disease; it has no localizing value.

The jaw jerk is variably present in normal individuals. It may be pathologically brisk as a result of lesions of both pyramidal pathways above the pons (i.e. a single lesion in the midbrain or lesions in both cerebral hemispheres). A *unilateral* upper motor neurone lesion above the pons does not affect the jaw jerk.

Note: An acute lesion of the upper motor neurone (usually traumatic or a stroke) causes immediate *flaccid* paralysis and *absent* reflexes but the plantar response is extensor. Usually after some days or weeks, the normal features of a pyramidal lesion develop (i.e. spasticity, hyperreflexia, etc.).

Note: Pyramidal lesions affecting the legs may cause involuntary flexor spasms when the legs are touched or become warm (e.g. in bed) and these are aggravated by urine infections and pressure sores. Severe lesions cause, in addition, spasms of the extensors and hip adductors. Either sort of spasm may be painful.

The lower motor neurone pathways

These start in the cranial nerve motor nuclei in the brainstem and in the anterior horn cells of the spinal cord (Fig. 1.1). The motor neurones emerge from the brainstem as cranial nerves and from the spinal cord as the anterior nerve roots which unite with the posterior sensory nerve roots to form the spinal nerves (Fig. 1.3) which, in the cervical and lumbosacral regions, form plexuses from which individual peripheral nerves arise. Cranial, spinal and peripheral nerves terminate at the motor end plates on skeletal voluntary muscles which are, in a sense, part of the lower motor neurone apparatus. A *myotome* is that group of muscles innervated by a single anterior spinal motor root (Table 1.2). A *motor unit* is the group of muscle fibres within a muscle which are innervated by a single motor neurone arising from one spinal anterior horn cell.

Lower motor lesions cause some combination of the following conditions:

Weakness and proportionate loss of skill

Weakness and proportionate loss of skill of those muscles supplied by the damaged nerve root, cranial or peripheral nerve, or generalized weakness if there is a more widespread disturbance of peripheral nerves (peripheral neuropathy, Chapter 14), nerve roots (radiculopathy, Chapter 14) or muscles (myopathy, Chapter 16). Neuropathic weakness is usually distal and myopathic weakness is usually proximal.

Wasting

Wasting of weak muscles appears in a matter of weeks after an acute root or peripheral nerve lesion and is characteristic of chronic lower motor neurone lesions. Wasting without weakness should be ignored if there are no other neurological signs since this can occur as a result of immobilization or cachexia, and is common in the elderly.

Asymmetrical muscle bulk is found in individuals who use one limb very actively (e.g. the dominant arm of plumbers).

Localized areas of subcutaneous fat may atrophy and give the false impression of muscle wasting (panatrophy of Gowers); the overlying skin and sometimes the underlying muscle may atrophy as well.

Pseudohypertrophy

Pseudohypertrophy (muscle enlargement with weakness) occurs in Duchenne and Becker muscular dystrophies (p. 423), myotonia congenita (p. 425) and very rarely in some peripheral neuropathies (p. 389).

Muscle tone

This is normal or reduced but is difficult to detect unless there is obvious weakness; certainly it is never increased.

Fasciculation

Fasciculation in muscles is due to random firing of motor units. Spontaneous and small individual contractions can be seen under the skin as irregular and continuous flickering movements. If noticed by the patient, particularly in the calves or small hand muscles, it is usually benign and of no consequence even if the contraction occasionally moves a joint in the hand; provided there are no other neurological signs, it can be ignored.

Otherwise fasciculation is due to a lesion of the lower motor neurone usually in the region of the anterior horn cell:
- motor neurone disease (Chapter 13)
- motor root compression (p. 320)
- polyradiculopathy (p. 389)
- poliomyelitis (p. 522)

A similar appearance can be seen in thyrotoxic myopathy (p. 437), gold toxicity (p. 548) and organic mercury poisoning (p. 547).

Reflexes

The abdominal reflexes are lost in lesions of the spinal cord and roots at their own segmental level (T7 to T12), the plantar response remains flexor or is absent, no primitive reflexes appear, and the tendon reflexes are depressed

Table 1.2 The spinal segment, motor nerve root and peripheral nerve supply to the major muscles

Muscle	C3	C4	C5	C6	C7	C8	T1	Nerve
Upper limb								
Trapezius	X	X						Spinal and spinal accessory
Diaphragm	X	X	X					Phrenic
Rhomboids		X	X					Dorsal scapular
Pectoralis major — clavicular head			X	X				Lateral pectoral
Supraspinatus			X	X				Suprascapular
Infraspinatus			X	X				Suprascapular
Deltoid			X	X				Axillary
Biceps			X	X				Musculocutaneous
Brachialis			X	X				Musculocutaneous
Brachioradialis			X	X				Radial
Extensor carpi radialis longus			X	X				Radial
Serratus anterior			X	X	X			Long thoracic
Teres major			X	X	X			Subscapular
Supinator				X	X			Posterior interosseous
Pronator teres				X	X			Median
Flexor carpi radialis				X	X			Median
Latissimus dorsi				X	X	X		Thoracodorsal
Pectoralis major — sternal head				X	X	X		Lateral and medial pectoral
Triceps				X	X	X		Radial
Extensor carpi ulnaris					X	X		Posterior interosseous
Extensor digitorum					X	X		Posterior interosseous
Abductor pollicis longus					X	X		Posterior interosseous
Extensor pollicis longus					X	X		Posterior interosseous
Extensor pollicis brevis					X	X		Posterior interosseous
Extensor indicis					X	X		Posterior interosseous
Flexor digitorum profundus I & II					X	X		Anterior interosseous
Flexor pollicis longus					X	X		Anterior interosseous
Flexor digitorum profundus III & IV					X	X		Ulnar
Flexor digitorum superficialis					X	X	X	Median
Flexor carpi ulnaris					X	X	X	Ulnar

	C3	C4	C5	C6	C7	C8	T1	
Abductor pollicis brevis						X	X	Median
Flexor pollicis brevis						X	X	Median (or ulnar)
Opponens pollicis						X	X	Median
Lumbricals I & II						X	X	Median
Adductor pollicis						X	X	Ulnar
Flexor pollicis brevis						X	X	Ulnar
Palmar interossei						X	X	Ulnar
Dorsal interossei						X	X	Ulnar
Lumbricals III & IV						X	X	Ulnar
Abductor digiti minimi						X	X	Ulnar
Flexor digiti minimi						X	X	Ulnar

Lower limb

	L1	L2	L3	L4	L5	S1	S2	
Iliopsoas	X	X	X					Spinal and femoral
Quadriceps		X	X	X				Femoral
Adductor femoris		X	X	X				Obturator
Tibialis posterior				X	X			Tibial
Tibialis anterior				X	X			Deep peroneal
Gluteus medius and minimus				X	X	X		Superior gluteal
Tensor fasciae latae				X	X	X		Superior gluteal
Extensor digitorum longus					X	X		Deep peroneal
Extensor hallucis longus					X	X		Deep peroneal
Extensor digitorum brevis					X	X		Deep peroneal
Peroneus longus					X	X		Superficial peroneal
Peroneus brevis					X	X		Superficial peroneal
Gluteus maximus					X	X	X	Inferior gluteal
Hamstrings					X	X	X	Sciatic
Flexor digitorum longus						X	X	Tibial
Gastrocnemius and soleus						X	X	Tibial
Small foot muscles						X	X	Medial & lateral plantar

or lost. The pattern of tendon reflex loss depends on which segment of the spinal cord, motor nerve root or peripheral nerve is involved since each tendon reflex depends on an afferent sensory nerve and root, the reflex arc at that level in the spinal cord, the efferent motor root and nerve, and the appropriate muscle group (Table 1.3 and Fig. 1.3).

General depression of reflexes occurs early in neuropathies when there may be little or no weakness but rather later, when muscles are obviously weak, in myopathies. The ankle reflex may be absent bilaterally in the normal elderly and some normal individuals have completely absent reflexes (particularly in association with the Holmes–Adie pupil (p. 178).

The tendon reflexes may be slow to relax in:
- hypothyroidism (p. 456)
- hypothermia (p. 486)
- beta-blockers

Table 1.3 Spinal cord, nerve root and peripheral nerve contribution to the tendon reflexes

Tendon reflex	Spinal cord/root level	Peripheral nerve
Biceps	C5/C6	Musculocutaneous
Supinator*	C6	Radial
Triceps	C7	Radial
Finger	C8	Ulnar and median
Knee	L3/L4	Femoral
Ankle	S1	Sciatic/tibial

* In fact mediated by the brachioradialis muscle which was once called supinator longus.

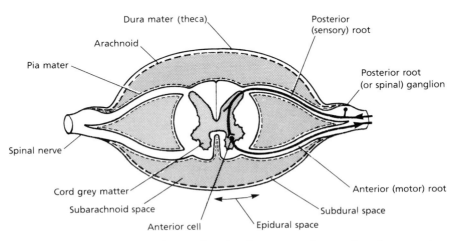

Fig. 1.3 Cross-section through the spinal cord to show its membranes, the reflex arc and the nerve roots.

A combination of upper and lower motor neurone features

This may be found in various circumstances:
- A primary neurological disorder of both systems, e.g. motor neurone disease (Chapter 13).
- A non-neurological disorder affecting both systems (e.g. diabetes, p. 453, AIDS, p. 526, syphilis, p. 515).
- Nerve roots and adjacent spinal cord affected by a single lesion, e.g. root compression at the C5 vertebral level may cause lower motor neurone root signs with C5 and C6 weakness, wasting, and loss of biceps and supinator jerks while cord compression at the same level may cause pyramidal signs in the legs and brisk triceps and finger jerks.
- An old and irrelevant disorder in one place and a new and relevant disorder in another, e.g. long after a lumbar disc prolapse or polio the ankle jerk may still be absent.
- Prolonged disuse may cause some muscle atrophy even in upper motor neurone lesions.

Note: In the initial stages, as an upper or lower motor neurone lesion develops, there may be only fragmentary features, e.g. merely an extensor plantar response in the former or absent reflex in the latter. One cannot expect, nor indeed wait for, a 'full house' of all the clinical features since by then it may be too late for effective treatment (see footnote to Table 1.1).

Testing muscle power is not always straightforward. A normal muscle may *appear* weak:
- if movement is painful (e.g. as a result of arthritis)
- in poor patient comprehension (or deafness)
- in generally ill patients
- in small children
- in the elderly
- if parkinsonism present and power takes time to build up (p. 280)
- if ataxia or postural loss present
- if sensory inattention or neglect present (p. 22)
- functional weakness (p. 38)

Note: Provided full power is reached, even for a moment, there is probably no organic weakness with the exception of intermittent weakness due to myasthenia (Chapter 15).

Weakness is graded as follows (MRC scale):

0: no muscle contraction visible or felt
1: flicker of muscle contraction but no movement of joint
2: muscle moves joint with gravity eliminated

3: muscle moves joint against gravity but not against resistance
4: muscle moves joint against resistance, as well as gravity, but less effectively than normal
5: normal power

Unfortunately grade 4 covers a wide spectrum of weakness from the examiner just being able to overcome a movement to easily being able to overcome it; in both cases the joint moves against gravity.

Note:
- hemiplegia is total paralysis of one side of the body (with or without face involvement)
- paraplegia is total paralysis of both legs
- monoplegia is total paralysis of one limb
- tetraplegia is total paralysis of all four limbs

Substituting 'paresis' for 'plegia' changes the meaning to partial paralysis. These terms are usually used when the weakness is 'upper motor neurone' in type but can be used for 'lower motor neurone' and 'myopathic' weakness.

The extrapyramidal motor system

This is less well localized and understood than the pyramidal system and is mediated at least in part by the basal ganglia. However, focal lesions here seldom produce identifiable and focal neurological features (see p. 25). Rather, 'extrapyramidal' disorders tend to cause a general disturbance of the extrapyramidal system; the clinical features are parkinsonism with poverty of movement and rigidity (p. 280) and/or involuntary movements such as tremor (p. 293), chorea (p. 293) and dystonia (p. 301).

The cerebellum

The cerebellum is involved in the smooth control of voluntary and involuntary movements (see also p. 199). A lesion in the cerebellar hemisphere and/or its connections with the brainstem causes:
- ipsilateral ataxia of the arm and/or leg with intention tremor and disorganization of large repetitive movements (this may be impossible to assess if the limb is very weak, postural sense is absent, the movements are interrupted by chorea, dystonia or myoclonus, and is difficult to test if the patient is blind, confused or has diplopia). Some asymmetry between the dominant and non-dominant limbs is normal

Note: Frontal lobe lesions can occasionally produce contralateral limb ataxia very similar to that caused by a cerebellar lesion.

- horizontal nystagmus
- dysarthria
- hypotonia (ipsilateral) but this is difficult to detect

Midline and diffuse cerebellar lesions tend to cause truncal ataxia more than limb ataxia, and not necessarily with any other 'cerebellar' features such as nystagmus.

The sensory system

Although sensory information from one side of the body is conveyed by the afferent sensory pathways to the contralateral cerebral hemisphere, the route taken (Fig. 1.4a and b) is a little more complicated than the descending motor system.

Posterior column sensation

Posterior column sensation (all of joint position or postural sense but only some vibration and touch sense) is conveyed by sensory peripheral nerves via the brachial and lumbosacral plexuses from the arms and legs, the spinal nerves, and the posterior spinal roots to the *ipsilateral* dorsal column of the spinal cord. The pathway ascends to the medulla where it crosses the midline to ascend in the medial part of the brainstem (medial lemniscus) to the thalamus, and from there via the internal capsule to the sensory cortex in the anterior part of the parietal lobe where, as in motor cortex, there is topographical organization (Fig. 1.5).

Pain sensation

Pain sensation (along with temperature and some vibration and touch sense) from the limbs and trunk separates from posterior column sensation on entering the spinal cord, ascends one or two levels, and then crosses the midline to ascend in the lateral part of the spinal cord (lateral spinothalamic tract) and then lateral brainstem to join up again with posterior column sensation at midbrain level.

Facial sensation

This is more complex (Fig. 1.4a). Touch and the afferent arm of the corneal reflex are carried by the trigeminal nerve into the pons where the pathway crosses the midline to ascend through the midbrain to the contralateral thalamus, and then to the face area of the sensory cortex. However, pain and temperature sensation pathways, after entering the pons, descend in the lateral part of the brainstem (adjacent to the ascending pain pathway

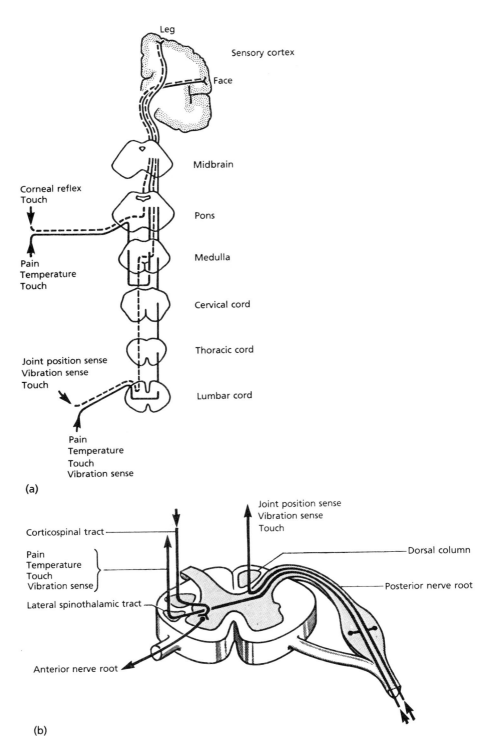

Fig. 1.4 (a) The sensory pathways. (b) Relationship between the sensory and motor tracts in the spinal cord.

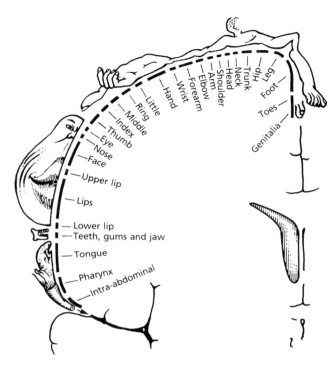

Fig. 1.5 Topographical organization of the sensory cortex in the cerebral hemisphere. (After W. Penfield and T. Rasmussen (1950) *The Cerebral Cortex of Man.* Macmillan.)

from the contralateral arm, leg and trunk), cross the midline in the lower medulla and upper cervical cord, and ascend in the medial part of the brainstem to the midbrain where they rejoin the touch pathways from the same side of the face.

Sensory testing is not easy and often exhausts both the patient and examiner. Useful points are:

• When mapping out cutaneous sensory loss, always work from the abnormal to normal area.

• Finger pulps are relatively insensitive to pain and touch so it is often better to test cutaneous sensation in the fingertips over the nailbed.

• Temperature sensation testing gives no more diagnostic information than testing for pain and is usually, therefore, a gimmick.

• Vibration sensation is often lost in the feet in the elderly and also early in generalized neuropathies.

• Sensation is normal in muscle disease, myasthenia gravis and motor neurone disease.

• Objective sensory loss can be quite difficult to find even when there are obvious sensory symptoms (particularly in multiple sclerosis and the Guillain–Barré syndrome).

• Cutaneous sensory loss will probably impair two point discrimination, stereognosis and graphaesthesia (p. 22). However, as long as there is some reasonable cutaneous sensation, then sensory inattention remains a valid way of testing for a contralateral parietal lesion (p. 22).

• Pain sensation is just that and must be tested by asking the patient if a disposable pin (dress pins are best, not hollow needles) or sharp end of a broken-off orange stick feels painful. On occasion sharp can be differentiated from blunt by touch sensation alone so that asking if it is the 'sharp end' or 'blunt end' is inappropriate.

Sensory symptoms include numbness (although patients may use this word to express weakness), loss of feeling (touch, pain, temperature, texture, etc.), tingling or pins and needles (paraesthesia), abnormal feelings such as water running down the skin and tight bands, enhanced pain sensation (hyperalgesia), touch which feels painful (dysaesthesia), and sometimes pain. Impaired vibration sense is unnoticed by the patient but joint position sense loss causes clumsiness, unsteadiness of gait and often a faulty perception of 'weakness' in the affected limb.

Patterns of sensory loss are helpful in localizing the site of a neurological lesion. Those for peripheral nerve and root lesions are illustrated in Chapter 14. Generalized neuropathies tend to cause sensory impairment symmetrically, first in the feet and then in the hands (p. 389), while central nervous system patterns of loss are illustrated in Figs 1.6–1.11.

A Charcot joint

This is a totally disorganized and destroyed joint which is painless. It is the consequence of repeated and usually mild injuries in the face of absent pain sensation. The knee and shoulder joints are the most commonly affected. The causes are:

• syringomyelia (p. 334)
• diabetic sensory neuropathy (p. 453)
• hereditary sensory neuropathy (p. 397)
• leprosy sensory neuropathy (p. 514)
• tabes dorsalis (p. 515)
• congenital indifference to pain

   Severe loss of pain sensation also leads to painless and unnoticed skin burns and deep and painless pressure sores on the feet and hands.

Lhermitte's symptom

This is a sudden electric shock-like flash or some other unpleasant feeling down the back and into the legs, occasionally into the arms, brought on by active or passive neck flexion. It is due to a lesion in the cervical spinal cord, often but not always multiple sclerosis (p. 344). Other causes include cervical spondylotic myelopathy (p. 327), other causes of cervical cord compression (p. 320), subacute combined degeneration of the spinal cord (p. 470) and acute radiation myelopathy (p. 334). It has also been described in some sensory neuropathies (cisplatin, p. 548, pyridoxine abuse, p. 470).

The cerebral hemispheres

Above the tentorium the brain mainly consists of the two cerebral hemispheres connected by the corpus callosum. Each hemisphere has four lobes (Fig. 1.12) whose functions when lost (or stimulated) are distinct enough to allow lesions to be approximately localized. Language function is in the dominant hemisphere which is the left in more than 95% of right-handed individuals and about 75% of left-handers, although in the latter dominance may not be very clearcut. Non-verbal and visuospatial functions are mostly located in the non-dominant hemisphere.

Frontal lobe lesions

These cause few, if any, clinical manifestations if they are anterior. Lesions in the very posterior part (i.e. the motor cortex) cause weakness, clumsiness

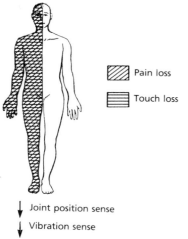

Pain loss

Touch loss

↓ Joint position sense

↓ Vibration sense

Fig. 1.6 Unilateral impairment of *all* modalities of sensation (light touch, joint position sense, pain and vibration) is due to a lesion in the contralateral thalamus or internal capsule. Contralateral parietal cortex lesions tend to cause less clearcut cutaneous sensory disturbance but loss of position sense along with 'cortical' sensory disturbance (astereognosis, inattention, etc. see p. 22).

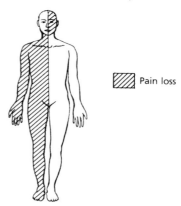

Pain loss

Fig. 1.7 Crossed sensory loss of pain (and temperature) is due to a lateral brainstem lesion involving the medulla (on the left in the illustration). This lesion interferes with the *descending* pain pathways from the ipsilateral face and the *ascending* pain pathways from the contralateral limbs and trunk (see also Fig. 1.4a).

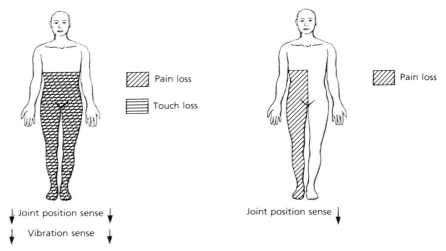

Joint position sense

Vibration sense

Joint position sense

Fig. 1.8 Bilateral loss of all forms of sensation with a sensory level (at about T6 in this illustration) is due to a spinal cord lesion (intrinsic or compressive) at about that level, or above. One would also expect a spastic paraplegia with a lesion at this level. Normal *sacral* pain sensation (so-called sacral sparing) is an unreliable indicator of an intrinsic cord lesion.

Fig. 1.9 The Brown-Sequard syndrome is the pattern of posterior column loss on one side and pain loss on the other due to a spinal cord lesion ipsilateral to the affected posterior column (i.e. the left in the illustration). In addition, there is upper motor neurone weakness of the leg ipsilateral to the lesion due to interruption of the descending corticospinal tract. It may be caused by trauma, tumour in or compressing the cord (p. 322), multiple sclerosis (p. 342), etc.

and other upper motor neurone signs (p. 4) in all or some part of the opposite side of the body depending on which area of the motor cortex is involved (Fig. 1.2). As well as, or instead of, such loss of motor function, frontal lobe lesions may cause partial motor seizures (p. 70) affecting the contralateral side, adversive seizures (p. 70), and sometimes complex partial seizures (p. 71). Frontal lesions may also cause difficulty in voluntary turning of the head and saccadic eye movement to the opposite side so that patients tend to 'look' towards the side of the lesion, at least when it is acute.

Lesions in Broca's area of the dominant frontal lobe cause language problems (p. 23).

More anterior frontal lesions may cause behavioural disturbance with apathy, loss of interest and concern, disinhibition and inappropriate jocularity. These features may be isolated or precede any dementia or physical disability, such as weakness, and must not be attributed to a psychiatric condition. Frequency and 'uncaring' incontinence of urine (and of faeces) occurs, but usually only with bilateral lesions (p. 31).

A frontal lesion may cause an ipsilateral palmomental reflex and a contralateral (or occasionally ipsilateral) grasp reflex; these reflexes can be present

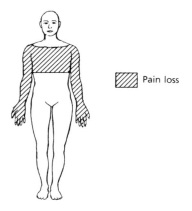

Pain loss

Fig. 1.10 A 'suspended' sensory loss (because there is normal sensation above and below) which is 'dissociated' (i.e. affects pain but not postural sense) must be due to a central cord lesion interrupting the pain fibres as they cross the midline, in the illustration from about C4 to T6 spinal cord level. It may, therefore, be due to syringomyelia (p. 334) or an intrinsic cord tumour (p. 322). Sometimes the sensory loss is asymmetrical in the sense that somewhat different spinal levels are involved on each side, and sensation can even be normal on one side.

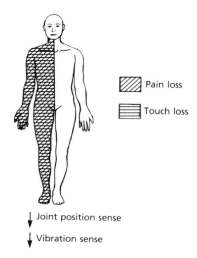

Pain loss

Touch loss

↓ Joint position sense

↓ Vibration sense

Fig. 1.11 Unilateral impairment of all modalities of sensation below the face is due to a lesion in the contralateral brainstem, thalamus, internal capsule or possibly parietal cortex. The face is not necessarily affected by a lesion in these sites since this depends on its exact location with respect to the facial sensory pathways (p. 15).

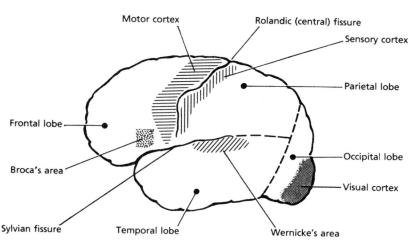

Motor cortex

Rolandic (central) fissure

Sensory cortex

Parietal lobe

Frontal lobe

Occipital lobe

Broca's area

Visual cortex

Sylvian fissure

Temporal lobe

Wernicke's area

Fig. 1.12 Localization of function in the dominant cerebral hemisphere.

bilaterally in the normal elderly as well as in diffuse cerebral disease. Mass lesions in or near the inferior frontal lobe may compress or invade the olfactory tract (to cause ipsilateral anosmia, p. 166) and optic nerve (to cause ipsilateral monocular visual failure and optic atrophy, p. 167).

A mass lesion between the frontal lobes (e.g. parasagittal meningioma) or bilateral ischaemia or haemorrhage (e.g. ruptured anterior communicating artery aneurysm) is particularly likely to cause urinary incontinence and motor disturbance in one leg, but very rarely in both legs (partial motor seizures or pyramidal weakness).

Parietal lobe lesions

Parietal lobe lesions, if anterior to involve the sensory cortex, cause sensory partial seizures (p. 70) and/or sensory loss on the opposite side of the body, the part depending on the site of the lesion (Fig. 1.5). Loss of touch, pain and vibration sense is patchy, inconsistent and mild; more obvious is contralateral loss of position sense, astereognosis (with eyes shut, inability to recognize objects held in the hand), impaired graphaesthesia (with eyes shut, ability to recognize numbers drawn on the palm) and impaired two point discrimination (normally less than about 2 mm on the finger tips). More posterior lesions cause sensory inattention (or suppression) and neglect on the opposite side of the body (which can be misinterpreted as weakness) particularly if the lesion is in the non-dominant hemisphere. Other non-dominant parietal features include constructional apraxia (inability to copy simple shapes), dressing apraxia (difficulty getting in and out of normal clothes), right-left disorientation, and getting lost in familiar places. Dominant parietal lobe lesions, particularly if inferior, cause language disturbance (p. 23), acalculia (impaired arithmetical ability), right-left disorientation, and finger agnosia (difficulty identifying individual fingers).

Note: Motor dyspraxia (or apraxia) is inability to perform a familiar movement even though comprehension, muscle power, sensation and coordination are all normal. It has no great localizing value, being a feature of frontal and parietal lesions on either side.

Occipital lobe lesions

These lesions (see also p. 169) cause a contralateral homonymous visual field defect which may involve the upper and lower quadrants (hemianopia) or just one quadrant (quandrantanopia). Bilateral lesions can cause cortical blindness which the patient may deny (the pupil responses are normal which sometimes leads to a mistaken diagnosis of confusional state or hysteria). More anterior lesions can cause contralateral visual inattention (or suppression), visual agnosia (inability to recognize objects despite normal visual acuity and language), prosopagnosia (inability to recognize familiar faces) and visual disorientation (inability to appreciate where objects are in relation to each other). Voluntary following (pursuit) movements of the eyes to the side ipsilateral to the lesion can be impaired. Partial seizures rather seldom arise from the occipital lobe (p. 70).

Temporal lobe lesions

Temporal lobe lesions have a marked tendency to cause seizures (usually complex partial, p. 71), memory loss, and language disturbance if in the dominant hemisphere (see below). Verbal and non-verbal (or visuospatial) memory is largely mediated by the dominant and non-dominant temporal lobes respectively with contributions from the medial thalamus and mamillary bodies. Although the dominant temporal lobe contains the auditory cortex, deafness does not result from a unilateral lesion. Bilateral temporal lesions can, however, cause cortical (or pure word) deafness; although patients can speak, write, read and respond normally to written commands and hearing and audiometry are normal, they cannot undertand spoken language and sometimes even non-verbal sounds such as the telephone ringing (auditory agnosia). Posterior temporal lesions may cause a contralateral upper homonymous quadrantanopia due to lower optic radiation involvement. In rare cases dominant temporal lesions cause a schizophrenic state.

Speech

Normal speech can be disrupted by a disorder of language function (dysphasia and aphasia are used interchangeably), articulation of words (dysarthria), sound production (dysphonia) and by abnormal intonation, rhythm and inflections in words and sentences (dysprosody).

Language function

Language function involves not just speech but also reading and writing which, when impaired, are called dyslexia and dysgraphia respectively. Dysphasia is seldom isolated; there is usually dyslexia and/or dysgraphia as well. All three parts of language function may be affected to different extents so their individual assessment is important. Dysphasia may be misinterpreted as confusion and confused patients may have mild word-finding difficulties.

Inability to name objects (nominal aphasia) is present in all types of aphasia, i.e. circumlocutions ('it's something you write with' instead of 'pen'), semantic errors ('caterpillar' instead of 'spider'), phonetic errors ('pin' instead of 'pen'). Other aspects of disturbed language function have more localizing value:

Lesions in Broca's area (Fig. 1.12)

These tend to cause non-fluent dysphasia with little if any spontaneous speech. Patients know what they want to say but cannot find the words, have relatively normal comprehension, and any words that are brought out come slowly, often with lack of prosody, but they may convey the correct meaning. Repetition is usually very slow, like the spontaneous speech.

Lesions in Wernicke's area (Fig. 1.12)

These tend to cause fluent dysphasia with normal prosody but the words are incorrect (paralogisms), non-existent (neologisms) and in an inappropriate order, giving the impression of nonsense speech or a foreign language (jargon aphasia). Comprehension is poor.

Lesions in the dominant inferior parietal lobe

Such lesions tend to cause conduction aphasia which is fluent with preserved comprehension. Repetition of words and phrases is impaired due to neural disconnection of Broca's from Wernicke's area. Dyslexia without dysgraphia may occur if there is a right homonymous hemianopia and the lesion also involves the splenium of the corpus callosum, so disconnecting the normal right occipital lobe from the cortical speech areas on the left.

In large dominant hemisphere lesions the dysphasia is global with impaired fluency, comprehension and repetition.

Dysarthria

Dysarthria is due to difficulty with the articulation of sounds to form words. If not obviously caused by a mechanical problem in the oral cavity (loose or missing false teeth, cleft palate, etc.), it must be due to weakness, incoordination, dystonia, chorea or myotonia of the muscles of the pharynx, palate, tongue, lips or face. The causes are, therefore, as listed below.

• Unilateral upper motor neurone lesions of the corticobulbar pathway tend to cause only mild dysarthria in proportion to any weakness of the bulbar muscles (tongue, palate, pharynx). In acute lesions (e.g. stroke) the dysarthria usually recovers because of the bilateral upper motor neurone innervation to the lower cranial motor nerve nuclei (p. 27).

• Bilateral upper motor neurone lesions of the corticobulbar pathways cause much more severe and persistent dysarthria, and even anarthria (complete inability to articulate words), as well as other features of a pseudobulbar palsy (p. 29).

• Unilateral or bilateral lesions of the 7th or the lower cranial motor nerves (i.e. 10th and 12th, a bulbar palsy, p. 29).

- Generalized neuropathies affecting the bulbar muscles (p. 389).
- Generalized myopathies affecting the bulbar muscles (Chapter 16).
- Myasthenia gravis affecting the bulbar muscles (Chapter 15).
- Involuntary movement disorders, e.g. Parkinson's disease (p. 280), dystonia (p. 301), chorea (p. 296).
- Cerebellar disorders (p. 199).
- Myotonic disorders (p. 424).

Dysphonia

Dysphonia is due to:
- vocal cord lesions (nodule, tumour, inflammation, etc.)
- vocal cord paresis (10th cranial nerve palsy, p. 195, recurrent laryngeal nerve palsy)
- weakness of chest muscles (myasthenia gravis, Chapter 15, generalized neuropathy, p. 389, etc.)
- dystonia (p. 301)
    The speech is soft or hoarse, as are individual sounds.

Dysprosody

This occurs in:
- non-fluent aphasia (p. 23)
- parkinsonism (p. 280)
- large *non-dominant* cerebral hemisphere lesions
- depression
- catatonia (p. 313)

Stuttering (or stammering)

This is usually a developmental abnormality. It can arise in aphasics and as a result of brain lesions in various places but has no localizing significance.

The basal ganglia region

The basal ganglia (caudate nucleus, globus pallidus and putamen together being referred to as the corpus striatum), internal capsule, thalamus and hypothalamus lie above the brainstem and below the cerebral hemispheres (Fig. 1.13). Destructive lesions in this area tend to cause contralateral motor and/or sensory loss due to involvement of the internal capsule and thalamus. Lesions restricted to the basal ganglia are unusual (more often involving the internal capsule as well to cause paralysis), so are seldom a cause of contralateral dystonia, chorea and tremor (Chapter 10). On the other hand, diffuse disorders of the brain and neurotransmitter systems often involve the basal ganglia to cause disorders of movement and posture (Chapter 10).

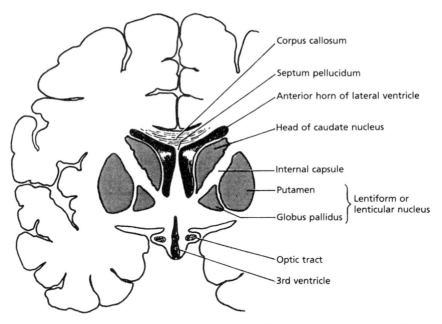

Fig. 1.13 Coronal section of the cerebrum just caudal to the optic chiasm. *Note*: Caudate and lentiform nucleus together are the corpus striatum.

Hypothalamic lesions

These seldom present to a neurologist since the consequences tend to be 'endocrine' with disturbance of appetite, thirst, temperature and weight control. A mass in the hypothalamus may compress the optic chiasm (p. 168) or obstruct the 3rd ventricle to cause hydrocephalus (p. 259).

Thalamic lesions

Such lesions are increasingly recognized as causing not just contralateral sensory loss (of one part, or usually of all the contralateral body including the face and affecting touch, pain and sometimes position sense) but also amnesia, particularly for short-term recall of verbal (dominant side) and non-verbal (non-dominant side) material. Bilateral lesions cause severe antero-grade global amnesia of the Korsakoff type (p. 468). Aphasia and contralateral neglect can also result from dominant and non-dominant thalamic lesions respectively. Finally, patients with thalamic lesions are often somnolent, obtunded and sometimes comatose.

'Thalamic pain'

'Thalamic pain' (better called central pain) is felt as a burning discomfort. It is a rare complication of a lesion anywhere in the central pain pathways from spinal cord to thalamus. Usually it starts some weeks after the onset of an acute lesion (e.g. stroke) causing either sensory loss which may have resolved by the time the pain appears, or causing *increased* pain perception which spreads locally and outlasts the stimulus (hyperalgesia). If the lesion is above the pons the discomfort is usually felt down the whole of the contralateral side of the body.

The brainstem

The brainstem is the Clapham Junction of the nervous system. Almost everything passes through it; the efferent corticospinal and corticobulbar tracts (p. 4) in the ventral part which are concerned with voluntary motor function of the bulbar, spinal, chest and limb muscles; the afferent sensory pathways (p. 15) in the central part concerned with the transmission of sensation from all parts of the body to the thalamus and then to the parietal cortex; and the efferent sympathetic pathways, also in the central part of the brainstem. A lesion in the brainstem is, therefore, likely to cause upper motor neurone signs below its level (i.e. the face is not involved if the lesion is below the facial nucleus in the pons), which may be bilateral (because the pathways are very close together in the brainstem) or contralateral; sensory loss of any or all modalities which is unilateral, crossed or bilateral below the level of the lesion (p. 15); and an ipsilateral or bilateral Horner's syndrome (p. 178). The level of the lesion is best determined by which cranial nerve nuclei are affected (they are mostly located in the dorsal part of the brainstem) and which functions specific to various parts of the brainstem are involved (Fig. 1.14).

Note: The jaw, upper face, palatal, pharyngeal, tongue, and laryngeal muscles have *bilateral* innervation from the corticobulbar pathways so that a unilateral upper motor lesion causes only transient, if any, contralateral weakness.

The midbrain

The midbrain contains the nuclei of the 3rd and 4th cranial nerves and, in association with the former, the nucleus for the parasympathetic nerve supply to the ipsilateral pupil constrictors. Lesions here will, therefore, cause diplopia and pupil dilatation. Also, vertical gaze is organized in the dorsal midbrain so that lesions may impair down-gaze and more often up-gaze (typically pineal region tumours, p. 274). In addition, there may be bilateral or contralateral weakness and sensory disturbance of the limbs and face, and bilateral or ipsilateral cerebellar signs due to involvement of the neural connections with the cerebellum.

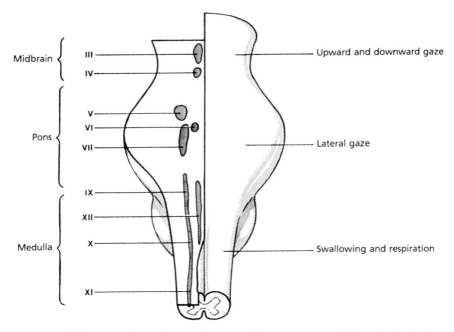

Fig. 1.14 The brainstem from above to show cranial nerve motor nuclei (on the left) and some brainstem functions (on the right).

The pons

The pons contains the motor nuclei of the 5th, 6th and 7th cranial nerves; the sensory nucleus of the 5th; the lateral gaze centres; the descending motor and sympathetic, and ascending sensory pathways. A lesion at this level may cause paralysis of the ipsilateral lateral rectus muscle (diplopia), ipsilateral face (affecting the forehead muscles as well as those below the eye because the lower motor neurones of the 7th cranial nerve are involved), and the ipsilateral jaw muscles although this is difficult to detect. Gaze may be impaired to the side of the lesion since the pontine gaze centre is concerned with moving the eyes and head to the same side (cf. frontal centre gaze centre, p. 20). Any Horner's syndrome (p. 178) is ipsilateral to the lesion and upper motor neurone weakness of the arms and legs is contralateral or bilateral. Corneal, touch and pain sensation is lost on the ipsilateral side of the face if the lesion is near the entry of the 5th cranial nerve. Any sensory disturbance in the limbs is contralateral or bilateral (p. 15). There may be ipsilateral limb ataxia due to disruption of the cerebellar-pontine connections. Vertigo and nystagmus also occur. Large pontine lesions may cause bilateral pin point pupils (sympathetic involvement), loss of consciousness and tetraplegia (see the 'locked-in' syndrome, p. 29).

Note: The medial longitudinal fasciculus connects the 3rd and 6th cranial nerve nuclei. A lesion causes an internuclear ophthalmoplegia, that is, paralysis of adduction of the ipsilateral eye on gaze to the contralateral side of the body. The abducting eye usually develops horizontal gaze nystagmus. This is an internuclear gaze palsy and normal lower motor neurone function of the ipsilateral medial rectus muscle is demonstrated by normal adduction when the patient is asked to converge the eyes.

The medulla

The medulla contains the motor nuclei of the 9th, 10th and 12th cranial nerves and a lesion here will cause weakness of the ipsilateral palate, tongue and vocal cord. There is likely to be dysphagia and dysarthria, particularly if the lesion is bilateral (p. 27); nystagmus (horizontal, vertical or rotatory, p. 193); ipsilateral Horner's syndrome, (p. 178); and, ipsilateral cerebellar ataxia. Vertigo, nausea, vomiting and hiccups may occur. Sometimes there is respiratory failure causing apnoea during sleep (p. 116). There is no facial weakness. Any limb weakness or sensory loss is contralateral, or bilateral if the lesion is both sides of the midline. However, the pain pathway from the face descends laterally and then crosses to ascend medially in the brainstem and any *pain* loss on the face is usually ipsilateral to the lesion, although it can be contralateral or bilateral (p. 15).

A *bulbar palsy* means weakness and wasting of the bulbar muscles (tongue, palate, pharynx) due to lower motor neurone lesions of the lower cranial motor nerves (10th, 12th) as a consequence of polio (p. 522), the Guillain–Barré syndrome (p. 398), motor neurone disease (Chapter 13), inflammatory or infective disorders around the brainstem (p. 497) and syringobulbia (p. 334). Similar 'bulbar' weakness may occur in some myopathies (p. 416) and myasthenia gravis (Chapter 15).

A *pseudobulbar palsy* means bilateral upper motor neurone weakness of the bulbar muscles. There is a brisk jaw jerk if the lesion is above the pons, and pyramidal signs in all four limbs because of involvement of the corticospinal tracts. The tongue is spastic and slow for repetitive movements. Emotional lability is common. The cause is either a single lesion in the midbrain or pons large enough to affect the descending motor pathways on both sides, (e.g. central pontine myelinolysis, p. 465) or several lesions bilaterally in the cerebral hemispheres or brainstem (usually due to stroke, p. 239, motor neurone disease, Chapter 13, multiple sclerosis, Chapter 12).

The *'locked-in' syndrome* is the combination of tetraplegia and mutism in an awake patient. It is caused by a large lesion in the ventral pons (usually infarction but sometimes haemorrhage, p. 227, trauma, central pontine myelinolysis, p. 465, etc.) which interrupts the corticospinal and corticobulbar tracts on both sides. The features are:
- Upper motor neurone paralysis of both arms, both legs, swallowing, speech, tongue and usually the face as well.
- Horizontal gaze paralysis. Vertical gaze and blinks are retained (because usually the midbrain is unaffected).

- Sensation is difficult to test and variably affected (unilateral or bilateral disturbance in face and limbs, corneal response variable).
- Ocular bobbing inconstant (p. 181).
- Pupil responses are usually normal.
- Hearing and vision are more or less normal as far as one can tell.
- Irregular, hyper or normal respiration but sometimes respiratory paralysis requiring ventilation.
- Normal consciousness (and EEG) because the dorsal pons and midbrain are intact.

Patients are often thought to be unconscious (cf. akinetic mutism, p. 126) but they are not and they can communicate by vertical eye movements and blinks. The code used (e.g. one blink 'yes', two blinks 'no', etc.) must be *consistent* and is best displayed by the patient's bed.

Most patients die in days or weeks. Some survive but very few recover useful function.

Neurological control of the bladder

Because the physiology of bladder control is complex and not well understood, it is best to use a simplistic model when localizing lesions in patients with urinary symptoms.

Contraction of the bladder and voiding of urine are mediated by a spinal cord reflex which can, up to a point, be voluntarily inhibited by descending pathways in the corticospinal tracts. As urine fills the bladder, the detrusor muscle, which makes up most of the bladder wall, is stretched and relaxes to accommodate the increasing volume of urine. This 'stretch' information is conveyed by parasympathetic nerves to the sacrospinal cord via the S2–S4 nerve roots. The efferent part of the reflex arc originates in the sacral cord and is conveyed by parasympathetic nerves in the same nerve roots which, by acetylcholine release at their terminations, cause contraction of the detrusor muscle; this increases bladder pressure and pulls up and opens the bladder neck. Simultaneously with detrusor contractions, the striated muscle of the external sphincter of the bladder at the origin of the urethra relaxes to allow urine to flow. The striated muscles of the external sphincter, and the associated pelvic floor muscles, are innervated by the pudendal nerves (also S2 to S4 spinal segments) and are under partial voluntary control so that bladder emptying can be interrupted or delayed until a convenient time.

Conscious sensation conveying bladder fullness, along with urethral sensation, is conveyed by the parasympathetic and pudendal nerves respectively, and the pathway ascends in the spinal cord to the cerebrum. As the bladder fills, the sensation changes from fullness to one of urgency to find somewhere to micturate, and then pain as the bladder becomes overfull.

The micturition reflex is under voluntary control which arises in the medial frontal lobes. The neural pathways descend in or near the cortico-spinal tracts to the sacral spinal cord and inhibit detrusor contraction while promoting contraction of the external bladder sphincter.

The role of the sympathetic nerve supply to the bladder via the hypo-gastric nerves is uncertain.

Frontal lobe lesions

These have to be bilateral or part of diffuse cerebral disease to cause urinary symptoms. The micturition reflex is normal and bladder emptying complete but there is little appreciation of bladder fullness. Voluntary descending and inhibitory control over bladder emptying is lost, which causes frequency but no particular urgency of micturition and eventually incontinence which may or may not distress patients depending on their mental state. In unconscious patients the mechanism of incontinence is similar.

Corticospinal tract lesions

These lesions have to be bilateral to affect micturition, usually in the spinal cord rather than the brainstem. As in frontal lesions there is interruption of descending voluntary control over bladder filling so that even small volumes of urine lead to uninhibited detrusor contractions with resulting frequency, urgency and eventually incontinence of urine. The bladder becomes small and 'spastic'. If the uninhibited detrusor contractions are met by contraction of the external sphincter (which may of course be partly voluntary since bladder and pelvic sensation can be normal) there is little or no urine flow; this is called detrusor–sphincter dyssnergia and leads to incomplete bladder emptying with residual urine.

Acute or subacute complete spinal cord lesions (usually traumatic or vascular) cause not just impairment of descending voluntary control but paralysis of the micturition reflex along with interruption of the ascending sensory pathways. As a consequence there is painless bladder over-distension, the external sphincter stretches and urine dribbles away; this is 'overflow' incontinence. After days or weeks the micturition reflex may recover to some extent and be activated by abdominal pressure, but voiding is seldom com-plete. Extreme bladder distension may cause sweating, flexor spasms in the legs, tachycardia and hypertension but still no pain because of the interruption of afferent sensory pathways to the brain.

Sacral root (S2 to S4) and pudendal nerve lesions, and autonomic neuropathies

These interrupt the micturition reflex and also usually impair the sensation of bladder fullness. This tends to cause painless over-distension of the bladder without either reflex voiding or normal sensory awareness and eventually 'overflow' incontinence as above. There is a large residual urine volume and the bladder is 'atonic'. Abdominal pressure can sometimes activate detrusor contractions.

   Urinary retention may, therefore, be due to:
- physical obstruction to flow:
  prostatic hypertrophy
  pelvic malignancy
- acute or subacute spinal cord lesion (Chapter 11):
  trauma
  infarction (p. 333)
  transverse myelitis (p. 332)
- sacral root lesion:
  compression (p. 320)
  inflammation (herpes simplex type 2, p. 523, herpes zoster, p. 523, etc.)
- autonomic failure (p. 403)
- anticholinergic drugs
- hysterical causes

Note: *Painful* over-distension of the bladder is almost always due to urinary outflow obstruction (e.g. enlarged prostate) which if unrelieved eventually causes the bladder wall to become stretched and 'atonic'.

Note: Urine infection causes inflammation of the bladder wall and sensitization of the stretch reflex, so leading to frequency and urgency of micturition along very often with dysuria. A neurogenic bladder is particularly likely to be associated with infection of excess residual urine, so making the urinary symptoms worse.

Note: Stretching of the pelvic floor muscles (e.g. post-parturition, uterine prolapse) weakens the external sphincter so that increasing the intra-abdominal pressure by coughing, straining and sneezing, etc. leads to the partial, or gross, escape of urine; this is 'stress' incontinence.

Note: Faecal impaction distorts the bladder neck and external sphincter so making any neurogenic bladder problems worse.

Diagnosis

An accurate history is, as usual, essential. Particular points to note are:
- is there frequency and urgency of micturition?
- incontinence, retention, or both at different times?
- is bladder sensation normal?
- is bladder distension painful?
- is urethral sensation to flowing urine normal?

- is perineal sensation normal?
- is there dysuria?
- is urinary incontinence precipitated by 'stress'?
- how much voluntary control over micturition is there?
- are there any other neurological features, particularly in the legs?
- are the bowels affected?
- is there impotence?

The examination is particularly concerned with any signs of corticospinal tract, sacral root and peripheral nerve dysfunction in the legs; evidence of autonomic failure (p. 403); a proper assessment of the abdomen; and a rectal/vaginal examination. Over-distension of the bladder can be felt on abdominal examination.

Investigation with cystometrography can be helpful in sorting out the nature of the problem but is rather less help in directing treatment. The bladder is catheterized and, while being filled with saline and then emptying, the bladder pressure and volume are recorded.

Note: Some patients, usually female, have frequency, urgency and occasionally incontinence of urine with no abnormal signs, neurological or otherwise. Disinhibited detrusor contractions are shown on cystometrography, so-called idiopathic detrusor instability. The cause is obscure; it is seldom identifiably 'neurological' and myelography to detect spinal cord or root compression is unrewarding.

Rectal continence and control are less well understood than that of the bladder. Incontinence of faeces is much less common than of urine and may not be a problem unless the stools are loose. The underlying mechanisms and causes are probably similar to urinary incontinence.

Note: Impaired rectal sensation may first be noticed because of inability to distinguish flatus from faeces.

Penile impotence is usually associated with the same neurological lesions and causes that lead to a neurogenic bladder (i.e. lesions of the corticospinal tracts, sacral roots and autonomic neuropathies) in addition to vascular, psychogenic, drug-induced and other non-neurological causes.

Localizing the lesion in some common clinical situations

Wasting of the small muscles in the hand

This may be merely due to disuse, usually as a result of old age or joint disease in the hand and wrist (e.g. rheumatoid or osteoarthritis). Any neurological cause cannot, because of the wasting, be due to a lesion above the anterior horn cells of the T1 (approximately) part of the spinal cord ipsilateral to the wasted hand because this is where the lower motor neurones to the small hand muscles arise (Table 1.2). A lesion above this would affect the pyramidal pathway which would not cause any wasting except as a result of long-term disuse. The possible neurological causes of wasting of the small muscles in the hand are, therefore:

- spinal cord at T1 level:
  trauma
  motor neurone disease (Chapter 13)
  syringomyelia (p. 334)
  tumour (p. 332)
  polio (p. 522)
- T1 nerve root (and lower brachial plexus):
  trauma
  malignancy/benign tumour (p. 320)
  cervical rib (p. 366)
  chronic meningeal infection (syphilis, p. 515, tuberculosis, p. 512, etc.)
- ulnar nerve, sparing abductor pollicis brevis which is supplied by the median nerve (p. 374)
- median nerve, sparing the dorsal interossei which are supplied by the ulnar nerve (p. 370)
- generalized neuropathies, usually causing bilateral wasting and weakness (p. 389)
- distal myopathies which are usually bilateral, e.g. myotonic dystrophy, distal muscular dystrophy (p. 416)

The exact site of the lesion is often revealed by the sensory findings, e.g. none in myopathies and motor neurone disease, characteristic distribution of sensory loss in ulnar nerve (p. 374), median nerve (p. 370) and T1 nerve root lesions (Fig. 11.3a), etc. Also the tendon reflexes in the arms are preserved with ulnar nerve and median nerve lesions and myopathies, but depressed or lost with spinal cord, root and brachial plexus lesions if the C5–C7 levels are affected as well as T1, and with peripheral neuropathies.

Absent ankle jerks

A unilateral absent ankle jerk, if not due to poor examination technique or ankylosis of the ankle joint, cannot be due to a lesion higher than the S1 segment of the spinal cord since it is a reflection of a lower motor neurone lesion to the ankle plantar flexors (Table 1.2); nor can it be due to a generalized peripheral neuropathy since it is unilateral. Therefore, it has to be due to a lesion involving the ipsilateral S1 spinal cord (e.g. as a result of trauma, motor neurone disease, Chapter 13, polio, p. 522, etc.), the S1 nerve root (e.g. as a result of lumbar disc compression, p. 326, tumour, p. 320), sciatic nerve (usually a traumatic lesion, p. 383), tibial nerve (again usually traumatic, p. 387), or the plantar flexor muscles of the calf (most unusual). More exactly where the lesion is can be simply determined with a pin because, with a spinal anterior horn or muscle lesion, sensation is normal but, with a root (Fig. 11.3b) or peripheral nerve lesion, there is a characteristic distribution of sensory loss.

Peripheral neuropathies (p. 389) and myopathies (Chapter 16) almost always cause *bilateral*, and often symmetrical, leg weakness, usually more distal in the former and proximal in the latter. In myopathies there is often some weakness of the arms as well whereas in neuropathies any weakness can be confined to the feet. The ankle jerks tend to be bilaterally lost early in neuropathies but later in myopathies. Radiculopathies (p. 389) tend to cause proximal weakness.

Upgoing plantar responses and absent ankle (and maybe knee) jerks

This pattern can be due to a single lesion at the conus medullaris (Fig. 11.1) which affects the pyramidal tract (to cause the upgoing toes) *and* the cauda equina (to cause the absent reflexes).

If not due to one lesion, then there must be lesions in both the upper and lower motor neurone pathways as a result of:
- vitamin B_{12} deficiency (subacute combined degeneration of the cord with a peripheral neuropathy, p. 470)
- Friedreich's ataxia (p. 336)
- tabes dorsalis (p. 515)
- motor neurone disease (Chapter 13), although usually the reflexes are brisk until the leg muscles are very wasted and even then they may still be brisk

Isolated weakness of one leg and/or foot

This can be a difficult diagnostic problem since the lesion may be anywhere from the contralateral motor cortex through the brainstem to the ipsilateral spinal cord down to the lumbar cord level (pyramidal features present), to the lumbosacral plexus and peripheral nerves (lower motor neurone features present). It may even, rarely, be due to myasthenia gravis (Chapter 15), and of course it could be hysterical.

The pattern of weakness can reveal where the lesion is since it may be consistent with upper motor neurone, anterior horn cell, nerve root, femoral nerve, sciatic nerve, or a more peripheral nerve lesion. Often information from outside the motor system is needed to localize the lesion further, e.g.
- partial motor seizures from a cortical lesion
- brainstem features (p. 27)

- local pain
- sensory features (if none, the problem might be motor neurone disease, Chapter 13)

Note: Parkinsonism, ataxia, impaired joint position sense, osteoarthritis and muscle claudication may all present with the *complaint*, but no actual, weakness of one leg.

Weak legs

Weakness of *both* legs, symmetrically or asymmetrically, may be due to:
- an upper motor neurone lesion which must be bilateral and usually is, therefore, in the thoracic or cervical spinal cord. With cervical lesions there may only be symptomatic weakness of the legs but usually there are signs in the arms (e.g. brisk or absent tendon reflexes). If in the brainstem, a lesion almost always causes other brainstem features (p. 27) and affects the arms as well. A single intracranial lesion has to affect the leg area of the motor cortex bilaterally to cause weakness of both legs or indeed pyramidal signs in both legs (p. 22).
- lower motor lesions which have to be bilateral and therefore involve the cauda equina (p. 316) or are generalized (e.g. peripheral neuropathies, p. 389).
- motor neurone disease (Chapter 13).
- muscle disease (Chapter 16) but usually the arms are involved as well.
- myasthenia gravis and the Lambert–Eaton myasthenic syndrome (Chapter 15).
- hysterical or malingering (p. 38).

The *complaint*, but no actual, weakness of both legs may be due to other neurological disorders such as parkinsonism (p. 280), impaired joint position sense, ataxia, myotonia (p. 418), dystonia (p. 301), chorea (p. 296), or the post-viral fatigue syndrome (p. 436) as well as non-neurological conditions such as muscle claudication, shortness of breath, general malaise, mental exhaustion and depression. On the other hand, patients who are found to have weak legs on examination may complain of no more than tiredness or may previously have been thought to have just a 'funny' gait.

Fatigue without weakness is not usually a symptom of a neurological disorder but rather of anaemia, renal failure, cardiac failure, affective disorder, poor sleep, etc. However, there are some rather subtle neurological causes of fatigue which can be easily missed:
- multiple sclerosis (Chapter 12)
- myasthenia gravis (Chapter 15)
- metabolic myopathies (p. 427)
- periodic paralysis (p. 432)
- inflammatory muscle disorders (p. 434)

- motor neurone disease (Chapter 13)
- claudication of the cauda equina (p. 328)
- post-viral fatigue syndrome (p. 436)

Poor balance

Balance deteriorates with age. Patients may complain of difficulty with balance due to a *central cause*:
- vertigo and labyrinthine dysfunction (p. 105)
- cerebello-pontine angle lesions (p. 194)
- cerebellar or cerebellar-brainstem connection lesions (p. 199)
- 'normal' pressure hydrocephalus (p. 262)
- parkinsonism (p. 280)
- postural hypotension (p. 102)

Or a *peripheral cause*:
- weak legs (p. 36)
- impaired joint position sense due to spinal cord or peripheral nerve/root lesions

Or, because of arthritis in the legs, hysteria or malingering.

Note: Early spinal cord lesions can cause cerebellar-looking ataxia in the legs even when joint position sense is normal.

Romberg's sign is elicited by asking the patient to stand still with the eyes shut. This ability to balance is very impaired if there is poor joint position sense in the lower limbs and can also be impaired with cerebellar lesions. On the whole, by the time the sign is definitely present there is obvious joint position sense loss in the toes or other neurological signs to localize the lesion.

Falls

Falls can be due to any number of underlying causes, not all of which are neurological. Often several are present in the same patient and the whole situation is exacerbated by loss of confidence and even agoraphobia following the first fall. There may be no obvious cause at all, particularly in the elderly.

Causes may be categorized as follows:
- loss of, or impaired, consciousness, e.g. seizures, syncope, etc. (Chapter 2)
- drop attacks (p. 222)
- vertigo (p. 105)
- weakness of the legs and/or feet (p. 36)
- myotonia of the legs (p. 424)
- parkinsonism (p. 280)
- 'normal' pressure hydrocephalus (p. 262)
- impaired postural sense in the feet due to spinal cord or peripheral nerve lesions

- cerebellar ataxia and imbalance (p. 199)
- involuntary movements occasionally (e.g. chorea, p. 296, or dystonia, p. 301, of the trunk and/or legs)
- drugs:
  psychotropic
  hypotensive (p. 102)
  alcohol (p. 542)
  causing vertigo (p. 105)
- joint instability and pain due to arthritis
- poor vision

Functional non-organic weakness and sensory loss

Hysterical (unconscious) and malingering (conscious) causes of weakness should be suspected if:
- voluntary effort is intermittent and full power is possible, even for an instant, with encouragement. However, a similar intermittent feel to weakness may be found if there is local pain and in myasthenia gravis (Chapter 13)
- the voluntary power tends to build up and be proportional to that put in by the examiner
- voluntary effort is inappropriate with simultaneous contraction of antagonists and agonists and spread of the effort to distant and irrelevant muscle groups along with excessive grunting and groaning
- the observed 'weakness' is inconsistent with what the patient can actually do, e.g. unable to lift either leg off the bed but can sit up unaided from the horizontal position and walk
- there are no other upper or lower motor neurone signs although this can be the case in myasthenia gravis (Chapter 15) and myopathies (Chapter 16)
- there are no pressure sores
- peripheral nerve conduction, central motor conduction time and EMG are normal (p. 55)

Hysterical and malingering causes of sensory loss should be suspected if:
- there is intermittent loss (e.g. with eyes shut, patients respond normally to the finger of their outstretched hand being touched and told to place it on their nose, but later appear to have cutaneous loss in the same finger)
- sensory loss is inconsistent with function, e.g. no position sense in the feet but normal gait
- sensory loss is clearly incompatible with normal sensory anatomy, e.g. extends to, rather than above, the jaw line unlike the expected trigeminal nerve distribution (p. 186)
- there is clear-cut nonsense behaviour, e.g. responds 'no' to being touched in the 'numb' area
- there are alternating bands of sensory loss and normality on the limbs

- vibration sense is lost only on one side of the sternum
- the patient is turned over and the sensory loss changes from one side of the trunk to the other
- the pattern of sensory loss is inconsistent and non-reproducible
- glove and stocking sensory loss is *not* particularly characteristic and is rather more often due to a peripheral neuropathy (p. 393)
- evoked somatosensory potentials and peripheral nerve conduction are normal (p. 55)

Note: There is often, but not always, a past history of other functional disorders or psychiatric disturbance and/or some potential for gain (e.g. discharge from the army). Sometimes there is a 'model' with a real illness (e.g. a friend with multiple sclerosis in a wheelchair).

Neurological investigations

General medical investigations (such as urine analysis, haemoglobin, etc.) are frequently required when investigating a 'neurological' problem, along with screening for syphilis and now AIDS. Biopsy of tumours, brain, muscle and peripheral nerve is considered in the appropriate chapters. The other 'neurological' investigations are:

- lumbar puncture and CSF examination (p. 39)
- skull X-ray (p. 44)
- myelography (p. 46)
- computerized tomography (CT) of the brain (p. 47)
- magnetic resonance imaging (MRI) (p. 47)
- cerebral angiography (p. 53)
- electroencephalography (p. 54)
- evoked potentials (p. 55)
- nerve conduction and electromyography (p. 55)

Lumbar puncture (LP) and CSF examination

The indications for lumbar puncture are discussed in the appropriate sections on meningitis (p. 493), subarachnoid haemorrhage (p. 230), multiple sclerosis (p. 348), dementia (p. 158), etc.

Technique (Fig. 1.15)

- Explain the procedure to the patient and why it is being carried out. Defuse patient's fears by reassurance. If the possibility of post-lumbar puncture headache is mentioned at all, it should not be emphasized.
- Lay the patient on the near edge of a firm bed, head to the left, and with the

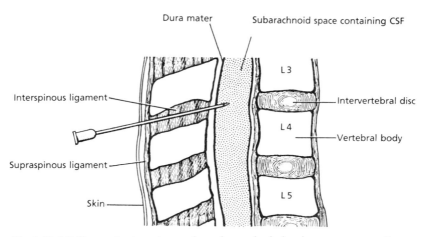

Dura mater   Subarachnoid space containing CSF

L3

Interspinous ligament

Intervertebral disc

L4

Vertebral body

Supraspinous ligament

Skin

L5

Fig. 1.15 Midline sagittal section to show the track of a lumbar puncture needle.

back and legs flexed as much as possible. The neck need not be flexed. The back must be perpendicular to the floor and the patient prevented from rolling forwards by pillows between the legs. The patient must be comfortable.
• Identify and mark the L3 vertebral spine which lies about on the line between the two anterior superior iliac spines.
• Wear sterile gloves (although many deem this unnecessary).
• Sterilize the lumbar skin and drape the area.
• Inject the skin and subcutaneous tissue down to the supraspinous ligament with about 2 ml of 2% lignocaine.
• While waiting for the local anaesthesia to develop (a few minutes) check the LP equipment; all components fit together, three-way tap works, the stylet tip is flush with the outer hollow needle with no ragged edge to it.
• Insert the lumbar puncture needle (20 gauge or the larger 18 gauge if difficulty is expected) in the midline in the L3/4 interspace and advance it in the sagittal plane, parallel to the floor, and slightly headwards. Resistance is felt as the needle penetrates the supraspinous ligament and then again at the dura (Fig. 1.15). Remove the stylet and CSF should flow out of the needle at which point the manometer is attached via the three-way tap.
• If the needle hits bone, or if there is root pain down the leg, it should be withdrawn to the subcutaneous tissue and reinserted.
• If fresh blood emerges from the needle, the LP may well be 'traumatic', particularly if the operator feels the needle is in the wrong place. This blood arises from the epidural venous plexus or occasionally from small blood vessels on nerve roots. Usually another disc space should be attempted.
• If CSF does not flow, despite the needle apparently being in the right place, rotate the open needle slightly but *never* withdraw it and reinsert without replacing the stylet first. Do *not* attempt to aspirate CSF.

- If the lumbar puncture fails, then attempt the L2/3 interspace, and then if necessary the L4/5 interspace. Higher than this the spinal cord may be injured and lower than this the dural sac containing CSF may have ended. Occasionally a lateral cervical approach under X-ray control is an alternative if lumbar puncture is impossible. Cisternal puncture should never be needed.
- Measure the CSF pressure after it has stabilized in a minute or so. It should show normal fluctuations with respiration, or if not with a cough.
- Empty the manometer into a sterile tube, and then fill two more, as well as a fluoride tube for glucose, directly from the needle to a total of about 10 ml. Label the sterile bottles first, second, third.
- Reinsert the stylet, remove the needle, put a plaster over the hole in the skin and advise the patient to lie down in any comfortable position for an hour or so before getting up.
- Take simultaneous blood glucose.
- Send specimens to the appropriate laboratory *at once*. If this is impossible, then refrigerate at 4°C.

Note: Do not repeat the lumbar puncture in the same interspace for one or two weeks, because the needle may enter not the subarachnoid space, but an epidural or subdural collection of CSF that has formed via a dural leak. Therefore, a lumbar puncture should not be done shortly before a lumbar myelogram.

Normal values

Pressure

The lumbar CSF pressure is always less than 250 mm of CSF, and usually less than 200 mm, if the patient is relaxed and the flow is free (i.e. fluctuation with respiration and coughing). Falsely low readings may be a consequence of removing too much CSF before the pressure is measured, a CSF leak around the needle, transtentorial herniation and brainstem coning (p. 257).

Protein

This is less than 0.4 g/l but some laboratories quote up to 0.6 g/l as normal. A very high CSF protein causes the CSF to clot (Froin's syndrome). CSF immunoglobulins and oligoclonal bands, see p. 348.

White cells

There should be no more than 5 lymphocytes per cubic ml and no polymorphs. For calculation of true white cell count in the presence of red blood cells, see p. 494.

Glucose

CSF glucose less than 50% of the simultaneous blood glucose is abnormal.

Blood

The CSF should be clear and contain no red blood cells although a few may be introduced by a mildly traumatic tap. If the CSF is bloody it should be centrifuged *at once* and the supernatant examined for xanthochromia (naked eye or better by spectrophotometry) which is due to the pigments derived from the breakdown of haemoglobin (it may also be found in jaundice or with a very high CSF protein).

A traumatic tap is suggested by decreasing concentration of red blood cells across the three sterile bottles and no xanthochromia because this takes a few hours to develop after red cells start to lyse. These features are not so reliable that one can always be absolutely sure about the presence or absence of subarachnoid haemorrhage; if in doubt, the lumbar puncture should be repeated.

Note: Normal ventricular and cervical CSF contains fewer cells, a total protein of up to 0.15 g/l, but the same glucose as lumbar CSF.

Complications

All complications are minimized if a diagnostic LP is performed only when the result is likely to influence patient management or if there is no simpler way to establish the diagnosis.

Headache

This is the most common complication and occurs after about 30% of diagnostic LPs. It is due to continuing CSF leakage through the dural hole. It starts within minutes or hours of standing up after LP and is a 'low pressure' headache which is usually present only on standing or sitting and is relieved by lying down. It may be accompanied by nausea, lightheadedness and occasionally vomiting. If there is any drowsiness, or if the pain comes on suddenly, then intracranial subdural or subarachnoid haemorrhage (see below) should be considered.

The risk of post LP headache can be reduced by using smaller needles (e.g. 22 gauge or even smaller) but these are tricky to insert and it is difficult to measure the CSF pressure and collect adequate volumes of CSF through them.

The treatment is bed rest (with paracetamol analgesia if necessary) until the headache goes, which usually takes a day or so. Prolonged headache is rare and, if not due to an intracranial cause, can perhaps be stopped by an autologous blood 'patch' in the epidural space or, as a last resort, by open surgery to seal the dural leak.

Transtentorial herniation and/or brainstem coning (p. 257)

This is the most serious complication but can be avoided by *never doing an LP if there is clinical evidence of raised intracranial pressure, focal cerebral, or posterior fossa signs.*

If there is raised intracranial pressure with shift of the intracranial contents, or obstruction to CSF flow, then removal of CSF, or continuing leakage of CSF after the LP, may lead to increasingly unequal pressures between the intracranial compartments and the vertebral canal, causing mass movements of the brain. However, even in the presence of raised intracranial pressure, *if* the CSF flow is free between all parts of the intracranial cavity and the spinal CSF compartment, then LP is safe but this can only be ascertained *by CT scan first.* Lumbar puncture is, therefore, contraindicated if the scan shows:
• an intracranial mass lesion, particularly in the posterior fossa (e.g. tumour, abscess, haematoma)
• obstructive hydrocephalus (p. 259)
• general brain swelling with obliteration of the CSF cisterns around the upper brainstem
i.e. LP is safe if the CT scan is normal even if the pressure is raised (e.g. in benign intracranial hypertension, p. 264).

In a patient with focal signs and/or in coma, and *if* bacterial meningitis is suspected and no CT scan is immediately available to exclude an intracranial abscess, then it is essential to treat at once with 'blind' antibiotics (p. 496) after collecting blood cultures, rather than risk a lumbar puncture and brain herniation.

Under some circumstances it may be crucial to obtain CSF for diagnostic purposes (usually microbiology) even if there is a risk of brain herniation. If so, this should be done in a neurology/neurosurgery unit able to handle the consequences.

Infection

Infection of the CSF, or an epidural abscess, are both extraordinarily rare. To reduce this risk, the needle should not be inserted through infected or inflamed skin.

Local lumbar back pain

This is common but usually settles down in a day or two unless a spinal haemorrhage has occurred (see below).

Spinal haemorrhage

Spinal haemorrhage (subdural, epidural or subarachnoid) is extremely rare and only likely if there are coagulation or platelet defects (including the use of anticoagulants at the time of, or an hour or so after, lumbar puncture); these should be corrected before the lumbar puncture. The consequences are severe back and/or root pain, spinal cord and/or root compression.

Intracranial subdural and subarachnoid haemorrhage

These are both very rare.

Epidermoid spinal tumours

These arose in children when hollow LP needles were used because epidermis was inserted in their tracks.

Epidural analgesia

Epidural analgesia may be complicated by:
- post-LP complications if the dura is penetrated (see above)
- transient hypotension, weakness of the legs, arms or diaphragm and retention of urine for some hours
- injection of anaesthetic into a spinal vein may cause seizures and drowsiness
- injection of anaesthetic into the subarachnoid space may cause paraplegia for some hours or days, and occasionally arachnoiditis
- nerve roots or spinal cord may be traumatized by the needle

Skull X-ray

CT scanning and MRI have not completely removed the need for a skull X-ray, particularly when the more sophisticated investigations are not quickly and readily available, and also when the skull X-ray can be informative:
- skull fractures
- size, shape and density of pituitary fossa
- bone tumours
- meningioma bone changes

For most purposes a single lateral view is sufficient but a full series includes occipito-frontal (posterior-anterior), Towne's (half-axial) and basal (submentovertical) views.

The following should be particularly looked for:
- shape of vault, symmetry and cranial fossae
- size, shape and density of the pituitary fossa
- evidence of raised intracranial pressure (p. 259)

- position of pineal gland if calcified
- intracranial calcification (see below)
- change in bone density (e.g. tumour, Paget's disease, p. 483, osteomyelitis, meningioma, p. 271)
- fractures, burr holes and other neurosurgical defects
- vascular markings (e.g. meningioma, p. 271)
- intracranial air (fracture, infection)
- sinuses (infection, tumour)
- post-nasal space (tumour, haematoma)
- craniocervical junction (dislocation, fracture, basilar invagination, congenital anomaly)

Special views and tomograms may be needed for the optic foramen, internal auditory meatus and the pituitary fossa.

Intracranial calcification may occur in the following conditions but is much easier to see on CT than skull X-ray:
- basal ganglia calcification (p. 293)
- tumour:
  meningioma (p. 271)
  oligodendroglioma (p. 272)
  craniopharyngioma (p. 274)
  teratoma (p. 274)
  epidermoid and dermoid tumours (p. 274)
- vascular lesions:
  carotid siphon atheroma
  arteriovenous malformation (p. 233)
  giant aneurysm (p. 231)
  Sturge-Weber syndrome (p. 234)
- infections:
  tuberculoma (p. 513)
  cytomegalovirus (p. 525)
  toxoplasmosis (p. 536)
  cysticercosis (p. 538)
  hydatid cyst (p. 539)
- others:
  tuberous sclerosis (p. 487)
- normal:
  pineal gland
  choroid plexus
  falx
  tentorium

The pituitary fossa may be enlarged as a result of:
- pituitary adenoma (p. 273)
- craniopharyngioma (p. 274)

- carotid siphon aneurysm (p. 231)
- 3rd ventricular dilatation
- empty sella syndrome. The CT shows only CSF density in the enlarged sella. This occasionally occurs after infarction of the pituitary gland but is a common incidental finding

Myelography

The spinal cord, nerve roots and foramen magnum region can be outlined radiologically after introducing iodinated contrast material into the CSF, usually by the lumbar route (occasionally by the cervical route to outline the upper border of a spinal block or to obtain more detail in the cervical region). The patient is tilted to run the contrast up and down the spinal canal and conventional X-rays are taken. Follow-up CT of regions of interest provides more detail of cord and root compression and, if done several hours post-myelogram, contrast may enter and outline a syrinx. The indications are discussed mostly in the section on spinal cord compression (p. 324).

Complications

These include:
- Those following lumbar puncture (see above).
- Spinal arachnoiditis months or years later but only if an oily non-water soluble contrast medium such as myodil has been used.
- Immediate or subacute deterioration of neurological function if there is spinal cord or root compression, and possibly in multiple sclerosis.
- Direct neurotoxicity of non-ionic water soluble contrast media which are now the most commonly used since they are much better at outlining nerve roots than the older oily media. Iohexol and iopamidol may be less neurotoxic than metrizamide. Symptoms appear a few hours after myelography, are maximal in 24 hours, and almost always resolve in a day or two:
  - seizures (generalized tonic-clonic, myoclonus, non-convulsive status epilepticus)
  - encephalopathy with generalized EEG slowing (confusion, headache, drowsiness, vomiting, hallucinations, aphasia, cortical blindness, asterixis, seizures and even coma)
  - increase in CSF cells (lymphocytes and/or polymorph neutrophils) and raised protein

Neurotoxicity is minimized by adequate hydration before and after myelography, and a head-up posture as far as possible during it and afterwards.
- Iodine 'allergy' is rarely a problem, i.e. urticaria, angioneurotic oedema, bronchospasm, fever, chills, pulmonary oedema, hypotension. Patients with known skin allergy to iodine, or a reaction to contrast in the past, should be given dexamethasone 4 mg oral 12 hours and again 2 hours pre-myelography.

Note: The CSF must *always* be examined for protein, glucose and cells and then stored because, if no compressive spinal cord lesion is shown, further analysis of CSF (e.g. cytology, oligoclonal bands, microbiology) may be important in the diagnosis of multiple sclerosis, malignant meningitis, etc.

Computerized tomography (CT) of the brain

CT is the most sensitive technique which is readily available for imaging the brain and intracranial CSF spaces, providing, in tomographic slices usually in the orbito-meatal plane, details of normal anatomy (Fig. 1.16), mass lesions (p. 268), hydrocephalus (p. 259), inflammatory lesions (p. 504), etc. CT of the optic nerves and orbit (Chapter 7) and spinal cord (see above) is also helpful. The indications for CT are described in the appropriate chapters.

The dangers are of excessive radiation, the risks of which are relatively small unless scans are frequently repeated (e.g. follow-up of hydrocephalus, cerebral abscess, etc.); general anaesthesia which is rarely needed except to control restless patients; and the systemic complications of intravenous iodinated contrast (see below) which may be used to enhance images by virtue of the fact that it leaks through defective blood brain barrier associated with many malignant and inflammatory lesions and is preferentially taken up in highly vascular lesions such as arteriovenous malformations. Iodinated contrast (or sometimes air) may be introduced intrathecally by LP to outline structures in the posterior fossa, and sometimes to locate the site of a CSF leak.

An additional intravenous contrast enhanced CT scan should not be routine but only performed to improve the information from an unenhanced scan if this is likely to alter the patient's management. In some situations only an enhanced scan is appropriate, e.g. if an intracranial tumour is suspected on clinical grounds. Intravenous contrast may, as well as causing 'allergic' reactions (p. 46) and sometimes neurotoxicity (p. 46), cause systemic toxicity (myocardial depression and cardiac failure, cardiac arrhythmias, acute renal failure) and possibly neurological deterioration if given soon after cerebral infarction.

Magnetic resonance imaging (MRI)

MRI is more expensive, slower, more claustrophobic and less readily available than CT but it does provide much better images of the brain and, increasingly, the spinal cord. However, the exact nature of the lesions shown still cannot be accurately deduced. There are no bone artifacts and any imaging plane can be selected. It is likely to complement rather than replace CT and myelography. Since there are no X-rays there are no dangers from irradiation. So far there does not appear to be any danger from the high intensity magnetic fields and the radio frequency waves that are used provided patients (and staff) do not have either on them, or near them, any ferromagnetic

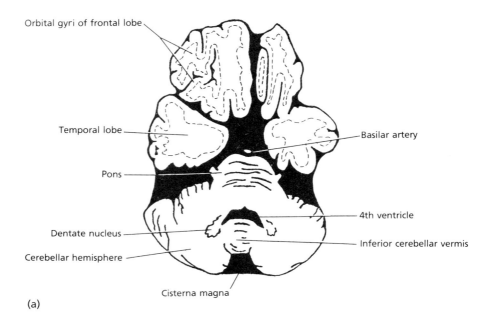

(a)

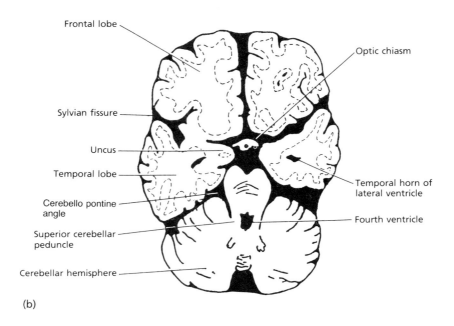

(b)

Fig. 1.16 Diagram to show normal brain structure as slices in the orbito-meatal plane.

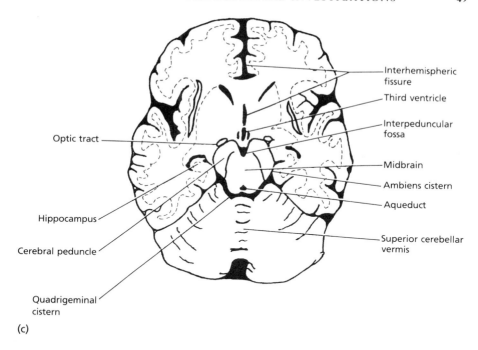

(c)

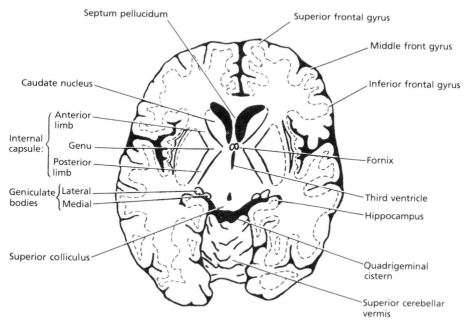

(d)

Fig. 1.16 *continued*

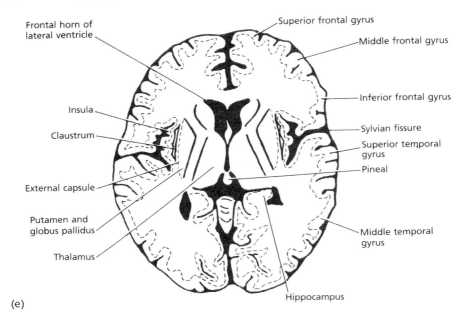

(e)

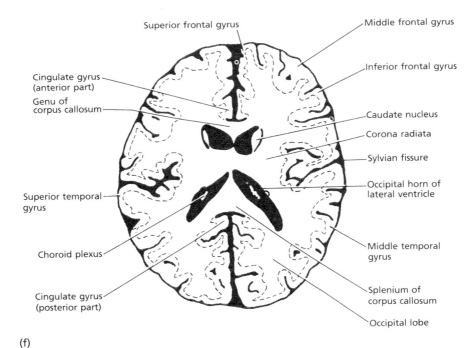

(f)

Fig. 1.16 *continued*

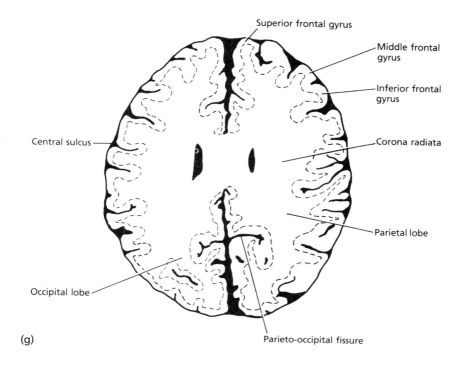

(g)

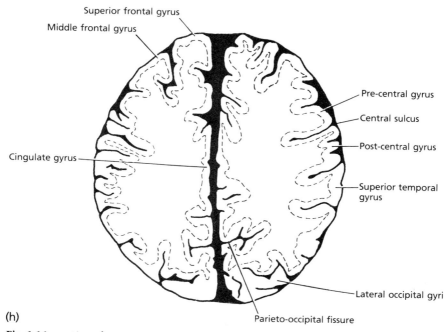

(h)

Fig. 1.16 *continued*

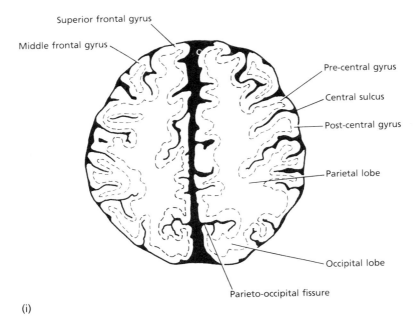

(i)

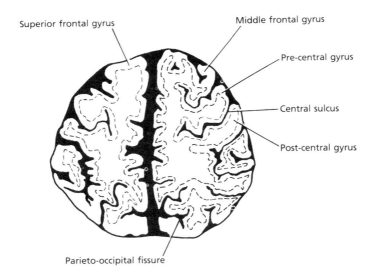

(j)

Fig. 1.16 *continued*

material to be attracted to the magnet (e.g. shrapnel, certain clips used in neurosurgery) or instruments containing switches activated by magnetic fields (e.g. certain pacemakers). MRI is particularly useful in:

- imaging the posterior fossa contents
- imaging the foramen magnum region
- diagnosis of syringomyelia (p. 334)
- diagnosis of multiple sclerosis (p. 350)
- diagnosis of dural sinus thrombosis (p. 224)
- diagnosis of vascular malformations (p. 233)
- spinal disease (p. 325)

Cerebral angiography

Arteries in the neck and head, along with the intracranial venous drainage system, can be displayed radiologically after the intravascular injection of iodinated contrast material. The non-ionic are less toxic than ionic formulations and cause less local discomfort and pain in the region of injection. Different techniques are used depending on local experience and the questions to be answered.

Arch angiography (aortography)

Transfemoral catheterization with injection of contrast into the arch of the aorta displays the aorta and major vessels in the neck, and sometimes the Circle of Willis at the base of the brain. The problems are overlap of simultaneously enhanced arteries (which can be overcome by taking views from different angles), lack of intracranial information, and no venous images.

Selective intra-arterial angiography

This type of angiography of carotid and vertebral arteries can be achieved after transfemoral catheterization and injection of contrast into the origin of each vessel (direct arterial puncture or catheterization from upper limb arteries are seldom used now). This technique provides more precise extracranial views than aortography as well as intracranial views, but does require more catheter manipulation if several arteries are imaged, and there is little information about the aortic arch and proximal parts of the arteries arising from it. Late views after injection provide venous images.

Intravenous digital subtraction angiography

This provides more or less the same information as conventional arch angiography but the images are less satisfactory. Although there may be fewer neurological complications (see below), large volumes of contrast have to be injected and this often causes local pain, 'allergy' (p. 46) and systemic toxicity (p. 47).

Intra-arterial digital subtraction angiography

This provides similar information to arch or selective intra-arterial angiograms depending on where the injection is made. Smaller quantities of contrast can be used, so reducing systemic and neurotoxicity at the expense of only a small loss of image quality (spatial resolution is less). It is particularly useful for spinal angiography and interventional procedures.

The most serious complication of any intra-arterial injection is stroke due to cerebral infarction in the territory of supply of the injected artery. It is rare (about 4% of all angiograms, permanent in 1%). It may be due to thrombosis on the catheter tip and embolization; dissection of the arterial wall by the catheter and subsequent thromboembolism; disruption of an atheromatous plaque with thrombosis or embolism; air embolism; and intravascular thrombosis due to a toxic effect of the contrast material. Vertebral angiography can cause transient cortical blindness. In addition there can be 'allergy' (p. 46), systemic (p. 47) or sometimes neurotoxicity (p. 46), the complications of general anaesthesia which is seldom used with the newer painless contrast materials, and haematoma formation at the arterial puncture site. Transfemoral catheterization may exacerbate peripheral vascular disease by damaging the arterial wall.

Electroencephalography (EEG)

Recording spontaneous brain electrical potentials over the scalp has been superseded in many areas of neurological diagnosis (particularly of intracranial mass lesions) but is still useful in:

- investigation and treatment of epilepsy (p. 79)
- diagnosis of coma (p. 129) and psychogenic pseudocoma (p. 126)
- diagnosis of encephalitis (p. 501)
- diagnosis of Creutzfeldt–Jakob disease (p. 531)
- diagnosis of subacute sclerosing panencephalitis (p. 525)
- diagnosis of excessive daytime sleepiness (p. 118)
  There are four main types of abnormality:
- A general excess of slow waves bilaterally in patients with metabolic encephalopathies (p. 129) and encephalitis (p. 501).
- A focal slow wave focus over a structural abnormality in one cerebral hemisphere, e.g. tumour, abscess, subdural haematoma, infarct or haemorrhage, all of which have to be fairly large to perturb the EEG.
- A focal or generalized spike or spike/wave discharge indicative of epilepsy (p. 79).

- Repetitive, generalized and stereotyped slow wave, sharp wave or triphasic complexes (so-called periodic complexes) in Creutzfeldt–Jakob disease (p. 531), herpes encephalitis (p. 501), subacute sclerosing panencephalitis (p. 525), lithium intoxication and post-anoxic brain injury.

Evoked potentials (EPs)

The evoked potential (or response) is the averaged EEG signal during a series of identical sensory stimuli (visual, auditory or somatosensory). The latency and amplitude of the EP are measured and abnormalities may provide evidence of a lesion in the relevant sensory pathway but do not reveal its nature. However, the EP can be normal even if the appropriate sensory pathway is damaged. It is *essential* that each laboratory provides age and sex specific normal values and that these are kept up to date by rigorous quality control. Exactly how 'normality' is defined (two or three standard deviations from the mean, etc.) has a profound effect on the test's sensitivity and specificity which again must be established by each laboratory.

EPs are particularly useful in the diagnosis of:

- A 'second' but subclinical lesion in multiple sclerosis, particularly in the visual pathway (by the visual evoked response) but this is being overtaken by MRI (p. 349).
- Acoustic neuromas using the auditory (brainstem) evoked response (p. 272).
- Brachial plexus lesions using the somatosensory evoked response from the hand and recording over the plexus, cervical spine and parietal area.
- Occasionally to confirm the presence of a lesion in a sensory pathway suspected on the basis of symptoms with unconvincing, or without any, clinical signs. Unfortunately the EP is often normal in this situation but a *definite* abnormality can be helpful (e.g. if uncertain about hysterical sensory, visual or hearing loss this would be ruled out by a technically well performed but abnormal EP).
- Monitoring of function during pituitary, spinal and other neurosurgery.

Note: Any cause of impaired visual acuity (e.g. cataracts) can affect the visual evoked potential.

Nerve conduction and electromyography (EMG)

Nerve conduction and EMG are mostly used in the diagnosis of peripheral nerve (Chapter 14) and muscle (Chapter 16) disorders and occasionally in the evaluation of generalized neurological diseases which have a peripheral neuropathy component (e.g. metachromatic leucodystrophy, p. 397, Refsum's disease, p. 478, etc.). The utility of, and indications for, the procedures are discussed in the relevant chapters. The techniques and normal values are described below.

Nerve conduction

Nerve conduction velocity must be measured at a standard ambient temperature and in a limb that is warm since the velocity declines in the cold.

Maximum motor nerve conduction velocity (MCV)

This is measured by supramaximal electrical stimulation at two points on the skin over a peripheral nerve trunk. The time taken from each stimulus to the beginning of the electrical response of the appropriate distal muscle recorded with a surface electrode (the compound muscle action potential, CMAP), or more painfully with a needle electrode, is noted. The difference between the proximal and distal motor latencies, along with the distance between the two points stimulated, allows calculation of the MCV over the intervening length of nerve (Table 1.4). *The distal motor latency* depends on the distance between the electrical stimulus and recording site, the distal MCV, neuromuscular transmission and muscle fibre conduction time (Table 1.5).

Table 1.4 Normal motor velocities (approximate)

Median nerve in forearm (to abductor pollicis brevis)	>45 m/sec
Ulnar nerve in forearm (to abductor digiti minimi)	>45 m/sec
Common peroneal nerve (to extensor digitorum brevis)	>40 m/sec
Tibial nerve (to abductor hallucis)	>40 m/sec

Table 1.5 Normal distal motor latency to onset of CMAP

Median nerve (wrist to abductor pollicis brevis)	<5 msec
Ulnar nerve (wrist to abductor digiti minimi)	<4 msec
Radial nerve (spiral groove to brachioradialis)	<5 msec

Note: MCV and distal motor latency should be the same on both sides so that an abnormality may be revealed by asymmetry between left and right, even when conduction velocity is normal.
Note: Laboratories must establish their own normal values and check them periodically.

The compound muscle action potential amplitude

This depends on the number of depolarized muscle fibres and is therefore reduced when the following occur:
- drop–out of motor fibres in the motor nerve (axonal neuropathy)
- fewer muscle fibres in a motor unit (denervated muscle)
- temporal dispersion of conduction velocities (axonal and, more commonly, demyelinating neuropathies)

The F-wave

This is a later potential than the CMAP and is due to antidromic proximal nerve impulses to the anterior horn cells followed by orthodromic motor conduction down the same nerve. An absent or delayed F-wave is therefore a result of lesions causing reduced proximal (to the stimulus) nerve or motor root conduction velocity; however, the F-wave can be normal with root lesions, particularly if mild or incomplete.

Repetitive nerve stimulation

This is used in the diagnosis of myasthenia gravis and the Lambert–Eaton myasthenic syndrome (Chapter 15).

Central motor conduction

Central motor conduction down the corticospinal tract can now be measured by electromagnetic stimulation of the motor cortex (or much less comfortably by electrical stimulation) and recording the compound muscle action potentials in distal limb muscles.

Sensory nerve action potentials (SAP)

These are measured in the hand by electrical stimulation over the digital nerves and recording at the wrist, and in the feet by stimulation over the sural nerve in the calf and recording below the lateral malleolus. Lesions of sensory nerves *distal* to the dorsal root ganglia lead to a reduction of SAP latency and particularly amplitude which are normally symmetrical on the left and right. By recording the SAP at two separate points over a nerve the sensory nerve conduction velocity can be calculated; also more simply by dividing the SAP latency by the distance between the stimulus and recording site (Table 1.6).

Table 1.6 Normal sensory action potentials

	Latency to peak	Amplitude
Median nerve (index finger to wrist)	3–4 msec	9–40 microvolt
Ulnar nerve (little finger to wrist)	2–4 msec	6–30 microvolt
Sural nerve (midcalf to below lateral malleolus)	2–4 msec	5–40 microvolt

Note: These values vary with age and depend on the distance between the electrical stimulus and recording site. Laboratories *must* provide their own control values.

Electromyography (EMG)

The EMG provides diagnostic information from muscles that are denervated (as a result of a lower motor neurone lesion) or myopathic, provided an abnormal site is sampled when the disease process is patchy. The EMG should, therefore, be sampled from several parts of the same muscle and the muscles selected on the basis of the clinical picture and diagnostic information required.

Note: An EMG must not be done from a muscle that is to be biopsied since it may distort the normal muscle fibre anatomy.

When a recording needle is inserted into normal muscle there is a brief electrical discharge (insertional activity) followed by silence. A weak voluntary contraction activates a few motor units and those near the needle tip are recorded. Their amplitude (100 microvolt–7 millivolt depending on the muscle) and number of potential changes (usually less than 4) are measured. As voluntary contraction increases, so more and more motor units are recruited until individual ones cannot be distinguished and the electrical activity becomes virtually continuous (the interference pattern is then said to be full).

In *denervated muscle*:

- insertional activity is increased
- spontaneous firing at rest; very brief low amplitude fibrillation potentials, positive sharp waves and large amplitude fasciculations
- reduced number of motor units so that recruitment and the interference pattern are incomplete
- surviving motor units may be larger than normal with more components (polyphasia) and of longer duration if there has been sprouting of motor nerve terminals and collateral innervation of denervated muscle fibres

In *myopathies* (p. 420):

- muscle is silent at rest except in polymyositis and some metabolic myopathies when fibrillations occur
- motor unit amplitudes are reduced. Also the units are of shorter duration and there is polyphasia. The muscle fibres in each motor unit are variably damaged in a patchy manner
- the interference pattern is full until muscle fibre loss is severe since the surviving motor units are polyphasic. The sound is a characteristic and abnormal crackling
- myotonic muscle causes characteristic high frequency waxing and waning discharges on needle insertion or voluntary muscle contraction

The interpretation of the EMG is subjective and operator dependent; it therefore requires considerable experience to do it well. Automated systems of motor unit and recruitment analysis are available but not yet widely adopted in clinical practice.

Neurological impairment, disability and handicap

Once a neurological diagnosis has been made, the progress of the disease and the effect of treatment are best monitored *not* by frequent and formal neurological examinations (for of what concern to the patient is the return of an absent or brisk reflex to normal?), but by asking the patient and his relatives how things are going and by attempting to measure something which is relevant, valid, reliable, sensitive to change, simple and communicable to others. Exactly what is measured depends partly on the disease and how an individual is affected by it (this will be referred to in later chapters when different diseases are discussed). There are also some general principles and measurements that can be applied to all neurological patients:

Impairment

Impairment is any loss or abnormality of psychological or physiological function or anatomical structure. Although this can usually be easily measured, it may not necessarily be of relevance to the patient. Examples are given in Table 1.7.

Table 1.7 Methods of measuring various impairments

Impairment	Measurement
Vision	Acuity, visual evoked potential (p. 55)
Strength	Myometer, MRC scale (p. 13)
Language	Functional communication profile, Frenchay Aphasia Screening Test
MS plaque	MRI (p. 47)
Consciousness	Glasgow coma score (p. 122)
Non-verbal memory	Rey figure recall
Absence seizures	Spike and wave on EEG (p. 72)
Nerve conduction	Nerve conduction velocity (p. 56)

Disability

Disability is any restriction or lack of ability (resulting from an impairment) to perform an activity in the manner or within the range considered normal.

Specific disabilities can be measured:

- of walking by a timed walk of 10 metres
- of manual dexterity by a standard nine-hole peg test
- of epilepsy by frequency of clinical seizures
- of migraine by number, duration and severity of headache attacks

A general level of disability can be measured by the widely used *Barthel index of activities of daily living* (Table 1.8).

Table 1.8 Barthel index of activities of daily living

Bowels	0	Incontinent or needs to be given enemas
	1	Occasional accident (i.e. about once a week)
	2	Continent
Bladder	0	Incontinent or catheterized and unable to manage catheter
	1	Occasional accident (less than one per day)
	2	Continent or, if catheterized, patient can manage catheter alone
Grooming	0	Needs help with personal care (e.g. doing teeth, hair, shaving, washing)
	1	Independent (even if implements provided by a helper)
Toilet use	0	Dependent on others
	1	Needs some help
	2	Independent on and off toilet, dressing and wiping
Feeding	0	Unable to feed self without help
	1	Needs some help (e.g. cutting, spreading) but can feed self
	2	Independent (if food provided in reach)
Transfer	0	Unable to transfer between bed, and chair, and no sitting balance
	1	Requires major help
	2	Requires some minor help
	3	Independent
Mobility	0	Immobile
	1	Wheelchair independent indoors
	2	Walks with the help or supervision of one person
	3	Independent (but may use an aid)
Dressing	0	Dependent on others
	1	Needs some help
	2	Independent, including buttons and zips
Stairs	0	Unable
	1	Needs help or supervision
	2	Independent up and down
Bathing	0	Dependent
	1	Independent in bath or shower, can get in and out and wash

The score can be summed (0–20) or each item considered separately. It is applied to what the patient actually does, not what someone thinks they ought to be able to do. This can be assessed from the patient's or relative's account without necessarily observing all the activities.

To some extent this scale is also to do with handicap since the score can be influenced by changing the patient's environment (e.g. by abandoning ties and using velcro instead of buttons).

Handicap

Handicap is the disadvantage for a given individual resulting from an impairment or disability that limits or prevents the fulfilment of a role that

Table 1.9 Modified Rankin scale

0	No symptoms
1	Minor symptoms which do not interfere with lifestyle
2	Minor handicap. Symptoms which lead to some restriction in lifestyle but do not interfere with the patients' capacity to look after themselves. There is no dependency on others
3	Moderate handicap. Symptoms which significantly restrict lifestyle and prevent totally independent existence
4	Moderately severe handicap. Symptoms which clearly prevent independent existence though not needing constant care and attention
5	Severe handicap. Totally dependent, requiring constant attention day and night

is normal for that individual. A simple measure of handicap that can be obtained even by telephone is the *modified Rankin scale* (Table 1.9).

This scale can be used to assess the whole patient including handicaps due to non-neurological impairments (e.g. arthritis, angina, breathlessness) or to assess just the neurological part of any overall handicap.

Disablement

Disablement is a generic term and refers to any experience identified by the terms impairment, disability and handicap.

Useful addresses of organizations which are not disease specific (for the latter see under the appropriate diseases)

Disabled Living Foundation, Equipment Centre
380–384 Harrow Road
London W9 2HU
Tel: 071-289-6111

Disability Alliance
25 Denmark Street
London WC2H 8NJ
Tel: 071-240-0806

Equipment for the Disabled
Mary Marlborough Lodge
Nuffield Orthopaedic Centre
Headington
Oxford OX3 7LD
Tel: 0865-750103

Medic-Alert Foundation*
17 Bridge Wharf
156 Caledonian Road
London N1 9UU
Tel: 071-833-3034

Offers a medic-alert emblem which allows identification of patients' medical
condition and information about them in an emergency 24 hours a day.

Spastics Society
12 Park Crescent
London W1N 4EQ
Tel: 071-636-5020

SPOD (Sexual & Personal Relationships of the Disabled)
286 Camden Road
London N7 0BJ
Tel: 071-607-8851

2　Blackouts, fits, faints and funny turns

Sudden attacks of loss of consciousness, altered consciousness, dizziness and vertigo are common. In the majority the main category of cause is obvious from the history.

The differential diagnosis includes other conditions discussed elsewhere:

- transient ischaemic attacks (p. 219)
- subclavian steal (p. 221)
- excessive daytime sleepiness (p. 114)
- transient global amnesia (p. 159)
- loss of consciousness during migraine (p. 137)
- intermittent obstructive hydrocephalus (p. 261)
- drop attacks (p. 222)
- hyperviscosity syndromes (p. 461)
- acute drug-induced dystonia (p. 302)
- breath holding attacks (p. 66)

Because a fall may *cause* a head injury, an unwitnessed head injury causing loss of consciousness and retrograde amnesia for the moments before the injury itself may lead to diagnostic confusion. Also one must remember that the elderly are very prone to fall, without loss of awareness, as a result of general imbalance and osteoarthritis perhaps combined with poor vision, as indeed is any patient with weak legs, loss of postural sensation in the legs, cerebellar problems of Parkinson's disease (p. 37).

Making the diagnosis

The specific clinical features of each type of attack are described later but the general approach to a patient with one or more 'funny turns' is essentially the same.

The *history* is crucial and every effort must be made to talk to an eyewitness, if necessary by telephone, unless the diagnosis is obvious. For each different type of attack, the details required include:

- date of first, date of last, frequency and any change in frequency, the longest and shortest gap between attacks
- general health in the days before and day of the attack
- *exact* position and activity at the onset, and time of onset
- precipitating factors; any relationship with posture, food, time of day, exercise, stress, alcohol, menstrual cycle, etc.
- exact description of attacks: warning symptoms, aura, pain in the chest or head, palpitations, duration, etc. Also from a witness: change of colour, abnormal movements, loss of consciousness, confusion, rigidity, and pulse. Afterwards: headache, confusion, bitten tongue, incontinence, muscle stiffness, skin purpura.

It is important to obtain details of general health, in particular cardiac or neurological symptoms; psychiatric problems; alcohol consumption and drugs; past history of migraine, head injury, febrile convulsions, epilepsy, etc.; and family history.

The *examination* must pay particular attention to:

- heart rate, rhythm, vascular bruits
- cardiac examination
- carotid sinus massage (but not if a localized carotid bruit) one side and then the other, and pressure on the eyes in children
- neurological signs; nystagmus, deafness, peripheral neuropathy, bodily asymmetry, etc.
- lying and standing blood pressure

Investigations are unnecessary in simple cases, such as vasovagal (p. 101) or micturition syncope (p. 103), but otherwise should include:

- full blood count
- blood sugar
- chest X-ray
- ECG (? heart block, sick sinus syndrome, QT interval, etc.)

Other investigations are dictated by circumstances. If a structural cardiac cause is suspected, then echocardiography; if epilepsy, perhaps a CT scan (p. 81) and EEG (p. 79); if vertigo, perhaps audiometry and caloric responses (p. 194), etc.

Ambulatory monitoring of the ECG for 24 hours (or longer) during normal and, if possible, precipitating activities is useful if the attacks are frequent enough to be captured. This is particularly so if the history suggests a cardiac arrhythmia, or the resting ECG is abnormal but not abnormal enough to be diagnostic (e.g. only first degree heart block), or nothing else can be found and the attacks are continuing. However, paroxysmal tachycardias can occur during tonic-clonic and complex partial seizures. Interictal cardiac rhythm disturbances are difficult to evaluate and are seldom serious enough to warrant therapeutic action, particularly in the elderly in whom asymptomatic arrhythmias are common; on balance, asymptomatic bradyarrhythmias are likely to be more relevant than asymptomatic tachyarrhythmias.

For undiagnosable attacks which are unacceptably frequent, ambulatory recording of the ECG and EEG simultaneously for several days may capture an attack; even admission to hospital for observation and EEG monitoring may be needed. It is also helpful to ask the patient to keep prospective notes about attacks and to teach relatives how to feel and count the patient's pulse. Certainly repeating the history and examination is useful and, as a very last resort, perhaps a therapeutic trial of anticonvulsants. The latter can, however, be misleading because of the placebo response, sometimes dangerous because of adverse effects, and may cause a patient to be inappropriately labelled as 'epileptic'.

There always remain some patients with occasional attacks for which no cause is ever found, even after months and years.

It is more important to diagnose and to treat quickly those conditions which are likely to cause death (e.g. cardiac bradyarrhythmias) than those which are not (e.g. complex partial seizures). Therefore, whilst there is no hurry for an EEG, an ECG is usually needed at once. If in doubt it is far better to wait and see rather than label attacks as 'vasovagal' (and inhibit further thought) or as 'epilepsy' (and damage the patients socially or by the adverse effects of inappropriate drugs; furthermore, stopping inappropriate anticonvulsants might even precipitate a withdrawal seizure in a non-epileptic).

Breath holding attacks are not epileptic. Occasionally babies and young children have episodes of sudden apnoea and deepening cyanosis lasting a few seconds. If more prolonged, the child may stiffen or even have an anoxic seizure. Attacks are spontaneous or precipitated by slight knocks or rage.

Epilepsy

An epileptic attack, or seizure, is a symptom not a disease. It is defined as an abnormal paroxysmal neuronal discharge in the brain causing abnormal function.

About 3% of the population have a non-febrile seizure at some time in their lives but the prevalence of *active* epilepsy is only about 5 per 1000, and of severely disabling epilepsy about 0.1 per 1000 (i.e. about 300 000 and 6000 cases respectively in the UK). Seizures start at any age but most commonly in the first two decades of life; the incidence of recurrent non-febrile seizures is about 50/100 000/annum. Anyone, given the right provoking circumstances (e.g. electroconvulsive therapy) may have a seizure, but epilepsy is used only to describe the condition of patients who have more than one non-febrile seizure. The vast majority of patients are mentally normal but presumably have a lower than average seizure threshold.

The causes of seizures

More or less any type of supratentorial brain damage may present with, or be complicated by, seizures. Therefore, *symptomatic* seizures have many possible causes:

Primary brain lesions

- intracranial tumours (p. 266):
  benign, malignant, primary or secondary
- infections (Chapter 18):
  encephalitis (p. 498)
  acute post-infectious encephalomyelitis (p. 502)
  abscess (p. 503)
  subdural empyema (p. 503)
  tuberculoma (p. 513)

syphilis (p. 515)
toxoplasmosis (p. 536)
cysticercosis (p. 538)
febrile convulsions (p. 76)
- trauma:
perinatal (immediate or delayed seizures)
head injury (immediate or delayed seizures) (p. 78)
supratentorial neurosurgical procedure
- vascular:
cerebral infarction (p. 246)
intracranial haemorrhage (p. 246)
cortical venous thrombosis (p. 225)
vascular malformation (p. 233)
hypertensive encephalopathy (p. 214)
collagen vascular disorders (p. 444)
Sturge–Weber syndrome (p. 234)
eclampsia
- miscellaneous:
multiple sclerosis (p. 345)
migraine (p. 137)
tuberous sclerosis (p. 487)
Ammon's horn sclerosis (p. 76)
progressive myoclonic epilepsies (p. 75)
xeroderma pigmentosum (p. 203)
Fahr's syndrome (p. 293)
pertussis immunization
burns encephalopathy in children

Systemic disorders

- metabolic and biochemical disorders:
metabolic encephalopathies (p. 124)
ischaemic/anoxic brain damage (p. 123)
hypomagnesaemia (p. 465)
lysosomal storage disorders (p. 477)
inborn errors of amino and organic acid metabolism (p. 480)
Leigh's disease (p. 482)
kernicterus
disorders of glycogen metabolism (p. 427)
mitochondrial cytopathies (p. 429)
pyridoxine deficiency (p. 470)
- drugs:
acrosoxacin
aminophylline
amphetamines

analeptics
anticholinergic drugs
antihistamines
baclofen
barbiturates*
benzodiazepines*
butyrophenones
cephalosporins
chlorambucil
chloroquine
cinoxacin
ciprofloxan
cocaine
cycloserine
cyclosporin
cytarabine
digoxin
disopyramide
domperidone
enoxacin
ephedrine
fluoxetine
general anaesthetics (althesin, ether, halothane, ketamine, methohexitone)
hypoglycaemic drugs
indomethacin
isoniazid
lignocaine
lithium
lysergic acid diethylamide (LSD)
maprotiline
methylphenidate
metronidazole
mexiletine
mianserin
monoamine oxidase inhibitors
naladixic acid
penicillin (intrathecal or high intravenous doses)
pentazocine
phencyclidine
phenothiazines
propoxyphene
sympathomimetic drugs (p. 294)

* Typically withdrawal seizures occur within a few days of suddenly stopping the drug which has been taken in high doses for a long time.

theophylline
thyrotrophin releasing hormone
thyroxine
tocainide
tricyclic antidepressants
zimeldine
• toxins:
alcohol* (p. 542)
lead (p. 547)
aluminium (p. 467)
tin (p. 547)
bismuth (p. 548)
carbon monoxide poisoning (p. 549)
iodinated radiographic contrast media, particularly intrathecal (p. 46)
organophosphorus compounds (p. 548)
plants (p. 552)

The classification of seizures

Patients with epilepsy may experience one or more different types of seizure
which are classified clinically and to some extent on the interictal EEG as
well:
• partial (or focal) seizures:
simple partial (motor, sensory, etc.)
complex partial
• partial seizures evolving to secondary generalized seizures
• primary generalized seizures:
absence seizures (typical and atypical)
tonic-clonic seizures (grand mal)
clonic seizures
tonic seizures
atonic (or akinetic) seizures
myoclonic seizures

Partial (focal) seizures

These have clinical and/or EEG evidence of origin in a localized part of the
cerebrum. A focal brain lesion (such as a tumour) is more likely to be the
cause than in primary generalized seizures but is not necessarily present, and
the epilepsy can certainly be 'idiopathic' rather than symptomatic of an
identifiable brain disorder.

Simple partial seizures occur with clear consciousness, whereas complex
partial seizures are accompanied by altered or impaired consciousness and
are more or less equivalent to what was called 'temporal lobe epilepsy'.

Partial and complex partial seizures may evolve into a tonic-clonic or other generalized seizure which is called 'secondary generalization'.

Primary generalized seizures

There is no preceding aura, the initial motor manifestations are bilateral, and at onset (and sometimes interictally) there are simultaneous and bilateral abnormal EEG discharges. Although there may be no clinical or EEG evidence of a focal origin, some such seizures are due to focal brain lesions (such as tumours). A secondary generalized seizure may be misclassified as primary generalized if the interictal EEG is normal and if a preceding partial aura has been forgotten by the patient as a result of amnesia induced by the seizure itself; such an aura may only come to light if a witness observes some characteristic feature (e.g. automatisms).

Simple partial seizures

Motor origin seizures

These usually arise from the motor or pre-motor cortex and are often called 'focal motor' or 'Jacksonian' seizures. The onset is with rhythmic twitching or jerking of one part of the body opposite the epileptic focus, often first the fingers, toes or face. This spreads over a minute or two, usually with increasing amplitude, to the rest of the body part and from one part to the next on the same side. As well as or instead of the twitching, there may be a sustained tonic or dystonic movement of one arm or leg. Also, there may be forced turning of the head and eyes to one side (usually to the opposite side to an electrical focus in the frontal lobe, so-called adversive seizures) with or without other motor manifestations. The seizures last seconds or minutes and, in severe cases, can be followed by temporary weakness (minutes or hours) of the involved part of the body (Todd's paresis).

Epilepsia partialis continua is rare. There is spontaneous and persistent regular or irregular muscular twitching of a limited part of the body for hours or days. Secondary generalization can occur. There is usually a focal brain lesion in the contralateral motor cortex, and often focal neurological signs. It is less violent than focal motor status epilepticus (p. 94). Medical and surgical treatment are seldom successful.

Cortical myoclonus is rare and is part of the spectrum of partial motor seizures, with or without secondary generalization, and epilepsia partialis continua. As such, it is due to an abnormal focal electrical discharge in or near the motor cortex. The clinical manifestation is one or more myoclonic jerks of a limb, or the face, on the contralateral side. It may be spontaneous or precipitated by action, muscle stretch and touch.

Sensory origin seizures

These usually arise from the sensory cortex. There are focal and spreading symptoms (like motor origin attacks) with tingling, dysaesthesia, burning, stinging and rarely pain. This must be differentiated from a migrainous aura which takes about 10 minutes to develop (p. 137) and focal ischaemia (p. 219) which affects all involved body parts more or less simultaneously.

Seizures originating in the occipital cortex cause simple (flashes, dots, dazzles) or complex (shapes, scenes, people) hallucinations contralateral to the epileptic focus. Sometimes objects appear larger than normal, too small, upside down or distorted. Rarely an intense visual memory occurs. As the hallucination develops the head and eyes may turn towards it.

Complex partial seizures

These usually arise in one temporal lobe (and are often called temporal lobe epilepsy) but can arise in adjacent areas of brain (e.g. frontal lobe). An old term is 'psychomotor epilepsy'. A huge variety of symptoms can occur but usually individuals experience only a small number in a stereotyped fashion. The attacks last seconds or minutes but sometimes longer, leaving the patient in a confused amnesic state, one form of non-convulsive status epilepticus (p. 97).

Autonomic features include nausea, an apprehensive feeling in the epigastrium rising to the throat, salivation, abnormal taste or smell, facial pallor or flushing, cardiac palpitations with tachyarrhythmias or more rarely bradyarrhythmias even with apparent disappearance of the wrist pulse (cf. Stokes–Adams attacks), discomfort in the chest, piloerection and 'goose flesh', penile erection and sometimes orgasm, abdominal pain, vomiting, incontinence of urine and less often faeces.

Psychic features include a dream-like feeling of unreality, déjà vu, fear, intense depression, unformed or formed memories, sexual fantasies, depersonalization and a feeling of being outside one's body or looking at oneself, distortion or change in shape of objects, anxiety, panic and distortion of time.

Motor features (automatisms) are not recalled by the patient and include grimacing, swallowing, lip smacking, chewing, rubbing the hands together, plucking at the clothes, muttering, vocalization, singing and more complex automatisms which are well co-ordinated but inappropriate (e.g. undressing, washing, etc.).

Other features include vertigo, distortion of sounds, abnormal sounds, inability to understand speech and sometimes a vivid visual memory or scenario. Directed aggression is extraordinarily rare although it is common for patients to be irritable and to resent external interference. During the attack the patients are blank, vacant or glazed. They appear confused and usually are unresponsive.

Note: Sudden inability to speak with normal consciousness, *speech arrest*, may be due to a seizure (usually dominant temporal or frontal lobe origin) and perhaps occasionally due to ischaemia in the dominant temporal lobe or brainstem. Dysphasic speech is less common during a seizure than during cerebral ischaemia.

Typical absence seizures (petit mal)

These are a manifestation of 'idiopathic' generalized epilepsy, start at the age of 4 to 12, and seldom persist over the age of 20. In many patients there are tonic-clonic seizures in addition or, if not, they appear in adolescence or later in about 30%.

There is no aura, and unless the children realize they have missed a small period of time, they may not be aware of the attacks at all. The attacks last seconds and afterwards the children are immediately alert and normal. A child suddenly stops any movement but does not fall, looks blank and glazed, is unresponsive, and there may be a few brief clonic movements of the eyelids or face. The attacks can occur many times a day and interfere with learning or become continuous, petit mal status (p. 97), causing a prolonged confusional state. During the attacks, and commonly between them, the EEG shows 3/second bilateral synchronous and symmetrical spike and wave discharges. The differential diagnosis includes complex partial seizures, 'day dreaming', or simply not paying attention at school. The prognosis and treatment of typical absence seizures are so different from those of complex partial seizures that they must be carefully distinguished by a history and the EEG even though to an outside observer they may look very similar.

Atypical absence seizures

These cause rather more involuntary movements with simple automatisms of the face, lips, eyes or hands, some minor clonic movements, and perhaps stiffening of the trunk. The child may fall and be incontinent. The EEG during an attack is more disorganized with widespread polyspike discharges and differentiation from complex partial seizures can be difficult. They are usually a feature of severe childhood epilepsies associated with brain damage.

Tonic-clonic (grand mal) seizures

These may or may not be preceded by an aura (i.e. a partial seizure as described above) which patients do not necessarily remember. The patient may cry out and then fall to the ground, rigid, jaw clenched, breath held, face contorted and frothing at the mouth. Within seconds this tonic stage is followed by rhythmic clonic jerking of the limbs, neck and back for several minutes. Cyanosis, incontinence of urine but rarely of faeces, and biting the side of the tongue or inside cheek are common. As the seizure subsides the patients relax, the colour returns to normal, but they usually remain unconscious with stertorous breathing for several more minutes. At this stage one may find extensor plantar responses, dilated pupils with impaired light response, absent corneal reflexes and no response to pain. On coming round patients are confused, irritable, drowsy and may want to sleep. Post-ictal headache, vomiting, muscle pain and stiffness, and purpura over the upper trunk are common. During the seizure the patients may injure themselves by falling against a hard object (NB head injury as a cause for persistent coma, p. 78) or into a fire, break teeth and occasionally sustain a crush fracture of a thoracic vertebra.

In some generalized seizures there is no tonic stage and the onset is with clonic jerking (*clonic seizures*), and in others the patient merely becomes rigid and crashes to the ground, being unconscious for only seconds or minutes (*tonic seizures*).

Atonic seizures almost always occur in children, not adults, and consist of a sudden collapse of muscle tone with falling to the ground or head nods, often with very brief unconsciousness.

Myoclonus (see also p. 307)

This may occur within the context of various epileptic syndromes. Cortical myoclonus has already been described (p. 70). Generalized myoclonic jerks are usually bilaterally synchronous and objects may be dropped from the hand. They can be isolated or accompanied by brief loss of consciousness and falling to the ground. They may be repetitive and precede a generalized tonic-clonic seizure. They are often experienced in the hour or so after waking up. They occur in 'idiopathic' epilepsy (see below), juvenile myoclonic epilepsy (p. 75), infantile spasms (p. 74), the progressive myoclonic epilepsies (p. 75) and the Lennox-Gastaut syndrome (p. 75). Treatment is with sodium valproate (p. 91), or if that fails with benzodiazepines, particularly clonazepam (p. 93).

Classification of the epilepsy syndromes

In the majority of patients, particularly children and adolescents (age 5–18), no definite cause is found and so they have 'idiopathic', 'constitutional' or 'cryptogenic' epilepsy. Even so, in many the cause of the seizures is probably a very small cryptogenic lesion such as a hamartoma, slow growing glioma (p. 271), vascular malformation (p. 233), long forgotten birth trauma or head injury; in others there is a definite familial tendency; and some others are probably due to Ammon's horn sclerosis (p. 76), perhaps as a result of childhood febrile convulsions, antenatal damage or birth trauma. Between the attacks most patients are entirely normal.

Seizures in 'idiopathic' epilepsy, or due to non-cerebral systemic disorders, tend to be primarily generalized, but when there is a structural and focal brain lesion the seizures are more likely to be partial (focal). However, this is only an approximate distinction and there is considerable overlap.

In some patients seizures occur only during sleep. On the whole the causes are similar to seizures which occur only while awake and those which occur while asleep and awake. Seizures soon after waking are a common feature of the 'idiopathic' primary generalized epilepsies (e.g. juvenile myoclonic epilepsy, p. 75).

In some women seizure frequency increases just before or during menstruation (*catamenial epilepsy*) perhaps because of water retention. Diuretics, acetazolamide (p. 94) and oral contraceptives may help, or anticonvulsants which, if used intermittently, do not lead to tolerance (e.g. clobazam, p. 93).

Reflex epilepsy

A few patients, who may or may not have seizures at other times, are particularly sensitive to having their seizures triggered by certain stimuli, most often flickering light (photic reflex epilepsy). Usually the seizures are primary generalized and the epilepsy is 'idiopathic'. This starts in childhood or adolescence and becomes less of a problem in adult life.

The most common trigger is television (particularly if the patient is close to the set or the picture is unstable) and others include certain video games, discotheque lighting, flickering sunlight, moving escalators and some nonvisual stimuli (e.g. noise, music, reading, certain specific mental activities, exercise). Sometimes the children appear to enjoy their seizures and seek out the stimuli or even induce them. In photic reflex epilepsy flickering light causes an epileptic response (photosensitivity) on the EEG although this can also be found in epileptic patients without photic fits.

Photic epilepsy can be abolished by covering one eye. Further advice is to view television from a distance and/or to have a small screen and to view in a well lit room. Anticonvulsants are only required if the stimulus cannot be avoided or if non-reflex seizures are also occurring.

Infantile spasms (West syndrome)

At about the age of 6 months a child starts having repetitive and sudden attacks of flexion of the neck, body and knees along with flexion and abduction of the arms (salaam attacks). Each attack lasts seconds. Soon various generalized seizure types occur, mental development stops and intractable seizures develop with hopeless mental retardation. The EEG may show hypsarrhythmia. Most of the children have some kind of previous brain damage (neonatal trauma, tuberous sclerosis, p. 487, etc.) but some are normal before the spasms begin. Conventional anticonvulsants have little effect but sometimes ACTH (i.m. 40–60 units daily) stops the seizures, at least for a few weeks.

Lennox–Gastaut syndrome

This syndrome is variably defined but probably represents a particularly severe form of epilepsy and mental handicap starting in childhood as a consequence of previous brain damage (prenatal or perinatal injury, etc.). There is a combination of myoclonic jerks, sudden atonic falls and head nods, tonic seizures and atypical absences which respond poorly to anticonvulsants. Primary generalized tonic-clonic seizures develop a little later. The EEG shows diffuse spike and wave at about 2 Hz. ACTH (see above) or a ketogenic diet (p. 95) may help in bad patches but are not successful long-term treatments.

Benign Rolandic epilepsy

This starts in childhood and remits in adolescence. It can be of dominant inheritance. While asleep there are focal motor seizures and occasionally secondary generalization. The EEG shows high voltage spikes over the Rolandic area (i.e. motor cortex).

Juvenile myoclonic epilepsy

Early morning generalized myoclonic jerks, tonic-clonic seizures and sometimes absence seizures start in late childhood, usually respond well to valproate, and seldom remit in adulthood. The EEG shows generalized epileptic discharges. It is an idiopathic epileptic syndrome, sometimes familial.

Progressive myoclonic epilepsies

These epilepsies are a heterogeneous group characterized by myoclonic seizures, tonic-clonic and other primary generalized seizures and progressive neurological dysfunction, particularly dementia and cerebellar ataxia. Most are autosomal recessive and the onset is usually in childhood or adolescence:
- Unverricht–Lundborg disease; no known biochemical disorder and widespread cerebral neuronal degeneration.
- Lafora body disease; PAS-positive inclusions in brain, liver, muscle and skin. Partial occipital seizures also occur.
- Sialidosis; there are excess urine sialic acid-rich oligosaccharides. Visual failure and macular cherry red spot also occur.
- Neuronal ceroid lipofuscinosis (p. 480).
- Mitochondrial cytopathies (p. 429).

Febrile convulsions

About 3% of children, aged from about 3 months to 5 years, have one or more generalized tonic-clonic seizures during the course of a febrile, usually viral, illness without evidence of intracranial infection or any other defined cause. A few children are obviously brain damaged (usually at or before birth); in some the febrile convulsion is the start of non-febrile epilepsy, or there is a family history of febrile convulsions. Prolonged febrile convulsions perhaps themselves cause brain damage, particularly Ammon's horn sclerosis (in the hippocampus of the medial temporal lobe, often unilaterally) with the later development of complex partial seizures.

Recurrent febrile convulsions occur in about one third of children after one attack but only about 5% go on to develop non-febrile convulsions (i.e. epilepsy), about five times the expected risk of normals. The risk of epilepsy is higher in a small subgroup with one or more of:
- febrile convulsion lasting more than 15–30 minutes
- focal features in the febrile convulsion
- multiple seizures during first attack
- neurological abnormalities or mental retardation
- family history of epilepsy
- onset within the first year of life

Children with a first febrile convulsion should be admitted to hospital for a lumbar puncture and the exclusion of meningitis, particularly if less than 2 years old. In subsequent febrile illnesses the child should be cooled with a fan and tepid sponging and given paracetamol early as an antipyretic. If a seizure occurs it should be treated with diazepam: i.v. 0.2 mg per kg or the i.v. solution given intrarectally 0.5 mg per kg. The latter can be managed by a sensible parent using a kit of ampoules of intravenous diazepam, a narrow syringe to draw out the solution without a needle, and some KY jelly to facilitate insertion of the syringe into the rectum. Alternatively, a Stesolid rectal tube may be used.

In the high risk group for eventual epilepsy, or if the febrile convulsions are very frequent, sodium valproate (p. 91) can be used as prophylaxis for one or two years, or some use phenobarbitone (p. 22) but this may cause behavioural problems.

Avoid whooping cough vaccination.

Memory, learning and concentration

Many epileptic patients have problems with memory, learning and concentration and some have severe disability. There are a number of possible causes, some of which are treatable:
- the static or progressive brain pathology causing the seizures
- anticonvulsant drug intoxication

- overt seizures interfering with schooling, learning and social development
- subclinical seizures interfering with learning and memory
- head injury and anoxia as a result of frequent seizures
- psychiatric and behavioural problems (see below)
- lack of expectation, social isolation

Psychiatric and behavioural problems

Patients with seizures are usually mentally and neurologically normal but a proportion do have psychological, behavioural and overt psychiatric difficulties. These can be hard to disentangle and are not necessarily more common than in the non-epileptic population, nor indeed than those who are brain damaged but non-epileptic. Particular predisposing factors include:

- Any brain damage, static or progressive, causing seizures may cause mental handicap, dementia, learning difficulties, behavioural problems and possibly schizophreniform psychosis if the temporal lobe is damaged.
- Seizures may cause short, repetitive or prolonged confusional and dreamy states, or be followed by confusion, so interrupting and disturbing normal concentration, learning and behaviour.
- Frequent seizures may interrupt schooling, work and concentration even if they are very mild or subclinical.
- Rarely aggressive behaviour can be part of the automatism of a complex partial seizure or occurs during the post-ictal confusional state.
- Falls during seizures may cause brain damage, embarrassment, etc.
- Anticonvulsants, particularly if several are used in high doses, can impair alertness, concentration, memory and learning; cause drowsiness, sometimes psychosis, irritability and hyperactivity, particularly in children on phenobarbitone.
- Social isolation as a result of prejudice, ignorance, inability to drive, stigma of the fits, physical appearance and employment difficulties.
- Hyposexuality and impotence may occur particularly in patients with complex partial seizures.

It is hardly surprising, therefore, that patients with seizures can become moody, anxious, withdrawn, depressed, irritable, aggressive, violent and suicidal. Nor is it surprising that hysterical pseudoseizures can occur as well (p. 111) and sometimes frank psychosis. These problems are difficult to sort out in an individual patient but it is important to:

- review anticonvulsants both from the point of view of toxicity and efficacy
- consider neurosurgery for medically uncontrolled seizures (p. 97)
- review the effects of any brain damage and cognitive problems
- treat major psychosis appropriately
- arrange social, work and marriage counselling as necessary

In some patients their behaviour improves when the seizures are relatively poorly controlled and deteriorates when they are well controlled.

The unconscious patient who is known to have epilepsy

Consider the following causes:
- deliberate or inadvertent overdose of anticonvulsants
- acute head injury
- chronic subdural haematoma (p. 235)
- progression of the underlying brain disorder
- non-convulsive status epilepticus (p. 97)
- other causes of coma (diabetes, etc., p. 122)

Note: After a single seizure the patient should be regaining consciousness in under an hour. If unconscious for longer then something else is going on.

Head injury and epilepsy

The more severe the brain injury, the more likely are seizures either early within the first week, or later. The risk of early seizures is greatest with:
- depressed skull fracture
- intracranial haematoma
- penetrating brain injury
- young children
- post-traumatic amnesia longer than 24 hours
    The risk of late seizures is greatest in the case of:
- early seizures
- depressed skull fracture
- intracranial haematoma
- dural tear

Note: The policy of prophylactic anticonvulsants for a patient after head injury or intracranial surgery but who has *not* had a seizure is popular but has no evidence to support it. It is probably best to await the first seizure, if any, and then treat using the customary guidelines (p. 82).

The diagnosis of the cause of the seizures

Once the distinction between seizures and another cause of altered consciousness has been made (p. 64) the question arises, 'what are the seizures due to?'.

Points to note in the history

- handedness
- pre-, peri- and neonatal health
- early development

- febrile convulsions
- possible absence attacks as a child
- head injury (skull fracture or unconsciousness)
- encephalitis, meningitis or other intracranial infection in the past
- drugs, alcohol, toxins
- behavioural and psychiatric problems
- family history of epilepsy

Points to look for on examination

- bodily asymmetry (thumbs, hands, feet, skull) indicating brain damage at birth or in the first few years of life contralateral to the small side (there may be brisk reflexes or a mild hemiparesis affecting that side as well)
- mental handicap
- abnormal neurological signs, raised intracranial pressure, etc.
- cranial bruit (? vascular malformation, p. 233)
- skin (vascular anomaly, p. 234, adenoma sebaceum, p. 487, etc.)
- skull; old or new injury, neurosurgical procedure

Routine investigations

Most patients presenting with one or more non-febrile seizures should have:
- full blood count and ESR
- liver function tests (?alcohol damage)
- blood glucose
- blood calcium
- syphilis serology but omit in children
- chest X-ray (?carcinoma bronchus, metastasis) but omit in children
- skull X-ray for intracranial calcification, shift of the pineal gland, fracture*, sinusitis*, osteomyelitis*, raised intracranial pressure*, bony changes of meningioma, asymmetry. Omit as a routine if CT is planned but some features(*) are not necessarily visible on CT.

   In acutely ill patients additional investigations are dictated by factors other than the seizures and include blood urea, electrolytes, CSF, CT scan, urine porphyrins, etc.

   In neonates particularly, consider blood glucose, electrolytes and magnesium, birth injury and intracranial haemorrhage.

   In children consider urine amino acids (p. 480).

Electroencephalography (EEG)

During most seizures the scalp EEG shows focal or generalized spike or spike/wave activity but this can be difficult to distinguish from movement and muscle artifact during tonic-clonic and other severe seizure types.

Immediately after the seizure the record usually shows generalized slowing. *Between* seizures, which is when most EEGs are performed, the record may be normal. However, the interictal record can be useful to:

- show focal spike, spike/wave or sharp waves suggesting a focal onset of the seizure and a possible focal cause for it
- show generalized spike/wave activity indicating a generalized epileptic disorder
- distinguish between absence seizures (3/second spike and wave) and complex partial seizures (normal, focal spike/wave or focal slowing over temporal or frontal lobe)
- show focal slow wave activity over a mass or large cerebral ischaemic lesion (but this is much better shown by CT)
- show generalized slow wave activity in metabolic and other generalized brain disorders

The distinction between seizures and something else depends far more on the history than on the interictal EEG since patients with definite seizures often have a normal record, and a few patients without seizures can have epileptic activity (i.e. spike or spike/wave) on the EEG. In a doubtful case a *very* abnormal EEG does increase the probability of epilepsy; however, mild abnormalities *must* be disregarded if the clinical history of seizures is uncertain.

A routine interictal EEG may be sensible in new cases of epilepsy and perhaps in some with a single seizure unless the attacks are obviously due to drug or alcohol withdrawal, metabolic disturbance or old head injury. It will:

- provide a baseline record
- localize an epileptogenic source sometimes
- help classify the seizure type
- suggest who should have a CT scan if this is not routinely available (i.e. if there is a focal spike/wave, sharp wave or slow wave focus)

Overbreathing, photic stimulation or sleep may provoke a seizure and will increase the chance of revealing abnormal seizure activity on the record.

An EEG *during* an attack is particularly useful but is rarely achieved during routine recording; artifact-free seizure activity confirms the epileptic nature of a particular attack but a normal record does *not* exclude the possibility. The chances of capturing a seizure are increased by ambulatory 24 hour (or more) monitoring of the EEG, and by telemetry (by cable or radio) of the EEG in a mobile subject preferably with simultaneous video monitoring to observe the seizure itself. These techniques for obtaining *ictal* EEGs are enormously important in:

- distinguishing real from pseudoseizures (p. 111)
- determining the frequency of subclinical epileptic activity which may, if frequent, impair memory and concentration
- diagnosing unusual symptoms in patients with seizures (confusional states, nocturnal enuresis, etc.)

- determining the side and site of the seizure focus when planning surgery (p. 97)

CT scan

This will reveal mass lesions, low density areas or focal atrophy (as a result of past stroke, head injury, congenital anomaly), large vascular malformations particularly if intravenous contrast is given which should be routine (non-enhanced scans are unnecessary in patients presenting merely with seizures). CT is most likely to be abnormal and helpful:
- in adults and neonates rather than children and adolescents
- for partial seizures
- if abnormal neurological signs exist
- if change in character of seizures occurs
- if very frequent seizures occur
- in acutely ill patients
- in cases of focal spike/wave, sharp wave or slow wave abnormality on the EEG

Note: The majority of CT abnormalities are 'atrophic'.

Ideally, a contrast-enhanced CT should be performed on all patients presenting with a seizure (unless caused by alcohol, drugs or metabolic disturbance), but if this is impractical it can be omitted if there has been just one seizure and there are no abnormal neurological signs, or if the seizures began in childhood.

MRI

This is seldom available at present but is more sensitive than CT in displaying small lesions and is particularly useful if seizures are intractable, CT with i.v. contrast is normal or a temporal lobe focus suitable for surgery is suspected.

CSF examination

This is only required if seizures present in the context of an acute cerebral illness (e.g. encephalitis, p. 498) provided there is no possibility of an intracranial mass; meningism indicating possible meningitis (p. 491) or subarachnoid haemorrhage (p. 228); first febrile convulsion to exclude meningitis (p. 76); and if the blood syphilis serology is positive.

There can be diagnostic confusion after a tonic-clonic seizure (particularly if multiple and prolonged) since occasionally this causes a mild CSF pleocytosis (usually less than 100 cells per cubic mm, either polymorphs or lymphocytes) lasting for a few days, and occasionally a slight rise in protein content.

When investigating prolonged or repeated tonic-clonic or motor seizures it must be remembered that they can result in any of the following:
- pyrexia, but seldom for more than 24 hours
- hyperglycaemia and, if seizure very prolonged, hypoglycaemia
- blood neutrophil leucocytosis
- increased blood lactate and metabolic acidosis (because of anoxia and increased muscle work)
- raised plasma creatine kinase, rhabdomyolysis, myoglobinuria (because of excess muscle activity)
- hyperuricaemia (because of excess muscle activity)
- renal failure (because of anoxia, hyperuricaemia, myoglobinuria)
- abnormal CSF (see above)

Treatment

Although about 80% of patients with a single unprovoked seizure will have a recurrence (mostly within a month and usually within the year), the overall prognosis is good. Only about 20% have a continuing and disabling lifelong problem, 10% have occasional seizures over many years, and 50% or so will, with treatment or perhaps even without, go into long-term remission.

Remission is *most* likely if:
- seizures start in childhood
- absence seizures (p. 00)
- benign Rolandic epilepsy (p. 00)
- one or a few generalized tonic-clonic seizures, which stop in 1 or 2 years
- no underlying cause

Remission is *least* likely if:
- seizures start under the age of one
- underlying brain lesion (e.g. tumour)
- neurological, mental or psychosocial handicap
- partial seizures (although secondary generalization may remit)
- very frequent seizures
- continuing seizures over several years

Most patients with seizures can be completely, or at least satisfactorily, controlled on one anticonvulsant.

First aid for tonic-clonic seizures

- place the patient on the floor or in a bed which he or she cannot fall off and let the seizure run its course
- remove any hard, hot or sharp objects which may cause injury

- loosen collar and cushion the head
- turn semiprone when possible
- as the tonic-clonic phase subsides, make sure the tongue is forward, remove any false teeth, clear the mouth of blood, mucous and vomitus
- insert plastic pharyngeal airway if available or necessary when the tonic-clonic movements subside
- stay with the patient until any post-ictal confusion subsides
- review or start anticonvulsants as appropriate

Do *not* try and restrain, nor force anything between the teeth in the tonic-clonic phase; a bitten tongue is more acceptable than broken teeth.

General policy

- Each tonic-clonic seizure requires first aid (see above) but even in less severe seizures the patient may require general looking after.
- Trigger factors (p. 74) should be avoided if they can be recognized and if it is feasible. Blanket recommendations (e.g. not to drink alcohol) are nonsense. Some patients are very sensitive to stress, overbreathing, late nights, alcohol, certain drugs (p. 67), etc.
- Treat any underlying cause if one can be found.
- Anticonvulsants are used as prophylaxis and have to be taken regularly for a long time. The decision to start is as much the patient's as the doctor's and one has to balance any advantage and its magnitude (reducing or stopping the seizures) with any disadvantage (adverse effects, nuisance of taking drugs, teratogenesis, cost, etc.).

One is *less* likely to start anticonvulsants if:

    trigger factors or an underlying cause can be dealt with (e.g. alcohol)
    infrequent sleep associated seizures only
    likelihood of poor compliance
    patient not driving or needing to drive
    work would not be jeopardized by another seizure
    seizures are mild (e.g. partial) and/or infrequent (e.g. less than one a year)
    myoclonic jerks only
    normal EEG

One is *more* likely to start anticonvulsants if:

    work would be jeopardized by another attack
    several tonic-clonic seizures in a short period
    very frequent partial seizures
    obvious epileptic activity on the EEG
    underlying brain lesion which cannot be treated (e.g. glioma)

- Explain to the patient (and the parents, other relatives, etc.) what is happening and discuss any modification of lifestyle which may be necessary (p. 99). Reassure that most patients with epilepsy are not brain damaged or 'mental'.

• See the patients quite frequently until the seizures stop or are optimally controlled and then review infrequently but regularly.

Which anticonvulsant?

There is little difference in anticonvulsant efficacy between phenytoin (p. 88), carbamazepine (p. 90), sodium valproate (p. 91) and phenobarbitone (p. 92) except in the treatment of typical absences and myoclonus (see below). Which anticonvulsant to use depends more on likely or actually experienced adverse effects and on cost (Table 2.1). For example, in children carbamazepine is probably the least likely to cause learning difficulties and in women one would probably avoid phenytoin because of occasional coarsening of the facial skin. It also depends on ease of use (a once daily regimen being most convenient) and on cost (phenobarbitone is extremely cheap). Second line drugs are primidone (p. 93), benzodiazepines (p. 93) and acetazolamide (p. 94). For typical absence seizures ethosuximide (p. 93) or sodium valproate are about equally effective but if, in addition, there are other seizure types then the latter is more appropriate. Myoclonus, if it requires treatment at all, responds best to sodium valproate or a benzodiazepine (clonazepam) but is often reduced in frequency by other anticonvulsants being used for other seizure types in the same individual.

General principles of anticonvulsant treatment

• Keep it simple: one patient, one drug and one doctor. Epilepsy is often a chronic condition and is best managed by the general practitioner with or without no more than one doctor in a hospital clinic. Several doctors cause confusion, tend to add one anticonvulsant to another, do anticonvulsant blood levels instead of listening to the patient, and avoid long-term commitment and responsibility.
• Most patients can be controlled on monotherapy. Combinations of anticonvulsants are probably no more effective, are likely to increase drug toxicity, produce unexpected and inexplicable anticonvulsant drug interactions, need complex dosing schedules making compliance difficult, and make drug levels almost uninterpretable. Combinations must be used with great caution and *never* in multi-drug formulations.
• Introduce the preferred drug in a low dose (Table 2.1) unless urgent treatment is required for status epilepticus or very frequent seizures (p. 95). Increase the dose slowly over a few weeks to reach the 'standard' dose (Table 2.1). If the seizures stop, do *not* increase the dose further. If they persist, go on increasing the dose slowly over weeks or months until they do stop, dose-related adverse effects appear, or the dose is about the likely safe maximum (Table 2.1). If the patient is compliant (check blood level) but seizures still continue at an unacceptable frequency (for the patient), particularly if there are adverse effects, then slowly introduce another anticonvulsant while

Table 2.1 Commonly used oral anticonvulsants

	Dose frequency per day	Total daily dosage (mg)			Children's standard dose (mg/kg/day)	Likely toxic blood level[††]		Tablet/capsule sizes	Cost of standard weekly dose (1990)
		Starting	Standard	Maximum[*]		mg/l	µmol/l		
Phenytoin	1–2	100	200–300	600	10	20	80	25, 50, 100	15 p
Carbamazepine	2–3	100	600	2000	30	10	40	100, 200, 400	121 p
Sodium valproate	2–4	400	800	2500	30	100	700	100, 200, 500	185 p
Phenobarbitone	1–2	30	90	600	5	40	170	15, 30, 60, 100	7 p
Primidone	1–2	62.5	500	1500	20	40[†]	170[†]	250	25 p
Ethosuximide	2–3	250	750	1500	30	100	700	250	156 p
Clonazepam	1–3	0.5	1.0	8	0.1	?	?	0.5, 2	62 p

[*] Some patients may achieve this dose without dose-related adverse effects but most will not; above this dose, anticonvulsant efficacy is seldom more and possibly less.

[†] Measured as phenobarbitone.

[††] A very approximate guideline; some patients tolerate higher levels, whereas others develop adverse effects below these levels.

Note: 1 Starting doses are given on the low side in a deliberate attempt to avoid unnecessary toxicity.

2 Liquid formulations available for all drugs except clonazepam.

tailing off and stopping the ineffective drug over a matter of weeks. If necessary, repeat this procedure until each first line anticonvulsant has been tried before resorting to combination therapy. After a change in dose a steady state takes 1–2 weeks to develop. Partial seizures are harder to control than primary or secondary generalized seizures but may be of less concern to the patient.

• Do not necessarily increase the dose after every seizure but take a longer term view and consider trigger factors, such as stress, or intermittent compliance.

• Use as infrequent dosing schedules as possible (Table 2.1), particularly since middle of the day doses can be forgotten or cause embarrassment.

• Avoid excessively high doses, particularly in combination therapy, since they are likely to cause toxicity and *may* increase seizure frequency.

• Do not change more than one thing at a time.

• Keep to the same formulation of a particular anticonvulsant.

• Stress the importance of regular pill taking to make assessment of efficacy and adverse effects practical, to improve efficacy, and to avoid withdrawal seizures as a result of suddenly stopping anticonvulsants. Missing the occasional dose is of no great consequence.

• There is considerable individual variation in efficacy and adverse effects for particular drugs, tolerance to adverse effects, the blood level for a particular dose of a drug, the blood level at which dose-related adverse effects appear, and the blood level at which seizures are controlled. This is partly due to the difficulty in measuring and interpreting blood levels. There is no blood level below which dose-related adverse effects never occur, nor below which seizures necessarily continue and, therefore, no lower limit to the 'therapeutic' range is quoted in Table 2.1.

• For patients on combination therapy, or high doses of monotherapy for many years, it is probably worth an annual check on haemoglobin (? folate deficient anaemia which if corrected does not impair seizure control) and plasma calcium and alkaline phosphatase (? osteomalacia).

• Relatively higher doses are required in children than in adults, whereas in the elderly relatively lower doses should be used. Liquid formulations may be helpful in children but often have a high sugar content (dental caries) and the swallowed dose can be erratic.

• Ask the patient to keep a diary of the seizure frequency and anticonvulsant dosage changes, also to keep a record of exact medication and doses to bring to each medical consultation.

• If drug toxicity appears inexplicably, consider:
  confusion with dose regimen
  return to proper compliance after not taking the drugs
  drug interactions (inhibition of anticonvulsant metabolic breakdown)
  loss of weight
  change in formulation
  change in hepatic/renal function or plasma proteins.

• When evaluating adverse effects it is better to listen to the patient and rely on the clinical picture than on blood levels. Some individuals develop adverse effects with very low doses (and blood levels).

• If two or more anticonvulsants are ineffective in combination, reconsider the diagnosis of epilepsy (could it be pseudoseizures instead of or as well as epilepsy?), consider surgery (p. 97) and possibly slowly reduce to one drug provided seizure control does not deteriorate.

• If seizures persist or became inexplicably frequent consider:
  poor compliance or misunderstanding
  malabsorption (diarrhoea, gastrectomy, etc.)
  weight gain
  change in renal or hepatic function, or change in serum proteins
  addition of drugs that lower seizure threshold (e.g. phenothiazines, see
      p. 67)
  drug interactions (e.g. withdrawal of a drug inhibiting metabolism of
      anticonvulsant)
  change of drug formulation
  pregnancy
  progressing neurological disease
  psychosocial problems
  trigger factors (e.g. stress, alcohol, etc.)
  pseudoseizures (p. 111)
  original diagnosis of epilepsy wrong
  onset of another cause of 'blackouts', e.g. syncope (possibly as a conse-
      quence of carbamazepine), occasionally anticonvulsant toxicity

• Before increasing the anticonvulsant dose double check on treatment regimen, drug formulation, patient understanding and compliance.

• If the patient becomes ill consider whether this might interfere with the anticonvulant effectiveness (e.g. diarrhoea) or whether the illness could be due to drug toxicity.

• Use plasma *drug levels* sparingly and *not* to force the patient into a so-called 'therapeutic range' when the seizures are already controlled, nor as a routine, and certainly not as a substitute for doing something useful. The blood level is the total concentration in the blood whereas the therapeutically effective portion is the proportion, often small, which is unbound to plasma proteins. Therefore, drugs (e.g. other anticonvulsants), pregnancy or illness (e.g. chronic renal failure) which affect plasma protein concentration or binding will reduce the validity of 'total' blood levels as a guide to toxicity.

  Drug levels can be helpful to:
  confirm the patient is taking any of the drug but are not a good guide to the
      exact dose
  confirm the clinical impression of toxicity and perhaps indicate which
      drug, if more than one is being taken, is the likely culprit

control intractable seizures
in making the decision to increase an already high dose
Plasma levels are most meaningful for patients taking phenytoin. Anticonvulsant levels in the saliva provide the best estimate of unbound, and therefore active, drug in the blood but are difficult to measure accurately and not widely available.

• Consider *slow withdrawal* of anticonvulsants over several months when seizure-free for two or more years. The risk of a recurrent seizure is about 20% in children and 40% in adults, which is double the risk compared with continuing anticonvulsants. Relapse usually occurs within 12 months of withdrawal which is the only certain way to determine whether treatment is still necessary and whether adverse effects really are or are not being experienced. The decision to withdraw, or to restart if there is a recurrence, must depend on the patient's feelings, work, driving licence, etc. Recurrence is *least* likely in the following cases:

onset of epilepsy in childhood (over the age of one)
a small number of generalized seizures over a short period
no neurological of psychiatric handicap
absence attacks only
normal EEG at the time of withdrawal
increasing length of remission
no underlying brain lesion

Anticonvulsant drugs and treatments

Phenytoin

Phenytoin is in many ways the easiest anticonvulsant to use since it can usually be given once daily, the drug levels correlate reasonably well with symptoms of toxicity, its metabolism is well understood, and it has been available for so long that there is extensive experience of its adverse effects. However, the main problem is that it is the one anticonvulsant showing clinically important saturation kinetics of its metabolism such that above a dose of about 200–300 mg daily a small increase in dose leads to a disproportionately large increase in blood level. At this dosage level increments should be very cautious, in 50 or even 25 mg steps, to avoid unexpected toxicity.

Dose related and reversible toxic adverse effects include:
• poor concentration and impaired learning
• drowsiness
• headache
• cerebellar syndrome (ataxia, dysarthria, nystagmus)
• diplopia
• nausea and vomiting

- psychosis*
- choreoathetosis*
- dystonia*
- slowing of cardiac conduction*
- effectiveness of oral contraceptives reduced (p. 99)
  Idiosyncratic adverse effects include:
- rash (10%), Stevens–Johnson syndrome
- gum hyperplasia
- coarsening of the facial skin, acne, hirsutism
- macrocytosis but rarely megaloblastic anaemia (in part folate responsive)
- osteomalacia/rickets
- systemic lupus erythematosus (p. 444)
- lymphoma-like syndrome
- chronic cerebellar atrophy (probably irreversible)
- chronic peripheral neuropathy (usually subclinical)
- serum sickness
- hepatitis
- IgA deficiency
- marrow suppression
- fetal malformation (p. 98)

The therapeutic (and toxic) effect is increased by concurrent administration of:

allopurinol
amiodarone
azapropazone
chloramphenicol
chlorpheniramine
chlorpromazine
cimetidine
co-trimoxazole
dextropropoxyphene
disulfiram
imipramine
isoniazid
metronidazole
miconazole
oral anticoagulants
phenylbutazone
sulphinpyrazone
sulphonamides
sodium valproate
sulthiame

* Rare.

thioridazine

viloxazine

Its effect is *reduced* by continuous nasogastric feeding, alcohol, carmustine, methotrexate, rifampicin, vigabatrin, vinblastine and possibly concurrent administration of antacids.

Phenytoin has an unpredictable effect on oral anticoagulant control; reduces the effect of cyclosporin, doxycycline, frusemide, quinidine and theophylline; reduces the level of thyroid hormones but TSH is unaffected and the patients are euthyroid; reduces insulin release, causing hyperglycaemia, and should be avoided in diabetics; and can increase plasma HDL cholesterol. Avoid in porphyria and exercise caution if liver disease is present.

Carbamazepine

Carbamazepine probably causes the fewest learning difficulties in children. However, some individuals are very sensitive to adverse effects, particularly in the first few weeks of treatment before autoinduction of its own metabolic breakdown occurs.

Dose-related and reversible toxic effects, particularly at the peaks of serum concentration, include:

- drowsiness, poor concentration, dizziness
- headache
- ataxia, nystagmus, dysarthria
- nausea, vomiting, diarrhoea
- diplopia
- dry mouth
- water intoxication*
- psychosis*
- choreoathetosis/dystonia*
- heart block, bradycardia*

  Idiosyncratic adverse effects include:
- rash (about 15%)
- light sensitive dermatitis
- marrow suppression
- fever
- lymphadenopathy
- osteomalacia/rickets
- pulmonary eosinophilia
- hepatitis

* Rare.

- systemic lupus erythematosus (p. 444)
- fetal malformation (p. 98)

Contraindications: heart block, porphyria, monoamine oxidase inhibitors. Exercise caution if hepatic disease.

The effect of carbamazepine is increased by:

- cimetidine
- danazol
- dextropropoxyphene
- diltiazem
- erythromycin
- isoniazid
- lithium
- verapamil
- viloxazine

Carbamazepine reduces the effect of oral contraceptives, doxycyline, haloperidol, theophylline; reduces thyroid hormone levels; has a variable effect on oral anticoagulant control but usually reduces the effect of warfarin; increases plasma HDL cholesterol; and tends to increase the effect of phenytoin.

Sodium valproate

This is a relatively new anticonvulsant and a number of adverse effects are still being discovered. It is particularly useful if a patient has both absence and tonic-clonic seizures since the only other alternative for the former (ethosuxamide, p. 93) is ineffective for the latter. It should be given on a full stomach to avoid gastric toxicity or the enteric-coated preparation used.

Dose-related and reversible adverse effects:

- anorexia, nausea, vomiting
- diarrhoea
- restlessness and irritability
- drowsiness
- postural and action tremor
- enuresis
- poor concentration and memory
- confusion
- psychosis

Idiosyncratic adverse effects include:

- increased appetite and weight gain
- hepatic failure (mainly in mentally handicapped infants)
- hyperammonaemia (particularly if ornithine carbamyltransferase deficiency, p. 480)
- pancreatitis

- alopecia and curly hair
- thrombocytopenia
- impaired coagulation/platelet function
- marrow suppression
- rash
- hypersalivation
- fetal malformation (p. 98)

Contraindications: liver disease, anticoagulants. Caution in small children, particularly with organic brain disease and taking several anticonvulsants. Before surgery, check coagulation and bleeding.

Sodium valproate has several unexpected and variable interactions with other anticonvulsants. Phenobarbitone levels rise and phenytoin levels fall but the free drug levels are variably affected. The therapeutic effect of sodium valproate tends to be less in patients taking other anticonvulsants.

Note: Valproate causes a false positive test for urine ketones, disturbs urine tests for amino acids and reduces thyroid hormone levels in the blood. Transient abnormalities of liver function tests are common soon after starting treatment and do not predict the occasional rare case of hepatitis.

Phenobarbitone

Phenobarbitone has the advantage of being cheap (Table 2.1) and it need only be given once or twice daily. Dose-related adverse effects include:
- poor concentration
- impaired memory
- dizziness, nausea, vomiting
- depression
- drowsiness
- ataxia, nystagmus and dysarthria
- psychosis*
- chorea/dystonia*

It tends to cause irritability, aggression and hyperactivity in children. Rare idiosyncratic adverse effects include skin rash, hypocalcaemia, folate responsive megaloblastic anaemia, subclinical peripheral neuropathy, marrow suppression, Dupuytren's contracture and possibly systemic lupus erythematosus (p. 444). It also increases plasma HDL cholesterol. Teratogenicity, see p. 98.

Phenobarbitone probably enhances the effect of sodium valproate and phenytoin but inhibits the effect of warfarin, quinidine, corticosteroids, oral contraceptives and some antibiotics. Levels are increased by sodium valproate.

Contraindications: porphyria.

* Very rare.

Primidone

Primidone is a second line anticonvulsant. Most of its therapeutic effect is through hepatic metabolic conversion to phenobarbitone and phenylethylmalonamide. It often causes adverse effects which are similar to those of phenobarbitone. Starting this drug must be very cautious since some patients react very adversely to it (Table 2.1).

Benzodiazepines

These are the first line intravenous or rectal treatment for status epilepticus (p. 94); useful as 'first aid' treatment for very frequent seizures short of status (given orally if practical or rectally if not: 5–20 mg diazepam, 0.5 mg/kg in children); and for febrile convulsions (p. 76).

Myoclonus tends to be reduced by benzodiazepines, and clonazepam is usually the drug of choice (valproate, p. 91, is an alternative).

Long-term oral therapy usually fails because tolerance develops in a matter of weeks, withdrawal can precipitate status epilepticus, psychological dependence occurs and adverse effects are a problem; sedation, fatigue, ataxia, dysarthria, irritability and confusion. Alcohol toxicity is potentiated. High doses in infants may produce drooling, disturbed swallowing and aspiration pneumonia. Intermittent oral treatment can be tried, although one has to be aware of withdrawal seizures, for any type of seizure which is tending to 'cluster' in defined periods (e.g. around menstruation) or if a lot of minor seizures (e.g. myoclonus, complex partial) are clustering over minutes or hours and building up towards a major generalized convulsion.

Dosage:
clonazepam 0.5–8.0 mg daily in 1–3 divided doses
clobazam 10–30 mg as a single night-time dose
diazepam 6–30 mg daily in 3 divided doses (less in the elderly)
nitrazepam 5–20 mg daily in 3 divided doses

Ethosuximide

This is used only for typical and atypical absence seizures but, if they are associated with generalized tonic-clonic seizures, an additional anticonvulsant or one that covers both seizure types is required, i.e. sodium valproate (p. 91). Adverse effects include:
• anorexia, nausea, vomiting
• headache
• drowsiness
• poor concentration and memory
• agitation
• hiccups
• skin rash

- marrow suppression
- psychosis
- systemic lupus erythematosus (p. 444)

Levels are increased by isoniazid. There are variable interactions with other anticonvulsants.

Acetazolamide

Acetazolamide is occasionally helpful in intractable epilepsy but tolerance soon develops. Intermittent courses for catamenial epilepsy are sometimes effective and it is said to be particularly helpful when overbreathing precipitates seizures. Dosage: oral, 250 mg twice daily up to 500 mg 3 times daily

Adverse effects: paraesthesia, anorexia, drowsiness, fizzy drinks taste flat and, rarely, agranulocytosis.

Vigabatrin

This is a new anticonvulsant which is worth trying for intractable seizures; oral 500 mg once daily increasing, if necessary, to 2 g twice daily. Adverse effects include drowsiness, dizziness, imbalance, irritability, headache, confusion, psychosis, weight gain and possibly brain microvacuolation.

Ketogenic diet

This helps a few children with severe epilepsy.

Pyridoxine-dependent seizures

In neonates and possibly infants, unexplained partial and generalized seizures (or even status epilepticus) which are unresponsive to conventional anticonvulsants can sometimes be stopped by pyridoxine (i.v. 100 mg or oral 50–100 mg daily). This is often a familial condition.

Obsolete drugs

These include ethotoin, methoin, methsuximide, methylphenobarbitone, phensuximide, sulthiame, troxidone.

Status epilepticus

This is an emergency and requires admission to hospital. It is defined as two or more epileptic seizures (convulsive or non-convulsive) without regaining consciousness between attacks, or any seizure lasting more than 30 minutes. In known epileptics the usual cause is stopping or changing anticonvulsants (or perhaps a head injury). If epilepsy *presents* as status, there is likely to be a serious underlying brain disorder (e.g. encephalitis, head injury, alcoholism).

About 10% die during convulsive status, more often of the underlying brain disorder than the seizures, although status can lead to cerebral anoxia, pulmonary inhalation, respiratory obstruction, injury, hyperpyrexia, pneumoperitoneum and direct damage to the brain (see also p. 76).

Management of convulsive status

- First aid (p. 82).
- Admit to intensive care unit, particularly for monitoring of drug-induced respiratory depression and hypotension, oxygen and ventilation if necessary.
- i.v. diazepam 10 mg over 1 or 2 minutes. Dose in children: 0.2–0.3 mg/kg. Sensible parents or spouses can give diazepam for intravenous solution by direct injection into the rectum (p. 76) using KY jelly and a narrow syringe: 10–20 mg in adults and 0.5 mg/kg in children. Stesolid rectal tubes are a good alternative. Beware respiratory depression, hypotension and over-sedation.
- Take blood for full blood count, ESR, glucose, liver function, electrolytes, anticonvulsant levels, toxic substances including alcohol.
- Secure a good i.v. line and keep open with 5% dextrose/saline. Be extremely careful to avoid inadvertent increase in rate of delivery if anticonvulsants are being added to the infusion rather than given as boluses; the latter method is preferable.
- Consider what the cause of the status and the epilepsy might be and investigate and treat appropriately. If in any doubt about alcoholism, give vitamin B_1 as i.v. Parentrovite forte 10 ml, or about hypoglycaemia, give i.v. 50 ml of 50% (50 g/dl) glucose solution. Previous epilepsy may be revealed by looking for drugs, prescriptions or appointment cards; telephoning relatives or general practitioner; medic-alert bracelet; facial features or gum hypertrophy in pheytoin takers.
- Monitor the following:
  conscious level (Glasgow coma score p. 122)
  seizure frequency
  pulse and blood pressure
  temperature
  respiration, blood gases, pH
  fluid balance, urea, electrolytes
  glucose
  blood levels of anticonvulsants
  ECG
  EEG
- At a very early stage continue or start (oral or via nasogastric tube) effective doses of anticonvulsants so that intravenous therapy can be stopped. If there is any doubt about gastrointestinal absorption, use i.v. boluses of intravenous phenytoin instead: loading dose 15 mg/kg (no more than 50 mg per minute) and then 5 mg/kg/day (see below).

- If within 5 minutes the seizures have not stopped, repeat 10 mg diazepam i.v. up to about 40 mg over 20 minutes.
- An alternative to diazepam is i.v. clonazepam (dose one tenth of diazepam) or i.v. lorazepam (4 mg in adults, 0.1 mg/kg in children).
- If the boluses of diazepam stop the seizures but they recur within 15–30 minutes, then use an intravenous infusion (otherwise proceed to paraldehyde, see below):

   Make up 100 mg i.v. *diazepam* in 500 ml of 5% dextrose or dextrose-saline and infuse at a rate to control the seizures, but no more than about 40 mg/hour which can cause suppression of respiration and hypotension. Use the diluted solution within four hours. An alternative is to use Diazemuls emulsion as an i.v. infusion.

   Clonazepam: make up 6 mg in 500 ml dextrose or dextrose-saline and use within 12 hours.

   Never give intramuscular benzodiazepines since absorption is erratic.
- If i.v. boluses of benzodiazepines are ineffective, then use a second choice anticonvulsant: paraldehyde, phenytoin, phenobarbitone or chlormethiazole.

   Paraldehyde: 5 ml into each buttock using a glass syringe (plastic can be used if the drug is drawn up and injected *immediately*). In children, dose is (age in years +1) ml up to a maximum of 10 ml. Repeat this dose every few hours as necessary but it is probably better under these circumstances to use an intravenous infusion and so avoid muscle necrosis: 6% solution in dextrose-saline (30 ml in 500 ml) up to 100 ml/hour. Respiratory depression can occur.

   Phenytoin: i.v. bolus (*never* i.m. or mixed in infusion bottle), max 50 mg/minute to avoid hypotension, up to a total of 15 mg/kg and flush through with normal saline. If the patient is already taking phenytoin the blood level should, if possible, be obtained first to avoid precipitating toxicity, although it is likely to be low given the patient is in status. Monitor the ECG because of the risk of cardiac conduction problems and watch for hypotension, respiratory depression and burning around the infused vein.

   Phenobarbitone: i.v. infusion, 100 mg/min, to a total dose of 10 mg/kg. Then continue, if necessary, to a total dose of 20 mg/kg at rate of 50 mg/min.

   Chlormethiazole: i.v. infusion as 0.8% solution in dextrose, 50–100 ml over 10 minutes and then up to 100 mg/kg/hour as necessary. It tends to cause prolonged sedation and respiratory depression.
- If all else fails, an anaesthetic dose of thiopentone must be given, along with assisted ventilation and perhaps paralysis, with continuous monitoring of the EEG to determine the efficacy of the treatment because the patient is paralysed and seizures cannot be seen.

   i.v. bolus 100–250 mg and then 50 mg every 2–5 minutes until the EEG is seizure-free. Then, maintenance infusion of 0.5–1.5 ml/min of a 0.5% solution in normal saline as required.

• Remember fluid balance, particularly if large volumes of intravenous fluids are being used as a vehicle for anticonvulsants.

Non-convulsive status epilepticus

Some patients, most already known to have epilepsy, may, without or after an obvious tonic-clonic seizure, lapse into a dreamy and confused state which often fluctuates and is accompanied by continuous generalized three/second spike and wave activity on the EEG (petit mal status) or more disorganized and sometimes focal epileptic activity over one or both temporal lobes (complex partial status). However, the distinction is often not clearcut. The patient is obtunded and more or less unresponsive; there may be automatisms in complex partial status and occasionally even psychotic symptoms. The patient is usually amnesic for most of the attack. The attacks can last hours or days and can usually be stopped at once with intravenous diazepam or clonazepam (p. 93) which should be followed by the oral anticonvulsant appropriate to the seizure type. The differential diagnosis includes hysteria, confusional states of any cause (p. 161), transient global amnesia (p. 159) and sometimes even an acute schizophrenic psychosis.

Surgery

Removal of a localized epileptic focus in the cerebral cortex can reduce or abolish seizures, allow anticonvulsants to be reduced or stopped, and improve behavioural disturbances. The best results are in children with a structural abnormality in one temporal lobe (e.g. Ammon's horn sclerosis, cryptic glioma, vascular malformation, hamartoma) which may not necessarily be found until the specimen is sectioned. Hemiparetic patients with cerebral palsy and epilepsy arising in one shrunken cerebral hemisphere can benefit remarkably by hemispherectomy or perhaps section of the corpus callosum, the latter to control secondary generalization. Gliomas presenting with seizures in adults are best left alone until other symptoms develop, particularly if the seizures can be controlled with anticonvulsants (p. 269).

Indications for surgery:
• Unsatisfactory control of seizures despite optimal anticonvulsant treatment.
• Seizures arise from a localized area of brain which can be demonstrated electrophysiologically (by routine EEG, sleep EEG, sphenoidal or better foramen ovale recordings, ambulatory or telemetered EEG, depth electrodes). Any cognitive or radiological abnormality (e.g. enlarged temporal horn, calcification on CT) should be consistent with the neurophysiologically identified focus. If there is cognitive impairment referable to the contralateral side, then temporal lobectomy is probably contraindicated for fear of producing global amnesia. If a discrete lesion can be shown radiologically by

CT or MRI, then more widespread EEG abnormalities are probably not a contraindication to surgery.

• The focus can be removed without serious neurological damage, e.g. shrunken hemisphere contralateral to a small hemiparetic side in a child with cerebral palsy, non-dominant temporal lobe. The anterior part of the dominant temporal lobe can be removed without causing aphasia or serious verbal memory disorder in some individuals. Dominance is determined by the intracarotid amytal test. Temporal lobectomy may cause an upper homonymous quadrantanopia and memory disturbance. More restricted temporal lobe resections are now possible which are less likely to cause amnesia, i.e. amygdalo-hippocampectomy.

Pregnancy

Seizures can start during pregnancy and occasionally do not recur subsequently. In epileptic patients pregnancy usually has no great influence on the seizures; they occasionally remit but in perhaps one third the frequency increases because of:

• non-compliance (often for fear of fetal malformation)
• sleep deprivation
• vomiting
• altered absorption, metabolism or protein binding of anticonvulsants
• the effect of pregnancy itself
• seizures in late pregnancy may be due to eclampsia or even cortical venous thrombosis (p. 225)

The usual principles of treatment apply (p. 82) plus:
• if possible, review need for and dose of any anticonvulsant *before* conception to establish excellent control or to withdraw unnecessary therapy
• there is no need to change medication after the first trimester for fear of any risk to the fetus from the drug which by then probably is minimal
• risk of fetal abnormality in epileptic mothers taking anticonvulsants is about double the normal (an increase from about 5% to about 10% for any abnormalities, many of which are trivial and some of which can be diagnosed by amniocentesis, e.g. spina bifida). This small relative risk is worth taking if the mother *definitely* requires anticonvulsants since tonic-clonic seizures can cause fetal anoxia. *Any* anticonvulsant is likely to be responsible, especially sodium valproate; if possible, therefore, replace this drug, or withdraw before conception and certainly try and avoid it in drug combinations
• have lower threshold for looking for fetal abnormalities by amniocentesis, etc.
• ensure regular folate supplementation during pregnancy
• breast feeding causes no problem for the baby
• withdrawal seizures do not seem to occur in the neonate
• vitamin K, 1 mg i.m. to neonate to prevent anticonvulsant-induced coagulation disorders (particularly from phenytoin and phenobarbitone)

• review anticonvulsants postpartum, particularly if the dose has been changed during the pregnancy

Oral contraceptives

These do not normally influence seizure frequency but occasionally and unpredictably anticonvulsants (particularly phenytoin, phenobarbitone and carbamazepine) accelerate the metabolism of oestrogens enough to cause midcycle breakthrough bleeding and rarely unexpected pregnancy. If even a small risk of pregnancy is unacceptable, the dose of oestrogen should be increased particularly if there is breakthrough bleeding, or alternative contraceptive methods used.

Living with epilepsy

Patients with active epilepsy require a lot of explanation and sensible advice concerning normal daily activities and only a check list is given here. Clearly the exact advice must depend on the individual circumstances, particularly the frequency of the seizures, the time of day they occur, their type, and any warning for long enough to be acted on.
• Discuss driving (see p. 556).
• Work and career planning; avoid potentially dangerous situations (e.g. fast moving machinery, working at height, near open water, with fragile equipment). On the whole it is best to tell employers the situation.
• School: the teacher should know that a child has epilepsy.
• Swimming: it is best to avoid it in the sea but under direct supervision in a swimming pool it is acceptable; a brightly coloured swimming cap is worth wearing. Wear a life jacket for water sports.
• Protect danger points in the home: fire and radiator guards, stairs, do not lock bathroom and toilet doors, care in the bath (shallow bath) or use a shower, care in the kitchen.
• Smother-proof pillows if nocturnal convulsions.
• Cycling is probably no more dangerous than usual (wear a helmet).
• Games and physical education are normally allowed.
• Sexual activity need not be altered.
• Epileptic mothers must be very careful with their babies. Breast feeding is not a problem. Keep tablets out of reach of children.
• Inheritance is not normally a problem although most patients worry about it. The risk of a child developing epilepsy is about 1 in 40 if one parent has idiopathic epilepsy and 1 in 4 if both parents have it, compared with 1 in 200 for the general population. If the parent has acquired epilepsy due to a known intracranial structural lesion, then the risk to the children is not increased.
• Alcohol, in moderation, is acceptable provided it does not trigger seizures in a susceptible patient.

- Late nights, television, video games, discotheques, as for alcohol advice.
- Carry a card, bracelet or necklace stating the diagnosis of epilepsy if the seizures are frequent (medic-alert, p. 62).
- Vaccination; do not vaccinate against pertussis or measles.
- Exemption from all prescription charges.

In general the diagnosis should be discussed openly with the patient, parents, spouse, teachers, employers, etc. Hiding the diagnosis merely contributes to any stigma which should be reduced at every possible opportunity. Over-protection, particularly of children, can be as bad as under-protection. The majority of patients with seizures are not mentally handicapped and lead normal lives. In some, however, there are serious neurological, social, behavioural, learning, psychological and other handicaps which require treatment in their own right.

Useful addresses

British Epilepsy Association
Anstey House
40 Hanover Square
Leeds LS3 1BE
Tel: 0345-089599

National Society for Epilepsy
Chalfont Centre for Epilepsy
Chalfont St Peter
Gerrards Cross
Bucks SL9 0RJ
Tel: 02407-3991

Syncope

Syncope is caused by a sudden drop in blood flow to the brain and has many causes (see below). This may lead to abrupt loss of consciousness without any warning (e.g. syncope due to aortic stenosis, complete heart block) but usually there is a preceding (or maybe *only*) feeling of faintness, light-headedness or dizziness (but not rotational vertigo), bilateral dimming or loss of vision, general weakness, nausea, hot and cold feelings, sweating and sounds seeming distant. Injury can result if the patient falls heavily. If the fall in cerebral blood flow is prolonged or severe, the patient becomes unconscious but usually for no more than a few minutes. There are no *focal* neurological symptoms (p. 220) except when a drop in blood pressure occurs in the presence of severe arterial disease in the neck or impaired cerebral autoregulation due to a previous stroke (p. 216). There may, depending on the cause, be additional symptoms such as chest pain (tachy- or bradyarrhythmias), palpitations (tachyarrhythmias), headache (migraine), etc.

During the attack the patient is floppy rather than rigid, and usually is pale. It can be difficult to feel the pulse and, even if it is attempted by a witness, information about its rate and rhythm is often unreliable. If the syncope is prolonged, particularly if the patient remains sitting upright, then an anoxic seizure can occur with rigidity, some tonic-clonic movements and even incontinence of urine (so-called convulsive syncope).

On coming round there is very little mental confusion or difficulty remembering the warning symptoms unless there has been a head injury. Sometimes after cough syncope the short paroxysm of coughing has been forgotten. The patient may flush but more often looks pale and washed out for some minutes.

Causes of syncope

- vasovagal syncope (p. 101)
- postural hypotension (p. 102)
- cardiac arrhythmia (p. 102)
- Valsalva manoeuvre (p. 103)
- structural cardiac disorders (p. 103)
- acute circulatory failure (p. 103)
- micturition syncope (p. 103)
- defaecation syncope (p. 104)
- carotid sinus syncope (p. 104)
- swallow syncope (p. 104)
- ice-cream syncope (p. 104)
- prostatic syncope (p. 104)
- cough syncope (p. 105)
- benign syncope in adolescent males (p. 105)
- hyperviscosity syndrome (p. 461)
- anaemia ? (p. 460)
- cervical spondylosis ? (p. 105)

Vasovagal syncope

This starts in childhood or adolescence, *very* rarely as an adult. Usually the children 'grow out' of it. It seldom occurs while lying down and is almost always precipitated by obvious and well recognized situations:
- the sight of blood, even on television
- acute pain (e.g. injury, injections, dental treatment, intestinal colic, vaginal examination, dysmenorrhoea, etc.)
- prolonged standing (school assembly, parade ground, etc.)
- heat and overcrowding

- acute emotional shock
- pregnancy

Usually the onset is rather gradual over a minute or so. There is marked pallor due to vasoconstriction in the skin, cardiac slowing, and a drop in blood pressure due to vasodilation in muscle and viscera. Consciousness returns in a minute or two.

Note: Some children are very sensitive to eyeball pressure which activates a profound vagal reflex, asystole for a few seconds, and then a reflex anoxic generalized tonic-clonic seizure.

Postural hypotension

This usually is obvious since the syncopal attack occurs on standing, particularly if the patient has been in bed or sitting for a prolonged period, or after a heavy meal. The symptoms resolve as soon as the patient lies down again. The postural fall in blood pressure can normally, but not always, be demonstrated in the clinic with a fall of systolic blood pressure of at least 30 mmHg, or to below 80 mmHg on, or within a minute or two of, standing up. Asymptomatic falls of this magnitude are, however, common, particularly in the elderly. The causes are:

- drugs:
  vasodilators (glyceryl trinitrate, prazosin, hydralazine, calcium blockers, etc.)
  hypotensives (methyl dopa, diuretics, ganglion blockers, etc.)
  L-dopa, bromocriptine
  tricyclic antidepressants, mianserin
  phenothiazines
- old age, particularly during an intercurrent illness with prolonged recumbency
- peripheral autonomic neuropathy (p. 392)
- central autonomic failure:
  Shy–Drager syndrome (multi-system atrophy, p. 291)
  Parkinson's disease (p. 280)
  spinal cord injury
  idiopathic 'pure' ortho-static hypotension (p. 404)
- tabes dorsalis (p. 515)
- hyponatraemia (p. 464)
- Addison's disease (p. 455)
- anaemia (p. 460)

Cardiac arrhythmias

These may cause chest pain and palpitations as well as the syncope. They are not usually related to posture nor precipitated by anything (except caffeine in tachyarrhythmias). During tachyarrhythmias there is seldom loss of consciousness whereas during bradyarrhythmias unconsciousness can be very sudden. Tachyarrhythmias can occur during complex partial seizures (p. 71) and cause chest pain, palpitations, pallor and flushing, sometimes even with an impalpable wrist pulse; therefore, if ECG monitoring is not combined with EEG monitoring, the wrong diagnostic conclusions can easily be drawn. Also, palpitations are common in panic attacks and overbreathing (p. 110). Following prolonged supraventricular tachycardia, polyuria occasionally occurs. The routine ECG may reveal the diagnosis and ambulatory ECG monitoring may be helpful if the attacks are frequent enough to be 'captured'.

Valsalva manoeuvre

Valsalva manoeuvre, either deliberately or during activities such as weight lifting, straining at stool, or playing a wind or brass instrument, is an obvious cause of syncope from the history.

Structural cardiac disorders

These may present with syncope, particularly during exercise. Many are associated with cardiac arrhythmias but the most likely cause of syncope is obstruction to blood flow or severe cardiac muscle failure:
- left ventricular outflow obstruction (aortic stenosis, hypertrophic obstructive cardiomyopathy)
- atrioventricular valve obstruction (myxoma, ball valve thrombus)
- severe impairment of ventricular function (usually due to ischaemic heart disease)

Acute circulatory failure

This may cause syncope but only as one component of an obvious clinical picture:
- central circulatory failure:
  acute myocardial infarction
  pulmonary embolism
  pericardial tamponade, etc.
- peripheral circulatory failure:
  rupture or dissected aortic aneurysm
  acute blood loss
  acute fluid loss (burns, vomiting, diarrhoea, etc.)

Micturition syncope

This occurs during or just after micturition and is seen in two main groups: healthy young men who, having got out of bed during the night, are standing up passing urine, and elderly men and women who often have evidence of vascular disease and postural hypotension. It is benign, seldom recurrent, and in males can be avoided by sitting down to urinate.

Defaecation syncope

This occurs in elderly patients with constipation and there is often coexisting ischaemic heart disease or postural hypotension. It may also occur after a rather sudden call to defaecate while asleep. Presumably a related form of syncope is that which can occur during manual evacuation, sigmoidoscopy or barium enema.

Occasional patients have short-lasting nocturnal attacks of abdominal colic, diarrhoea, vomiting and syncope and the cause is obscure.

Carotid sinus syncope

In some individuals a few seconds' gentle massage of one or other carotid sinus (behind the angle of the jaw) produces abnormal slowing of the heart (asystole of more than 3 seconds), sometimes an abnormal drop in blood pressure (greater than 50 mmHg systolic) and occasionally both. It is *rarely* symptomatic and few patients have syncope induced by pressure on the neck, e.g. from head turning, tight collar. Symptomatic patients are middle-aged or elderly and there may be associated sinoatrial or ischaemic heart disease.

Swallow syncope

Swallowing can activate a vagal reflex to cause bradycardia or atrioventricular block and syncope, and very rarely a tachyarrhythmia. There is often a structural abnormality of the oesophagus (carcinoma, achalasia, stricture, diverticulum or hiatus hernia) and sometimes digoxin toxicity, ischaemic heart disease, or glossopharyngeal neuralgia (p. 147). Sometimes there is no apparent cause.

Ice-cream syncope

Cold foods, particularly ice-cream, held in the mouth can provoke a vagal reflex and syncope in some susceptible children, and occasionally in adults.

Prostatic syncope

This is precipitated by rectal examination, particularly if the patient is standing, and is probably due to a vagal reflex bradycardia and hypotension.

Cough syncope

This occurs during prolonged and paroxysmal bouts of coughing, usually because of chronic bronchitis. The patient may have no recall of the coughing bout so the diagnosis comes from a witness. There is seldom any cardiac or neurological disorder and the exact cause is uncertain.

Benign syncope in adolescent males

Adolescent males, but rarely females, may faint after they have been lying or sitting for a period of an hour or more, particularly in the evening. The loss of consciousness is sudden, it occurs a few seconds *after* standing up, and postural hypotension does not appear to be the cause. It does not occur after rising in the morning. Attacks are infrequent and remit in a matter of months.

Cervical spondylosis (p. 328)

This is often invoked as a cause of syncope, vertigo and non-specific dizziness in the elderly. Although 'dizziness' on looking up is a common and almost universal symptom in the elderly (perhaps as a result of kinking and obstruction of the vertebral arteries against vertebral osteophytes), it is extremely unusual to be able to demonstrate *symptomatic* obstruction of vertebral artery flow by this mechanism. Perhaps symptoms are more likely if there is widespread arterial disease in the neck or in the Circle of Willis compromising collateral blood flow to the brainstem.

Note: Spondylosis on neck X-ray is so common in the elderly that symptoms should not be ascribed to it without good reason.

Vertigo

Vertigo is the subjective hallucination of movement, usually a feeling of rotation but sometimes a feeling of side-to-side motion. With the eyes open the environment appears to be moving. It is, therefore, quite different from the symptoms of syncope (p. 100) and is certainly not merely non-specific 'dizziness'. Often there is associated nausea, vomiting and difficulty with balance. Usually vertigo is made worse by moving.

The cause is either central within the brainstem or peripheral within the vestibular nerve or inner ear. This differentiation depends not so much on the character of the vertigo as on associated features such as deafness, diplopia, etc. and on the context and character of the attacks (such as benign positional vertigo, p. 107). Horizontal or rotatory nystagmus (p. 193) occurs in both, but tends to outlast the symptoms in brainstem lesions, and vertical nystagmus occurs only with brainstem lesions.

Central vertigo

Brainstem lesions (p. 29) may cause episodic or prolonged vertigo but, unless there are other definite brainstem features, it is difficult if not impossible to localize lesions, e.g. diplopia, dysarthria, pyramidal and cerebellar signs, etc. Usually hearing is normal. If nystagmus is present and *persists* after the symptoms have resolved, the lesion is likely to be central. Causes include:
- multiple sclerosis (p. 345)
- vertebrobasilar TIA (p. 220), brainstem (p. 239) or cerebellar stroke (p. 223)
- subclavian steal (p. 221)
- vascular malformation (p. 233)
- basilar migraine (p. 138)
- Arnold–Chiari malformation (p. 202)
- syringobulbia (p. 334)
- drugs (anticonvulsants, alcohol, barbiturates)

Vertigo can be a feature of complex partial seizures but almost always with other more typical symptoms (p. 71) and is rarely, if ever, a result of cervical spondylosis (p. 327).

Peripheral vertigo

The clues to localization are other features such as deafness, tinnitus and pain or fullness in the ear. The causes are:
- vestibular nerve lesions:
  meningitis (p. 495)
  acoustic neuroma (p. 272) and other cerebello-pontine angle tumours (p. 194) rarely cause vertigo, particularly if there is no deafness, but more often unsteadiness of gait
  ototoxins, e.g. aminoglycosides, frusemide, etc. cause imbalance rather than vertigo
- inner ear lesions:
  'viral' labyrinthitis (p. 106)
  Menière's disease (p. 107)
  benign positional vertigo (p. 107)
  benign recurrent vertigo (p. 107)
  head injury
  infection (otitis media, syphilis, etc.)
  vascular lesions

'Viral' labyrinthitis

'Viral' labyrinthitis (or vestibular neuronitis) is an acute or subacute attack of vertigo and imbalance, often with nausea and vomiting, which lasts several days and is followed by a feeling of imbalance and some positional vertigo for a matter of weeks. In the early intensely symptomatic stage there is horizontal nystagmus. Audiometry is normal but there is usually unilateral canal paresis on caloric testing. The viral origin is unproven but the syndrome can occur in epidemics; sometimes the cause may be 'vascular' in the brainstem or inner ear.

Exactly similar *symptoms* can occur in multiple sclerosis (p. 345) and cerebellar strokes (p. 223) although there are usually signs, often subtle, of the central origin. Whether the term 'viral' labyrinthitis should ever be used is debatable since it so often hides either diagnostic incompetence or ignorance. It is better to refer to 'vertigo, cause not yet diagnosed', unless it is epidemic.

Menière's disease

This starts in middle age with progressive, although fluctuating, sensorineural deafness and tinnitus (often unilateral, at least at first) with occasional bouts of acute and sometimes disabling vertigo lasting several hours, or occasionally a few days. There may be a feeling of fullness in the affected ear(s). It is due to dilatation of the membranous labyrinth.

Benign positional vertigo

This is vertigo precipitated by movement of the head, usually when it is turned to one side or the other immediately after lying down in bed. If the precipitating posture is maintained the vertigo resolves in some seconds and is not reproduced by repeating the same posture within the next few minutes. Usually the problem resolves in a few weeks. It can often be provoked by Hallpike's manoeuvre: tilting the patient quickly from sitting to supine and turning the head to the left and right over the end of the couch causes vertigo and rotatory nystagmus after a latent period of a few seconds. This rapidly fatigues and does not recur if the test is quickly repeated. There may be a canal paresis on caloric testing (p. 194). Between attacks the patient is normal or has only mild and non-specific 'dizziness'.

It can occur within days or weeks of head injury, in the aftermath of 'viral' labyrinthitis (see above), or for no obvious reason. The cause is a disturbance in the inner ear. Brainstem and cerebellar lesions can produce similar symptoms but the vertigo and nystagmus do not fatigue if the posture is maintained or repeated.

Benign recurrent vertigo

This is sudden attacks of vertigo and nystagmus lasting minutes or hours, sometimes followed by imbalance and positional vertigo for days or weeks. There are no other symptoms and no cause is found. Audiometry and caloric tests are normal. It can occur at any age.

Treatment

There is no effective prophylactic treatment so that long-term drug therapy is not indicated. For disabling attacks themselves, various vestibular sedatives may help, but only for the duration of the symptoms:

prochlorperazine   20 mg, then 5–10 mg 8-hourly, oral, as necessary
                    12.5 mg i.m. 6-hourly as necessary
                    25 mg suppository repeated every 8 hours as necessary
cinnarazine   15–30 mg 8-hourly, oral
betahistine   8–16 mg 8-hourly oral

All these drugs can cause sedation, drowsiness, dry mouth, headache and blurred vision.

Metabolic conditions

Hypoglycaemia

This is almost always intermittent and the clinical picture includes:
- adrenergic features:
  sweating
  tachycardia and palpitations
  pallor
  tremor
- neurological features:
  confusion, amnesia
  visual blurring, diplopia
  light-headedness, dizziness,
  incoordination
  headache
  clouding and loss of consciousness

Sometimes there are only *focal* neurological features (e.g. hemiparesis, aphasia, dysarthria) without the adrenergic symptoms, so the attacks masquerade as TIA (p. 219) or stroke (p. 236); generalized tonic-clonic seizures; or obscure episodes of confusion, bizarre behaviour and personality change. Peripheral, mainly motor, neuropathy and dementia are very rare and late. Blood glucose levels do not seem to correlate with which hypoglycaemic symptom(s) will occur.

Diagnosis is easy if there is an obvious cause for hypoglycaemia (see below), almost always being treatment of diabetes with hypoglycaemic drugs. It is most difficult with insulinoma and factitious hypoglycaemia.

The constellation of symptoms tends to be stereotyped in an individual and attacks usually occur before food (particularly during the night or before breakfast), or after exercise, and are relieved by glucose. The diagnosis is best confirmed by finding a blood glucose of less than 2.5 mmol/l as near the *onset* of the attack as possible since later it may normalize spontaneously. This can often be done at home by the patient or relative using a glucose monitoring kit. Failing this, three consecutive overnight fasts should precipitate hypoglycaemia, with or without symptoms, in the face of an inappropriately high plasma insulin if there is an insulinoma. In diabetics with early morning focal or non-focal neurological attacks, one usually finds an excessively low blood glucose during the night.

Causes of hypoglycaemia

- oral hypoglycaemic drugs/insulin:
  diabetics
  factitious
- insulinoma
- other tumours:
  sarcoma (abdominal, retroperitoneal, pleural)
  hepatoma
  adrenal carcinoma
  terminal cancer
- excessive alcohol consumption (p. 542)
- hypothyroidism (p. 456)
- Addison's disease (p. 455)
- hypopituitarism (p. 273)
- late dumping
- cerebral malaria, quinine, quinidine (p. 534)
- hepatic encephalopathy (p. 467)
- sepsis

Phaeochromocytoma

This may present with paroxysmal attacks of severe pounding headache, sweating, palpitations, apprehension and tremor. Faintness and loss of consciousness are unusual. During the attack the patient is usually pale and the symptoms last for a matter of minutes. About half the patients have sustained hypertension and in the attack there is a severe rise in blood pressure.

The diagnosis depends on finding excess catecholamines or their metabolites in a 24-hour urine specimen, particularly if taken immediately after an attack. The urine must be kept cool and then assayed for vanilylmandelic acid, metanephrines, adrenaline and noradrenaline. If normal, but clinical suspicion is high, the test should be repeated. The assays can be interfered with by the patient taking methyl dopa, monoamine oxidase inhibitors or phenothiazines; consuming bananas, coffee, tea or chocolate; and withdrawal of clonidine. Catecholamines may also be measured in the plasma.

Carcinoid syndrome

This is due to the secretion of 5-hydroxytryptamine and other metabolically active substances from a carcinoid tumour (usually metastatic in the liver or primary in a non-gut site such as the bronchus). Attacks (lasting minutes, hours or even days) of hot flushing, palpitations, tachycardia and hypertension are characteristic. There may be faintness as well. Attacks of wheezing, diarrhoea, colic, nausea and vomiting also occur. The diagnosis is made by finding excess 5-hydroxyindole acetic acid in a 24-hour urine specimen but the assay can be interfered with by excess consumption of bananas, pineapple, walnuts or phenothiazines.

Systemic mastocytosis

This is a proliferative disorder of mast cells in the skin and other tissues. Excessive secretion of histamine causes attacks of flushing, hypotension, palpitations, diarrhoea, abdominal colic, vomiting, headache, shortness of breath and chest pain. Usually there are obvious skin lesions (urticaria pigmentosa) and biopsy reveals excessive numbers of mast cells.

Psychogenic attacks

There are various more or less reasonably well defined types of 'blackout' or 'funny turn' which are caused by non-organic psychological mechanisms; frequently they coexist and overlap in the same individual. They do not occur during sleep.

Panic attacks

Acutely or chronically anxious patients may have sudden attacks of *severe* anxiety with panic, apprehension, 'butterflies in the stomach', fear or even terror, palpitations, sweating, tightness in the throat, shortness of breath, chest pain, 'dizziness' and unsteadiness along with the features of overbreathing (see below). The attacks last minutes and the diagnosis is usually obvious from the description and the context. There is no altered consciousness and the symptoms subside once the provoking situation is removed.

Chronically anxious patients often complain of a multitude of vague symptoms which do not make any sense from the point of view of organic disease: dizziness, stabbing head pains, flitting pins and needles, etc.

Functional overbreathing

Overbreathing causes respiratory alkalosis and, eventually, pins and needles around the mouth and in the fingers and toes; dizziness and faintness but rarely loss of consciousness; and occasionally tetanic cramps in the hands and feet. Very rarely the sensory symptoms are unilateral, making for confusion with TIA (p. 219). Overbreathing can occur in the context of acute anxiety or a panic attack but sometimes there is no overt stress of psychopathology. The diagnosis is supported if the symptoms can be reproduced by asking the patient to overbreathe in the clinic. Treatment is explanation, reassurance, avoidance of provoking factors and sometimes advice to rebreathe into a paper bag.

In patients with epilepsy, overbreathing may precipitate a seizure (this being a standard way of attempting to activate the EEG) which may explain why stress is such a common precipitant of seizures and how functional overbreathing can so easily be confused with epilepsy.

'Pseudoseizures'

Consciously (malingering) or subconsciously (hysteria) some people have attacks which look superficially like tonic-clonic seizures or syncope, or even like status epilepticus. Females are more often affected than males; commonly the patient has behavioural or psychiatric problems, and sometimes it is epidemic (particularly in institutions or closed communities). Some patients have, in addition, organic neurological problems such as genuine seizures or mental handicap.

It may be possible to precipitate attacks by suggestion. To the trained observer the attacks do not look genuine in a way that is difficult to describe. Unconsciousness is unreal and attempting to open the patient's eyes may lead to voluntary contractions of the orbicularis oculi and upward deviation of the eyes (Bell's phenomenon, p. 191). Allowing the limp hand to fall on the face may be resisted. Abnormal movements tend to be non-specific 'trembling' or wild asynchronous purposeful and histrionic 'thrashing about'. There are none of the rhythmic clonic movements of a seizure. The eyes may be forcibly deviated towards the ground, but to whichever side the patient is laid on. Cyanosis and pallor do not occur but going red in the face is common. Tongue biting, other injury, and urinary incontinence are rare but possible, while faecal incontinence probably never occurs. There is no genuine post-ictal confusion. During the attack the plantars are flexor, pupil reactions normal and the corneal reflex is retained. The pulse is regular although sometimes there is a tachycardia.

Differentiation from seizures is supported by a normal EEG during or immediately after an attack (if necessary using telemetry and video recording) and a normal prolactin level 20 minutes post-attack compared with a baseline immediately pre-attack, or at the same time on a non-attack day. After a tonic-clonic seizure the serum prolactin usually at least doubles and/or rises to greater than 700 mu/l. This rise is less consistent but can occur after complex partial seizures, but is unusual after partial seizures. A *definite* rise makes a pseudo-tonic-clonic seizure unlikely and no rise at all makes a pseudoseizure somewhat likely, particularly if it appeared to look superficially like a tonic-clonic seizure. Twenty-four hours after a tonic-clonic seizure the plasma creatine kinase is sometimes raised but this never happens after lesser seizures or pseudoseizures. In the end there is no single diagnostic 'test' but rather a number of pieces of circumstantial evidence.

In children seizures can be fabricated by the parents, usually the mother, and this is difficult to discover unless there is a third party present at the time when a seizure was said to have occurred.

Agoraphobia

This may present to a neurologist with 'dizziness', panic attacks (p. 110) or overbreathing (p. 110) and the diagnosis depends on connecting these symptoms with the feared environment.

Depression

This usually presents with headache (p. 143), atypical facial pain (p. 147) or pseudodementia (p. 153) but can also cause faintness, dizziness and lack of coordination.

Post-concussional syndrome

Non-specific dizziness is common after head injury and can be psychogenic. Positional vertigo (p. 107) is organic.

3 Sleep disorders

Excessive daytime sleepiness (EDS)

Sleepiness during normal waking hours is unexceptional after disturbed night-time sleep, after heavy meals or alcohol and in quiet, relaxed or monotonous surroundings. However, there are several reasonably well-defined causes of *persistent* and *excessive* daytime sleepiness:

- narcolepsy syndrome (p. 114)
- sleep apnoea (p. 115)
- intracranial disease (p. 117)
- general medical disorders (p. 117)
- drugs (p. 117)
- menstrual hypersomnia (p. 118)
- Kleine–Levin syndrome (p. 118)

The term narcolepsy should be used only to refer to the narcolepsy syndrome (see below).

Narcolepsy syndrome

This is the most common cause of EDS (about 50/100 000 population), equally frequent in males and females. About two thirds of cases are sporadic and one third familial. It is strongly associated with the HLA DQw1/ DR2 locus on chromosome 6, but this haplotype is present in 25% of the UK population. The cause is unknown. Occasionally it is associated with multiple sclerosis (Chapter 12).

The onset is between the age of about 15 and 35 and the problem becomes lifelong. There are five components to the syndrome which are not necessarily all present in all patients although the combination of EDS and cataplexy is essential for a definite diagnosis:

- *Repetitive and irresistible sleep episodes* during normal waking hours. These can occur in 'normal' circumstances (sitting comfortably after dinner) but characteristically also occur in 'abnormal' circumstances (e.g. standing, talking). They last seconds or minutes. Often the patient has prolonged periods of inattentiveness during which some behaviours are automatically carried out. The patient may pass into rapid eye movement (REM) sleep within 10 minutes of sleep onset, but not all do this.

> *Note*: Sleep onset REM also occurs in depression, after sleep deprivation and in young children.

EDS often precedes other components of the narcolepsy syndrome by months or years.

- *Cataplexy* is episodes of sudden loss of muscle tone with weakness which last seconds, usually precipitated by sudden increase in alertness (e.g. laughter, anger). Possibly prazosin makes it worse.

- *Sleep paralysis* is the frightening sensation of being unable to move at the moment of going to sleep or waking up. It can occur in normal people.
- *Hypnagogic hallucinations* are vivid, and often frightening, visual or auditory hallucinations at the onset of sleep (and occasionally on waking). They can also be caused by beta-blockers and occur in normal people.
- *Disturbed nocturnal sleep*, restlessness, and frequent wakening.

All these symptoms may cause emotional problems, poor work record, accidents and marital breakdown.

Treatment

Daytime sleepiness is helped by dexamphetamine; oral, 5 mg daily, gradually increasing to as much as 60 mg or even 120 mg daily if necessary in 2–3 divided doses; or mazindol, oral, 2 mg daily, gradually increasing as necessary to 12 mg daily in 2–3 divided doses. Although adverse effects are common (sweating, irritability, restlessness), dependence in these patients is unusual.

Cataplexy and sleep paralysis respond to clomipramine, oral 10–25 mg at night, increasing if necessary to 150 mg daily in 2–3 divided doses. Unwanted effects include anticholinergic symptoms, cardiac arrhythmias, hypotension, seizures, drowsiness, weight gain and impotence.

Clomipramine and dexamphetamine can be used together if both daytime sleepiness and cataplexy are a problem. In a few patients protriptyline, up to 60 mg daily in 3 divided doses, may alleviate both symptoms.

Useful address

UK Association of Narcolepsy
South Hall
High Street
Farningham
Kent DA4 0DE
Tel: 0322-863195

Sleep apnoea

This is conventionally described as cessation of airflow at the nose and mouth during sleep for more than 10 seconds, more than 5 times per hour. Symptoms are rare unless apnoeas occur more than 10–20 times per hour. Sleep apnoena is almost always due to upper respiratory tract obstruction when nasal and oral airflow cease while respiratory efforts continue. Central failure of the involuntary and automatic respiratory centre of the brainstem is much less common; airflow ceases as does respiratory effort. Disentangling these two types (or their relative contributions) is not always easy, particularly since during sleep the brainstem response to pH and $Paco_2$ is reduced, and the pharyngeal muscles become flaccid.

Central non-obstructive sleep apnoea

This can occur in brainstem lesions (tumour, infarct, MS, etc., p. 203) particularly if the lower medulla is involved, and with neuromuscular ventilatory failure, particularly with paralysis of the diaphragm (p. 417). During sleep, when the voluntary cortical respiratory mechanisms are not in operation, hypoventilation with hypoxaemia, respiratory arrest and even death can occur. EDS usually is not a problem but morning headache is. Some kind of mechanical ventilatory support may be needed at night.

Obstructive sleep apnoea

Snoring is common, particularly in men, and is due to pharyngeal wall collapse and airflow obstruction during sleep. Under certain circumstances this can become pathological, symptomatic and sometimes life-threatening:

- malformation of the nose, jaw or pharynx
- tonsil or adenoid enlargement
- macroglossia
- massive obesity (Pickwickian syndrome)
- Down's syndrome
- acromegaly (p. 458)
- hypothyroidism (p. 456)
- Shy–Drager syndrome (p. 291)
- achondroplasia (p. 484)

All these conditions tend to narrow the upper airway so that respiratory obstruction and apnoea occur during sleep. However, many other patients have no obvious cause. The syndrome occurs in children and adults, can be familial, and is much more common in males.

The cardinal symptom is loud and persistent snoring, which usually started in childhood and adolescence, along with frequent and prolonged periods of sleep apnoea (up to one minute or more), during which arterial oxygen saturation falls and cardiac arrhythmias are common, and often ending with a loud snort or gasp with brief arousal. Sleep is restless, sleep-walking common, enuresis fairly frequent and the patients are usually difficult to rouse. Morning headache is common. Alcohol and other sedatives exacerbate the problem, as may a temporary increase in airway obstruction from an upper respiratory tract infection.

During the day the patients are often tired, lethargic, irritable and fall asleep in inappropriate circumstances, probably because of inadequate night-time sleep. Periods of subwakefulness and confusion are common and work record declines. Hypertension and obesity are also common, and in severe cases cor pulmonale develops.

Treatment

- Any airway obstruction should be dealt with on its merits (tonsillectomy, etc.).
- Reduction of any excessive weight, sedative or alcohol consumption sometimes helps.
- Protriptyline (10–20 mg at bedtime) can occasionally help the EDS component but has much less effect on the apnoea.
- Continuous positive airway pressure through the nose during sleep can be very successful.
- Tracheostomy is now rarely needed. It relieves both the obstructive apnoea and EDS but is a final resort because of the potential complications and aesthetic concerns.

Intracranial disease

This seldom presents with EDS and there is little or no diagnostic problem. Possibilities include:
- raised intracranial pressure (p. 256)
- hypothalamic tumour (p. 26)
- post head injury
- encephalitis (p. 498)
- Whipple's disease (p. 463)
- sarcoidosis (p. 472)

General medical disorders

These seldom present with EDS although it is a frequent symptom in established disease:
- hypothyroidism (p. 456)
- renal failure (p. 465)
- hepatic encephalopathy (p. 467)
- hypoglycaemia (p. 108)
- Prader–Willi syndrome

Drugs

- sedatives, hypnotics and tranquillizers
- tricyclic antidepressants, mianserin, trazodone
- antihistamines
- anticonvulsants
- opiates
- methysergide

- lithium
- indomethacin
- abuse of amphetamines or other stimulants

Menstrual hypersomnia

A rare condition of adolescence in which EDS is related to the days before and after the onset of menstruation. Oestrogens appear to be effective.

Kleine–Levin syndrome

Periods of days, several times a year, of sleepiness for which there may be partial amnesia. These periods are preceded or followed by excessive or abnormal eating. Somewhat similar features can occur in Whipple's disease of the nervous system (p. 463) and organic hypothalmic disorders such as tumours.

The diagnosis of excessive daytime sleepiness

This depends almost entirely on the history and it is crucial to question the bed partner or parents about excessive snoring. General, upper respiratory and neurological disorders must be excluded and the main differential diagnoses are complex partial seizures (p. 71) and hypoglycaemia (p. 108).

Investigations in a sleep laboratory are not always needed. An audio (with or without video) recording of nocturnal snoring, apnoea and restlessness can be as useful as, and often easier to obtain than, a sleep recording of heart rate, EEG, eye movements, respiratory muscle activity, nasal airflow, and Pao_2 by ear oximetry. Inappropriate HLA status more or less rules out the narcolepsy syndrome.

If excessive daytime sleepiness is not obviously due to sleep apnoea and if there are no other clinical features of the narcolepsy syndrome, then EEG recording to detect the rapid onset of REM sleep may help make the diagnosis of the narcolepsy syndrome.

Insomnia

Normal daily sleep requirements vary from 3–12 hours and become less with age. Difficulty going to sleep, and frequent and early waking are far more common than EDS and have probably affected everyone. *Abnormal* difficulty in sleeping (insomnia) may be caused by:
- anxiety
- depression
- interference with sleep by physical symptoms such as pain, cough, itching, dyspnoea, restless legs, nocturia, etc.

- schizophrenia
- hypomania
- sleep reversal, e.g. in elderly demented patients, during intercurrent physical illness in the elderly, encephalitis lethargica (p. 290), South African trypanosomiasis (p. 536)
- drugs, e.g. excess alcohol consumption, stimulants such as caffeine, amphetamines, nicotine and withdrawal from sedatives and hypnotics

Insomnia is more common in females and in old age.

Treatment

Treatment is of the underlying cause with general advice concerning privacy, quiet and a warm comfortable bed, avoidance of sleep during the day, avoidance of coffee, tea and alcohol before going to bed, relaxation techniques, and a warm milky beverage at bedtime. A dull book or sexual intercourse may also help.

Night sedation should be avoided if possible or used only for a matter of days or weeks to cover periods of anxiety, bereavement, etc. No more than the lowest effective dose should be used. Stopping benzodiazepines usually leads to a few nights of disturbed sleep, anxiety, restlessness, palpitations and sometimes withdrawal seizures.

- alcohol, one measure of an acceptable spirit helps some patients
- temazepam, oral, 10–60 mg at bedtime (moderately short duration of action)
- triazolam, oral, 0.125–0.5 mg at bedtime (quick onset and very short acting but may cause daytime anxiety and agitation)
- diazepam, oral, 2–30 mg at bedtime (rather long acting)
- promethazine is useful in children, oral, 6–12 months: 10 mg, 1–5 years: 5–15 mg, 6–10 years: 10–25 mg, adults: 25–50 mg
- chloral hydrate is particularly useful in children and the elderly, oral, 30–50 mg/kg in children, 500–2000 mg in adults
- chlormethiazole is particularly useful in elderly confused patients, oral, 200–400 mg or more if necessary. Adverse effects include sneezing, headache and conjunctival irritation.

In the elderly, small doses of hypnotics can cause excessive daytime sleepiness, lethargy, falls, incontinence and confusion. Even in normal adults mental functioning may be impaired the morning after taking a hypnotic and driving performance may be affected.

Parasomnias

Sleepwalking

This occurs in about 15% of children but is rarely a serious problem. Usually it disappears in adulthood. There is little associated dreaming and, if wakened, only mild disorientation. In adults there may be background emotional stress.

Night terrors

Night terrors are not epileptic. Some children (and occasionally adults) go through a period of a few years when they wake in the night screaming, terrified, confused and possibly hallucinating. They do not recognize their parents and may mumble incomprehensibly. There is a rapid pulse, piloerection and a look of terror. In the morning they have no recall of the attack.

Bruxism

Bruxism (nocturnal teeth grinding) occurs in children but rarely in adults when it may be related to stress or head injury.

Head banging

Head banging during sleep is a childhood phenomenon with no obvious cause.

Nocturnal 'myoclonus'

Nocturnal 'myoclonus' (or periodic movements in sleep) are rather stereotyped and abrupt withdrawal movements followed by a brief tonic contraction which occur intermittently throughout the night, usually in one leg but sometimes in the arm. This is most common in the elderly, is not epileptic and is usually of no consequence except in severe cases when the movements can disrupt sleep and possibly cause excessive daytime sleepiness. It can be associated with the restless legs syndrome (p. 306)

Benign hypnagogic myoclonus

See p. 308.

Restless legs syndrome

See p. 306.

Sleep paralysis

See p. 115.

4 Coma and brain death

Coma, semi-coma, stupor and obtunded are imprecise words since, like blood pressure, consciousness is a continuous variable from a state of normality to unresponsiveness to all sensory stimuli. Therefore, conscious level should be measured on a standard scale, the best of which is currently the Glasgow coma score (GCS) (Table 4.1)

The three subscores should always be expressed separately (max. GCS 4, 6, 5) but can be summed as well (max. GCS 15).

Table 4.1 Glasgow coma score

Eye opening:	
nil	1
to pain (applied to limbs)	2
to voices (including command)	3
spontaneously (with blinking)	4
Motor response:	
nil	1
arm extension to pain (nail bed pressure)	2
arm flexion to pain (nail bed pressure)	3
arm withdraws from pain (nail bed pressure)	4
hand localizes pain (supraorbital or chest pressure)	5
obeys commands	6
Verbal response:	
nil	1
groans (no recognizable words)	2
inappropriate words (including expletives)	3
confused speech	4
orientated	5

Note:
● The *best* response must be used since one side of the body may be weak and so confound the assessment.
● Verbal response may be depressed inappropriately to the level of consciousness by aphasia, intubation and facial injury.
● Sensory loss (e.g. from cervical cord injury) may confound eye opening to pain in the limbs and motor response to nail bed pressure.
● Eye opening may be interfered with by orbital swelling or 3rd nerve palsy.
● Arm movements may be impaired by local trauma or a cervical cord lesion.

Causes of coma

Consciousness depends on integration of the reticular activating system in the brainstem with the cerebral cortex. It is, therefore, impaired by lesions in the posterior fossa (within, or compressing the brainstem); supratentorial lesions large enough to cause brain shift and transtentorial herniation and brainstem compression (p. 257); and diffuse bilateral disturbance of the whole brain.

Posterior fossa lesions

- Within the brainstem (p. 203):
  haemorrhage, spontaneous or traumatic (p. 227)
  infarction (p. 222)
  tumour (p. 266)
  infection/abscess (p. 503)
- Compressing the brainstem, often with obstructive hydrocephalus:
  cerebellar tumour, haemorrhage, infarct, abscess (p. 199)
  cerebello-pontine angle mass (p. 194)

Brainstem signs and impaired brainstem reflexes appear early (particularly abnormal eye movements and pupil responses). Limb signs are bilateral (symmetrical or asymmetrical) and often rather subtle (extensor plantars, reflex change) rather than obvious (hemiplegia).

Supratentorial mass lesions

- tumours (p. 266)
- intracranial haemorrhage spontaneous or traumatic (p. 227)
- cerebral infarction (p. 222)
- subdural/extradural haematoma (p. 235)
- abscess (p. 503)
- pituitary apoplexy (p. 273)

Limb signs are asymmetrical (hemiparesis) and, if consciousness is not too deep, focal and lateralizing cognitive signs are also obvious (e.g. aphasia). As consciousness deepens, as a result of transtentorial herniation, a unilateral third nerve palsy may occur, because of medial temporal lobe herniation, along with ipsilateral hemiparesis due to compression of the opposite cerebral peduncle against the tentorial edge. Further herniation causes impaired up-gaze and perhaps Cheyne–Stokes respiration with small reactive pupils, then medium-sized and fixed pupils with dysconjugate eye movements and decerebrate rigidity, and finally fixed dilated pupils with no reflex eye movements and no response to pain.

Diffuse brain lesions

- ischaemic/anoxic damage:
  cardiac arrest

anaesthetic accident
head injury
blood loss/shock
subarachnoid haemorrhage (p. 228)
intracranial venous thrombosis (p. 224)
collagen vascular disorders (p. 444)
'hyperviscosity' syndromes (p. 461)
thrombotic thrombocytopenic purpura (p. 462)
disseminated intravascular coagulation (p. 462)
hypertensive encephalopathy (p. 214)
drowning
fat embolism (p. 487)
respiratory failure
decompression sickness (p. 485)
acute mountain sickness (p. 485)
irradiation (p. 486)
• metabolic encephalopathies:
hepatic encephalopathy (p. 467)
renal failure (p. 465)
dialysis dementia (p. 467)
endocrine:
   hypothyroidism (p. 456)
   hyperthyroidism (p. 456)
   Addison's disease (p. 455)
   Cushing's syndrome (p. 455)
   hypopituitarism (p. 273)
hypo/hyperglycaemia (p. 108)
hypo/hypernatraemia (p. 464)
hypo/hypercalcaemia (p. 457)
hyperammonaemia:
   hepatic failure (p. 467)
   portacaval shunt, surgical and rarely congenital (p. 467)
   ornithine transcarbamylase deficiency (p. 480)
   argininosuccinic aciduria (p. 481)
   citrullinaemia (p. 481)
   argininaemia (p. 481)
   carbamylphosphate synthetase deficiency (p. 481)
   lysinuric protein intolerance (p. 481)
   Reye's syndrome (p. 483)
   sodium valproate (p. 91)
   systemic carnitine deficiency (p. 429)
   amino and organic acidurias (p. 480)
   asparaginase toxicity
porphyria (p. 398)

mitochondrial cytopathies (p. 429)
Leigh's disease (p. 482)
- infection:
encephalitis/meningitis (p. 498)
cerebral malaria (p. 534)
septicaemia (e.g. typhoid, p. 509)
pneumonia
- drug intoxication:
benzodiazepines
opiates
hypoglycaemic drugs
barbiturates
anticonvulsants (p. 88)
- toxins (see also Chapter 19):
alcohols (p. 542)
organic solvents (p. 546)
carbon monoxide (p. 549)
metals (p. 547)
- miscellaneous:
post-ictal (p. 73)
Wernicke's encephalopathy (p. 468)
neuroleptic malignant syndrome (p. 289)
hypothermia (p. 486)
burns encephalopathy in children
hypereosinophilic syndrome (p. 459)

Before consciousness is lost there is usually a preceding confusional state without focal cognitive or limb signs (so the causes of this form of coma are similar to those of confusional states, p. 162). Generalized rather than partial seizures (tonic-clonic and myoclonic) are common. Bilateral extensor plantars with generalized limb hypotonia develop and any disturbance of brain-stem reflexes is late; however, in sedative-induced coma, eye-movement reflexes are abolished rather earlier and before the pupil responses disappear. Raised intracranial pressure and cerebral oedema are common in ischaemic/anoxic and metabolic encephalopathies. Asterixis (p. 296) is a feature of hepatic, renal and respiratory failure.

Many metabolic encephalopathies cause *intermittent* confusion and coma, often precipitated by stimuli such as alcohol (hepatic failure), chest infections (respiratory failure), high protein meals (hyperammonaemia), drugs (porphyria), etc.

Note: Hypoglycaemia can sometimes cause *focal* signs (p. 108).

Differential diagnosis

Coma may be confused with:
- 'locked in' syndrome (p. 29)
- persistent vegetative state (p. 126)
- non-convulsive status epilepticus (p. 97)
- catatonia (p. 313)
- hysterical pseudocoma (p. 126)

In a sense, the *persistent vegetative state* (coma vigil, akinetic mutism) is one form of coma since, although spontaneous eye opening and blinking are usually present (GCS 4), the eye movements are roving and there is no intelligible verbal response (GCS 1 or 2) nor any indication of cognitive function; the limbs may be spastic or flaccid and can often localize pain (GCS 5). There is no response of eye movements to command (cf. the 'locked-in' syndrome, p. 29) even though it is usually clear from the startle response that the patient can hear. Patients grimace, swallow and breathe spontaneously and brainstem reflexes are usually preserved. The EEG is diffusely slowed. This state is a consequence of severe traumatic or ischaemic/anoxic brain injury and appears as consciousness lightens and the patient comes off the ventilator. Full recovery never occurs and death follows in months or years.

In *hysterical pseudocoma* the patient looks 'asleep' rather than unconscious, there are no abnormal neurological signs, respiration is normal and menace causes blinking if the eyes are open. Eye opening itself may be resisted and the limbs tend to resist being moved. If the arm is allowed to fall towards the face it does not land on it. There may be an obvious response to pain, the corneal responses are normal, and it is very difficult for any conscious patient to tolerate the inside of the nostril being tickled with cotton wool or the external auditory canal being irrigated with ice-cold water for caloric testing. The EEG is normal.

Note: In confusional states (p. 161) and non-convulsive status epilepticus (p. 97) the patient is not unconscious but has an abnormal Glasgow coma score.

Finding the cause

The cause may be obvious (e.g. head injury, cardiac arrest), confounded by other factors (e.g. alcoholic intoxication with a head injury), or rare and obscure (e.g. porphyria). As usual the diagnosis depends mainly on a good history and clinical examination backed up by sensible investigations.

History

This is almost always obtainable from someone, although obviously not the patient, e.g. relatives, friends, police, ambulancemen. It is crucial to obtain any hospital records and information from the general practitioner, if necessary by telephone (to find the general practitioner's name, telephone the local Family Practitioner Committee, or in Scotland the Health Board, giving the patient's name and date of birth). Also, note any drugs, prescriptions, syringes or medic-alert bracelet in the patient's clothes or house.

Important issues to consider are:
- known general medical disorders (e.g. diabetes, renal failure)
- recent symptoms (headache, fever, etc.)
- speed of onset of coma
- recurrent coma (e.g. metabolic encephalopathy, p. 124)
- seizures
- known medications or access to drugs
- recent head injury (subdural haematoma, p. 235)
- foreign travel (malaria, p. 534)
- suicide note
- alcoholism
- where patient found (e.g. in a caravan or boat with carbon monoxide poisoning, p. 549)

Examination

After establishing an airway, if necessary by intubation (see below), it is essential to quickly assess the respiratory and cardiovascular status and record the GCS before doing a careful neurological and general examination.

Neurological examination must concentrate on:
- Focal neurological signs; focal cognitive deficits indicating a left or right cerebral hemisphere lesion before the patient is too unconscious to be assessed (e.g. aphasia); limb signs which can be assessed by response to pain (pressure on the nail bed and Achilles tendon), spontaneous movements, muscle tone, tendon reflexes, plantar responses; facial weakness may be detected during a grimace or by a weak cheek blowing out during expiration.
- Brainstem signs and reflexes, e.g. pupil size and reaction to light are crucial. Small pin-point pupils are seen in pontine lesions and opiate overdose; large fixed pupils in extensive brainstem lesions, anoxia, sedative overdose, anticholinergic poisoning or eyedrops; unilateral fixed dilated pupil in third nerve palsy.

Note: The light unresponsive pupil of a blind eye should react to consensual light stimulation (unlike in a third nerve palsy). The optic disc may well be pale with chronic blindness, depending on the cause.

Eye movements may be conjugate or dysconjugate and must be tested for response to head movement provided there is no neck fracture (doll's eyes manoeuvre, p. 179) and, if necessary, to ice-cold water caloric stimulation (p. 194); if the brainstem is intact, the eyes move towards the irrigated ear. If the ear drum is perforated, use a cold draft from the piped oxygen supply. If the external ear is blocked (wax), the test may be impossible. Corneal and gag responses should also be tested.

- Meningism (p. 492) may indicate meningoencephalitis, subarachnoid haemorrhage, a posterior fossa mass or, possibly, traumatic injury to the neck.
- Papilloedema, or a tense anterior fontanelle in infants, indicates (but their absence does not exclude) raised intracranial pressure. Do *not* dilate pupils because this makes continuing assessment of their size and light response impossible (see above).
- Early in metabolic encephalopathies (particularly in hepatic, renal and respiratory failure) there may be a 'flap' of the outstretched hands (asterixis, p. 296).
- Respiratory pattern abnormalities are not particularly helpful. In metabolic coma respiration is normal, deep and regular due to acidosis, or Cheyne–Stokes. Brainstem lesions tend to cause irregular and chaotic breathing, hyperventilation and, in medullary lesions, gasping respiration.

General examination must concentrate on:
- signs of trauma, e.g. head (bleeding/CSF from ears or nose), abdomen
- temperature (fever or hypothermia)
- evidence of a convulsion; bitten tongue or cheek, skin petechiae
- breath odour; ketones, alcohol, hepatic foetor
- needle marks from medication, drug abuse
- colour; cyanosis, cherry red from carbon monoxide poisoning, jaundice
- stigmata of liver disease (spider naevi, gynaecomastia, hepatomegaly, etc.)
- gums (phenytoin adverse effect)
- skin blisters are a non-specific sign of prolonged coma

Investigations

Blood

Blood must be taken at once for glucose, full blood count, urea and electrolytes. Depending on the situation, screening for drugs and toxins may be required as well as liver function tests, alcohol level, blood cultures, thyroid function and blood gases. Other biochemical investigations may need to include:
- plasma calcium and phosphate
- blood ammonia (normal < 50 µmol/l)
- plasma cortisol (? Addison's disease)

- urine porphyrins
- plasma lactate (? mitochondrial cytopathy)
- urine orotic acid (? ornithine transcarbamylase deficiency)
- blood/urine amino acids (? aminoacidurias)

Note: In liver failure the liver function tests can be normal but ammonia levels are usually raised.

Note: Alcohol is an unlikely cause of coma if the blood level is less than 200 mg % (44 mmol/l).

Chest X-ray

This is not so urgent but may be needed as a baseline in case of later pulmonary complications.

Skull X-ray

Skull X-ray is important if there is any hint of skull trauma. Fractures can be easier to see than on CT.

CT scan

CT scan must be done urgently if there is any sign of a focal supratentorial or a brainstem lesion, or if there is evidence of raised intracranial pressure.

Note: A unilateral supratentorial lesion which does *not* cause lateral displacement of the brain is an unlikely cause of coma.

Lumbar puncture

This is safe if there are no focal signs of a mass lesion, nor raised intracranial pressure, and is urgent if there is *any* suspicion of meningoencephalitis. It will also confirm subarachnoid haemorrhage if CT is not available (p. 223), but note that a cerebellar haemorrhage can present with *acute* headache and a stiff neck and then a lumbar puncture is dangerous (p. 228).

Electroencephalogram

This may be useful to confirm a generalized encephalopathy (widespread bilateral slow waves). *Focal* slow waves suggest a focal mass lesion indicating the need for a CT scan if one has not been performed already. In metabolic and drug-induced coma the slowing of the EEG may occur early while symptoms are still mild. Also, the EEG may reveal non-convulsive status epilepticus (p. 97).

Note: A flat (iso-electric) EEG does not necessarily indicate brain death since it can occur in reversible drug-induced coma.

Electrocardiogram

Electrocardiogram may reveal a relevant arrhythmia or recent myocardial infarction.

Note: There may be more than one cause of coma in an individual patient.

Treatment

Emergency treatment

- Place on side, no pillow, head slightly down so that saliva dribbles out of the mouth, and check the airway. Clear the airway if necessary with swabs or suction.
- Insert a pharyngeal airway or, if cough reflex is inadequate or the patient is hypoventilating, intubate and ventilate as necessary.
- Check blood pressure and pulse and restore circulatory function as necessary.
- Set up intravenous line and take blood for full blood count, urea, electrolytes, glucose, liver function, drugs and toxins, etc.; also, store plasma and serum in case they are needed later for diagnosis.
- If any possibility of hypoglycaemia, give 50 ml of 50 g/dl (50%) glucose i.v.
- If any possibility of alcoholism, give i.v. or i.m. 10 ml Parentrovite forte (p. 469).
- If any possibility of opiate overdose, give naloxone, i.v. 0.8–2 mg repeated at intervals of 2–3 minutes to a maximum of 10 mg if conscious level and respiratory function do not improve within minutes; if necessary, by i.v. infusion to maintain therapeutic effect because of short half life.
- Neurological and general medical examination (including temperature) and careful check for injuries (head, neck, abdomen, etc.).
- Catheterize bladder and record fluid balance.
- Further investigations as indicated, e.g. chest X-ray, skull X-ray, ECG, CT scan, EEG, etc.
- Treat the underlying cause.

Longer term management

- care of airway and chest; physiotherapy, suction, etc.
- turn 2-hourly to prevent pressure sores
- bladder care
- eye care

- mouth care
- bowel care; enemas as necessary
- fluid balance, feeding (nasogastric tube or parenteral)
- monitor respiration, pulse, blood pressure, temperature, Glasgow coma score, neurological state
- passive limb movements to avoid contractures
- avoid sedative drugs if possible

Brain death

Patients with severe and irreversible brain damage may survive with a normal circulation for weeks or even months provided they are mechanically ventilated. However, if the brainstem is dead, recovery never occurs and the heart will stop eventually; therefore, mechanical ventilation can be withdrawn even if the heart is still beating. The UK guidelines for brainstem death are practical and reliable; provided the necessary preconditions are met, no patient has survived, even with continuing ventilation, once the brainstem has been shown to be dead.

Preconditions

1 Absolutely no doubt that the patient's condition is due to *irremediable* structural brain damage. The diagnosis of a disorder which can lead to brain damage must be fully established; this is usually a head injury or spontaneous intracranial haemorrhage, but it can be cerebral anoxia (post cardiac arrest, drowning, etc.) when very great care and time are required to be certain that the damage really is irremediable.

If in any doubt about the irreversibility of brain damage then do not disconnect the ventilator.

2 The patient is deeply comatose (no eye opening, motor or verbal response; GCS 1, 1, 1) with no suspicion that the cause is depressant drugs (e.g. narcotics, tranquillizers, hypnotics, alcohol). Primary hypothermia, metabolic and endocrine causes must be excluded and there should be no profound abnormality of blood electrolytes, glucose or acid-base balance.

3 The patient is being maintained on a ventilator because spontaneous respiration had previously been inadequate or ceased altogether. Muscle relaxants and other drugs must be excluded as the cause and, if used, any residual effect must be ruled out by showing adequate neuromuscular transmission (e.g. spinal reflexes, electrical stimulation of peripheral nerves).

Tests for confirming brain death

1 *All brainstem reflexes must be absent*:
- Fixed pupils with no response to bright light. Paralytic eye drops, eye

injury and 2nd or 3rd cranial nerve lesions can cause problems here. The pupils are not necessarily dilated in brainstem death.

- Absent corneal reflexes.
- Absent vestibulo-ocular reflexes on irrigation of each ear in turn with 20 ml ice-cold water (check for wax or perforation of the drum first).
- No motor response within the cranial nerve distribution (head, eye or face) elicited by adequate stimulation of any somatic area (nail bed, supraorbital and Achilles tendon pressure should all be tried on each side).
- No reflex response to touching the pharynx nor to a suction catheter passed into the trachea.

2 *Apnoea.* No respiratory movements when the ventilator is disconnected and the Pa_{CO_2} reaches 6.65 kPa, preferably checked by direct measurement. To avoid anoxia during disconnection, the patient should be ventilated with 100% oxygen for 10 min first and then, during disconnection, 6 l/min 100% oxygen delivered through a tracheal catheter. If just before disconnection the Pa_{CO_2} is less than 3.5 kPa, then 5% CO_2 in oxygen should be delivered via the ventilator until this level is achieved, usually in less than 5 min.

Note:

- The tests should all be repeated after an interval, the length of which depends on the clinical situation.
- The tests must be performed by two experienced clinicians.
- Body temperature must be greater than 35°C.
- Spinal reflexes may persist even when the brain is dead (e.g. deep tendon reflexes).
- Decerebrate or decorticate posturing and epileptic seizures are all incompatible with brainstem death.
- An isoelectric EEG is not required since this can be followed by recovery in sedative overdose.

5   Pain in the head and face

Headache

Headache is a common symptom in general practice (about 2% of all visits) and neurology clinics (about 20% of new patients). The causes are:

- migraine (p. 137)
- migrainous neuralgia (p. 141)
- psychiatric and psychological conditions:
  tension headache (p. 142)
  depression (p. 143)
  anxiety
  hysteria and malingering (p. 143)
  hypochondriasis
- infection:
  meningitis (p. 491)
  encephalitis (p. 498)
  subdural empyema (p. 503)
  osteomyelitis of the skull
  post-herpetic neuralgia (p. 523)
  non-specific effect of fever
- trauma:
  head injury
  post-traumatic headache (p. 145)
  subdural haematoma (p. 235)
- raised intracranial pressure (p. 256)
- vascular disease:
  subarachnoid haemorrhage (p. 228)
  primary intracerebral haemorrhage (p. 227)
  cerebral infarction (and TIA) (p. 222)
  giant cell arteritis (p. 450)
- arterial hypertension (diastolic blood pressure at least 120 mmHg, p. 214)
- low pressure headache: post lumbar puncture (p. 42)
- hypercapnia (respiratory failure, sleep apnoea, p. 115)
- acute mountain sickness (p. 485)
- polycythaemia rubra vera (p. 458)
- 'hyperviscosity' syndrome (p. 461)
- hypothyroidism (p. 456)
- acromegaly (p. 458)
- premenstrual tension
- pain as a result of disorders of the:
  eyes (p. 147)
  ears

skull
sinuses
neck
teeth
parotid gland
temporomandibular joint
carotid artery (p. 147)
- miscellaneous paroxysmal headaches:
post-ictal headache (p. 73)
cough headache (p. 143)
benign orgasmic cephalgia (p. 143)
phaeochromocytoma (p. 109)
colloid cyst of the 3rd ventricle (p. 275)
ice-cream headache (p. 144)
exercise headache (p. 144)
thunderclap headache (p. 144)
cephalgia fugax (p. 144)
exploding head syndrome (p. 144)
- drugs and toxins:
alcohol (p. 542)
caffeine (particularly withdrawal)
vasodilators (e.g. glyceryl trinitrate, dipyridamole, calcium blockers)
sympathomimetic drugs (p. 294)
hypoglycaemic agents
chronic carbon monoxide exposure (p. 549)
anti-infective drugs (e.g. cycloserine, ethionamide, griseofulvin, rifampicin)
anti-inflammatory drugs (e.g. indomethacin, phenlybutazone, quinidine)
specific drugs:

amiodarone	monoamineoxidase A inhibitors
benzodiazepines	omeprazole
bezafibrate	phenytoin
carbamazepine	quinine/quinidine
cimetidine, ranitidine	simvastatin
clofibrate	theophylline
danazol	tricyclic antidepressants
ethosuxamide	vigabatrin
gemfibrozil	zimeldine
lovastatin	

By far the most common causes of headache in general practice, or the out-patient clinic, are migraine and various forms of psychogenic and tension headaches. Even in neurology clinics less than 5% of headaches are due to serious intracranial structural disease and most of these have additional and obvious neurological features (e.g. seizures).

Migraine is rarely, if ever, a symptom of structural intracranial disease such as an arteriovenous malformation (p. 233), tumour (p. 236) or aneurysm (p. 231).

The diagnosis of headache

Often the cause is obvious and incidental to the main clinical problem (e.g. fever). Although the differential diagnosis is long, finding the cause of headache is not difficult and depends primarily on the history, occasionally on the examination, and exceptionally on investigation.

For each type of headache, and patients may have more than one, important points in the history are:
- When did it first start?
- Is it intermittent, or persistent?
- If intermittent, how frequent is it?; the longest period of freedom; the shortest period of freedom; the date of the last episode?
- What is it like? Is it stereotyped? Is there a prodrome? Is the onset sudden or insidious? Where is the pain and any radiation? Are there any associated symptoms (e.g. vomiting, diplopia, visual changes)? How long does it last?
- How severe is it? Kept from sleeping, woken from sleep, time off work or school, consumption of analgesics?
- Is severity or frequency changing?
- What precipitates or exacerbates it?
- What improves it?
- Is it related to time of day, food, alcohol, stress, menstruation, etc.?
- Are there other neurological symptoms?
- Are there any psychiatric or psychological factors?
- What does the patient think it is due to?
- General health?
- Past history (head trauma, sinusitis, migraine, cancer, etc.)?
- Family history (migraine, other headache)?
- Drugs and toxins?
- Occupation?

Examination of the whole patient, including blood pressure, is as important as the neurological examination which, apart from the occasional surprise (e.g. papilloedema), is usually normal unless there are additional neurological symptoms. A thorough examination can be remarkably therapeutic, particularly if it has never been done properly before. Auscultation for cranial bruit is particularly impressive but one is never heard since headache alone is so rarely caused by an arteriovenous malformation (p. 233).

Investigations depend on the history and examination and are mostly unnecessary. If the headache is persistent and obscure, a skull X-ray is advisable (in mild psychiatric conditions it can be therapeutic). CT scan is necessary if there are focal neurological symptoms or signs, raised intracranial pressure, an abnormal skull X-ray, or if the headache is persistent and the cause obscure. Occasionally severe occipital pain may be due to an Arnold–Chiari malformation (p. 202) which can be excluded by MRI, or if necessary by myelography. In the elderly, giant cell arteritis (p. 450) is easily forgotten but easily treatable; the ESR usually is very high. For reasons of self-aggrandizement and financial gain some neurologists order an EEG.

Migraine

Migraine is an ill-understood but well recognized and common syndrome of recurrent and stereotyped headaches with characteristic features, and often with a family history. About 20% of the population will have migraine at some time in their lives. It is often difficult to determine where migraine ends and tension headaches begin; frequently patients have both.

Classical migraine

There is a prodrome of spreading and intensifying focal neurological symptoms (possibly due to intracranial vasoconstriction or spreading neuronal depression) which reaches its maximum in about 10 minutes and resolves slowly in a total of about 20–30 minutes. Occasionally it persists for hours or days.

The symptoms are usually visual with 'dazzles', 'flashing lights', 'shimmering', 'watery patches', 'zigzag lines' or 'blind patches' (often a homonymous hemianopia) spreading across the vision of one or — much more often — both eyes. The positive symptoms are present with the eyes open or shut. Sometimes there is numbness or paraesthesia on one or both sides of the body, mild hemiparesis or language disturbance. Very rarely syncope or a seizure occurs.

Headache normally starts as the neurological symptoms resolve, but can be concurrent with them, and is unilateral or generalized. It is often severe and prostrating, lasts several hours or rarely days, and may be accompanied by nausea or vomiting. Photophobia, phonophobia, facial pallor, intolerance of certain odours, irritability, mild confusion and anorexia are common. Patients may seek relief by lying down in a darkened room and going to sleep.

Note: A few migraine patients 'seem to know' for several hours when an attack is imminent. The symptoms are vague and include elation, hyperactivity, hunger and thirst.

Common migraine

This is similar to classical migraine but there is no prodrome or focal neurological symptoms. Some patients have both classical and common migraine.

Hemiplegic migraine

This is a very uncommon variant of classical migraine. Hemiplegia, and often other severe cerebral hemisphere disturbances, start with or during the headache and may outlast it by hours or days. It is often familial.

Basilar migraine

Basilar migraine is another uncommon variant, usually in adolescent girls. The prodromal symptoms are of brainstem disturbance with diplopia, ataxia, dysarthria, vertigo, bilateral sensory or motor symptoms, and sometimes syncope. The neurological symptoms may outlast the headache.

Ophthalmoplegic migraine

This condition is extremely rare. The pain is around one eye and is accompanied by an extraocular muscle palsy (usually third cranial nerve) which may last days. Unless both eyes are affected at separate times, other painful orbital (p. 174) or retro-orbital (p. 184) conditions must be excluded by CT, angiography, etc.

Transient migrainous accompaniments

Transient migrainous accompaniments (migraine equivalents) are typical prodromes of classical migraine but with no headache. Unless there is a past history of classical migraine with a similar prodrome, but *with* headache, the diagnosis is difficult.

Retinal migraine (p. 222)

Note: In very severe attacks of migraine there can be a modest increase in neutrophils or lymphocytes in the CSF, a mild fever and rarely coma. Other causes for such changes must be carefully excluded, e.g. infectious meningitis (p. 491), cerebral vasculitis (p. 444), metabolic encephalopathies (p. 124), etc.

Natural history

Migraine usually, but not always, starts in adolescents or young adults and the attacks tend to become less frequent and less severe in the elderly; sometimes the headache component disappears. Rarely it can cause cerebral infarction (p. 215). The severity and frequency of the attacks are variable (from more than one a week to more than a year between attacks) and usually unpredictable. In some patients there are definite precipitating factors:

- Food is often claimed but seldom proven (chocolate, milk, cheese, citrus fruit, fish, etc.) A true food allergy is much discussed but probably does not exist.
- Hunger
- Alcohol (e.g. red wine)
- Stress, or relief from stress
- Pregnancy, the puerperium, and the contraceptive pill (but sometimes the attacks are less frequent)
- Menstruation
- Exercise
- Head injury (sometimes only mild as in 'footballer's migraine' when heading the ball can be enough to precipitate an attack)

Treatment

Explanation and reassurance are the most important aspects of treatment and may be all that are required.

For the attacks

Lying down in a dark room, simple analgesia (aspirin, paracetamol) and going to sleep may be enough to control most headaches. If nausea is a problem or vomiting interferes with the absorption of analgesics, then metoclopramide (10 mg oral) is given at the first symptom of an attack. This drug is not just an antiemetic but promotes gastric emptying and peristalsis, which are both reduced during a migraine attack, and so increases absorption of aspirin.

If vomiting cannot be prevented with an oral antiemetic, then a suppository should be given (prochlorperazine 25 mg) or an intramuscular injection (metoclopramide 5–10 mg; prochlorperazine 12.5 mg).

Ergotamine helps some patients and should be given as early as possible in an attack, along with an antiemetic if necessary since it can cause nausea, vomiting and abdominal pain. Too much (more than 12 mg/week oral or 6 mg/week aerosol) causes peripheral ischaemia and digital gangrene. Chronic treatment in even a more modest dosage can cause dependence so that stopping the drug provokes headache. It should be used *sparingly* and only in patients who definitely respond to it, and no more than 3 mg by mouth or 6 mg per rectum per attack (usually 1 mg is quite enough).

Contraindications include pregnancy, breast feeding, peripheral vascular disease, ischaemic heart disease.

Preparations include:
- cafergot: oral, ergotamine tartrate 1 mg, caffeine 100 mg; suppository if vomiting cannot be controlled: ergotamine tartrate 2 mg, caffeine 100 mg

- migril: oral, ergotamine tartrate 2 mg, cyclizine 50 mg, caffeine 100 mg
- medihaler ergotamine; an aerosol delivering 0.36 mg/puff, maximum 3 puffs per attack
- lingraine: sublingual ergotamine tartrate 2 mg

Prophylaxis

The requirement for prophylaxis depends on the attack frequency and severity of the headache, how much the migraine interferes with the patient's life, the patient's attitude towards daily medication, and tolerance to the adverse effects of the drugs which are proposed. Any prophylactic drug should only be used for a few months, and not years, and regular attempts made to withdraw it. Some patients respond to one drug, others to another, others to none; on balance, the order in which to try the various possibilities is: aspirin, propranolol, pizotifen, promethazine, verapamil, amitriptyline, clonidine and methysergide. If a drug is helpful, it will be obvious in a few weeks and a placebo effect, which in migraine amounts to 30% reduction in attack frequency, must be remembered. A diary card to record attack frequency is useful.

- Remove precipitating factors if identifiable and possible.
- Relaxation training possibly.
- Treat anxiety or depression if relevant.
- Aspirin; oral, 600 mg daily.
- Beta-blockers; propranolol is most often used starting at 10 mg twice daily and increasing to full beta-blockade if necessary.
- Pizotifen: oral, 0.5 mg 3 times daily or 1.5 mg at night, increasing to 2 mg 3 times daily if necessary. Anticholinergic adverse effects, weight gain and drowsiness may be troublesome.
- Promethazine: oral, 10–25 mg at night.
- Verapamil: oral, 40 mg 3 times daily increasing to 160 mg 3 times daily if necessary. May cause constipation, headache, nausea, vomiting, flushing, hypotension, bradyarrhythmias.
- Amitriptyline: this may be effective independent of any antidepressant effect: oral, 50 mg at night increasing to 150 mg if necessary.
- Clonidine: 50 µg twice daily increasing to 75 µg twice daily if necessary. This can aggravate depression and insomnia and must not be stopped suddenly for fear of rebound hypotension.
- Methysergide: oral 1 mg at night, increasing to 2 mg 3 times daily (with food) if necessary, is probably the most effective, but also the most toxic drug. This anti-serotonergic drug has many immediate adverse effects (gastrointestinal symptoms, drowsiness and muscle cramps) and if given for more than about 6 months at a time can cause fibrosis of the retroperitoneum, pleura, mediastinum and heart valves. However, it can be extremely effective in short courses.

Do not use more than one drug for prophylaxis at a time: if one fails it should be stopped and another tried. Many patients have tension or other forms of psychogenic headache as well as migraine, making management particularly difficult.

Useful addresses:

The Migraine Trust
45 Great Ormond Street
London WC1N 3HD
Tel: 071-278-2676

British Migraine Association
178a High Road
Byfleet
Weybridge
Surrey KT14 7ED
Tel: 0932-352468

Migrainous neuralgia (cluster headache)

These are stereotyped and recurrent attacks of pain in and around one eye (almost always the same one) with no aura. The pain is occasionally precipitated by alcohol or glyceryl trinitrate, but not between clusters. It starts fairly suddenly, often at the same time of day or, more often, night and is extremely severe, lasts about an hour, and is usually accompanied by ipsilateral conjunctival injection, lacrimation, rhinorrhoea and nasal stuffiness. Despite the name, patients do not usually have common or classical migraine.

The attacks tend to occur one or more times daily for several weeks with months or years of intervening freedom (hence the term cluster headache). Males are affected more than females (6:1) and the age of onset is 20–50.

During the cluster, and sometimes for longer, there can be an ipsilateral Horner's syndrome (p. 178). Other signs (e.g. facial numbness, extraocular muscle palsy) should prompt the search for an underlying structural cause which is most unusual (e.g. sphenoid wing meningioma).

Treatment

Some patients obtain relief by inhalation of 7 l/min of 100% oxygen through a face mask for a few minutes. Others find that sublingual ergotamine helps (p. 140). However, the pain is usually too severe and too brief for such strategies and prophylaxis during the cluster is required.

- ergotamine (suppository a few hours before expected attacks, but cautions as above, p. 139); omit one night every week or so to check if cluster has stopped
- methysergide (p. 140)
- pizotifen (p. 140)
- corticosteroids (prednisolone 60 mg daily for a few days, then tailing off)
- ipsilateral sympathectomy (chemical or surgical stellate ganglion block)

Chronic migrainous neuralgia

Some patients have attacks similar to migrainous neuralgia but they occur day after day for months or years. Females are more often affected than males. As well as the above prophylactic treatments, the following are sometimes helpful:

- Indomethacin: oral, up to 250 mg daily in 2–3 divided doses.
- Lithium carbonate: oral, 0.25–2.0 g daily. Monitor blood level and avoid greater than 1.2 mmol/l on samples taken 12 hours after the preceding dose. Dose-related adverse effects include tremor, brisk tendon reflexes, rigidity, ataxia, dysarthria, nystagmus, nervousness, confusion, drowsiness, coma, seizures, anorexia, vomiting, diarrhoea, polyuria, polydipsia, oedema, weight gain, uraemia, hypothyroidism. Caution if renal, thyroid or cardiovascular disease or taking carbamazepine (p. 90).
- Operations as for trigeminal neuralgia are of uncertain benefit (p. 146).

Psychiatric and psychological conditions

Tension headache

This is very common but only a small proportion reach a neurologist, usually because the patients believe they have a brain tumour or their general practitioners want reassurance that they do not. They do not *start* after late middle age when other causes of headache are more likely (giant cell arteritis, p. 450, raised intracranial pressure, p. 256, depression, p. 143, etc.).

The headache is usually bilateral frontal, occipital or generalized and is felt as a 'pressure', 'dull ache' or 'tight band' around the head. It can be mild or severe. It tends to occur at times of stress, towards the end of the day, and on exposure to glare or noise. It may persist all day and last for days or months on end. Seldom does it wake the patient from sleep. There is no nausea unless analgesia-induced and no focal neurological symptoms. Often there are associated complaints of poor concentration, memory loss and non-specific 'dizziness'. Any underlying stressful cause can appear to be superficially 'good' rather than 'bad', e.g. a more senior job, getting married. Sometimes the cause seems to be excessive scalp or neck muscle contraction.

Treatment

- explanation and reassurance that the cause is tension headache and not a brain tumour, meningitis, etc.
- avoidance of relevant stress if practical
- relaxation programmes
- mild analgesics
- mild tranquillizers (diazepam) for short periods if anxiety and agitation are major components

Depression

Headache is a common component and sometimes the other symptoms are occult.

Note: Depression is a common symptom of giant cell arteritis (p. 450).

Hysteria and malingering

The complaint of headache is common in both and the diagnosis depends on the history, the patient's situation, the possible advantages to the patient, and the absence of any organic features.

Miscellaneous paroxysmal headaches

Cough headache

Most headaches are worsened by coughing, but particularly those due to raised intracranial pressure (p. 256) in the posterior fossa or an Arnold–Chiari malformation (p. 202). However, in some patients, usually adults, coughing induces a sharp pain in the head (often occipital) followed by a dull ache and no cause can be found. Sneezing, laughing and straining may cause similar headache. These headaches tend to resolve spontaneously but, if they do not, then a posterior fossa tumour or Arnold–Chiari malformation must be excluded by CT, which if negative should be followed by MRI or myelography.

Benign orgasmic cephalgia

Acute, severe, explosive generalized or occipital headaches (usually at the moment of orgasm during sexual intercourse or masturbation) are more common in men than women. They last minutes or hours. They can start inexplicably at any time of life, do not necessarily occur at every orgasm, and usually remit spontaneously.

Prophylaxis with propranolol may help; oral, 40–80 mg daily or more if necessary. Indomethacin is an alternative.

Headache can be a hysterical symptom to avoid sexual intercourse which itself can occasionally cause subarachnoid haemorrhage (p. 228); this causes a headache which is much more prolonged than benign orgasmic cephalgia, and is also likely to be accompanied by a stiff neck. Muscle tension headache, occipital radiating to the neck, is common but comes on more slowly than orgasmic cephalgia and starts before orgasm.

'Ice-cream' headache

This occurs within a minute or less of swallowing ice-cream or ice-cold water.

Exercise headache

This is a debilitating generalized headache which can occur during or after quite moderate exercise and it sometimes sounds migrainous. It can occur out-of-the-blue, or after head injury and usually resolves in a few weeks. Sometimes it is hysterical. Propranolol before exercise may help, as may indomethacin.

Thunderclap headache

Occasional patients experience one or more attacks of sudden and severe headache, sometimes with vomiting, and with no obvious precipitants. These may last up to a day or so. Clinically, they cannot be distinguished from subarachnoid haemorrhage (p. 228), and, therefore, CT and CSF examination may be required, at least on one occasion to exclude sub-arachnoid bleeding.

Cephalgia fugax (ice pick headache, benign paroxysmal cranial neuralgia)

These are sharp, very brief, stabbing and sometimes severe pains which occur in various parts of the head. There may be 1–20 attacks per day coming in bouts lasting days or weeks. There is seldom any underlying cause although this symptom is described by some patients with migraine or severe and obvious extracranial occlusive vascular disease.

Exploding head syndrome

Some patients are occasionally woken as they fall off to sleep by the hal-lucination of a sudden and loud noise or 'bang' in the head, perhaps a flash of light, but no pain. It is benign.

Post-traumatic headache

Immediately after a head injury there is a headache, but as the soft tissue damage resolves so the headache normally gradually disappears. In some patients, even after a mild injury, the headache persists for months or years and in others it reappears a few weeks after the injury and persists. If there are other neurological features within the first 3–6 months (e.g. drowsiness, confusion) then a chronic subdural haematoma (p. 235) is a possibility. However, the vast majority of patients have no focal neurological features although they may complain of various combinations of poor concentration, non-specific dizziness, irritability, fatigue and sometimes positional vertigo (p. 107). Under these circumstances investigations are fruitless. Treatment is reassurance and the normal management of any associated anxiety or depression. Some patients develop headaches with obvious features of tension headache, migraine or neck pain related to whiplash injury of the cervical spine and these can be treated accordingly. Post-traumatic headache is not necessarily related to litigation, nor does it necessarily resolve when any compensation is settled.

Pain in the face

Any cause of headache (p. 134) may cause pain referred to the face. Additional causes are:
- trigeminal neuralgia (p. 145)
- atypical facial pain (p. 147)
- cerebello-pontine angle tumour (p. 194)
- fifth nerve neurofibroma (p. 272)
- isolated trigeminal sensory neuropathy (p. 187)
- Gradenigo's syndrome (p. 188)
- nasopharyngeal tumour
- cervical spondylosis (p. 327)
- post-herpetic neuralgia (p. 523)
- dissection of the internal carotid artery (p. 214)
- tabetic lightning pains (p. 516)
- angina (usually felt in the neck and jaw rather than the face)

Trigeminal neuralgia (tic douloureux)

These are agonizing lancinating pains in the face lasting a few seconds to about a minute, almost always on one side, which are usually triggered by touching the affected area, cold winds, eating, brushing the teeth and sometimes even by talking. There may be one or many such attacks per day. It is rare in the ophthalmic division of the fifth cranial nerve and usually radiates from near the corner of the mouth to the same side of the face, ear, eye and head. It comes in 'bouts' lasting days or weeks and may leave a background burning or aching throughout the 'bout'. Intervening periods of freedom can be months or years.

It usually starts in late middle age and the cause is unknown; there are no neurological signs or other features in the history to suggest any underlying structural lesion. Very occasionally a cause comes to light by a careful neurological history (e.g. previous neurological episodes such as optic neuritis) and examination (e.g. facial numbness, absent corneal reflex), a skull X-ray or the passage of time:
- multiple sclerosis (this causes bilateral trigeminal neuralgia much more often than in idiopathic cases, Chapter 12)
- cerebello-pontine angle tumour (p. 194)
- fifth nerve neurofibroma (p. 272)
- basilar artery ectasia (p. 212)

Treatment

Carbamazepine is very effective and should be started in a dose of 100 mg twice daily oral, and fairly quickly worked up to as much as 600 mg 3 times daily to control the pain, provided adverse effects (p. 90) are tolerable. Attempts to withdraw the treatment should be made every week or two so that the drug is not continued unnecessarily through a spontaneous remission.

Phenytoin is the second choice, oral, 100 mg twice daily up to 600 mg daily; adverse effects, p. 88. Clonazepam, oral, 0.5–2.0 mg daily; adverse effects, p. 93; or baclofen, oral, 5 mg 3 times daily working up to 30 mg 3 times daily over a week or two if necessary may help; adverse effects, p. 352.

If medical treatment fails (which is unusual), or is effective but at the price of unacceptable adverse effects, and the patient is prepared to accept the possibility of a numb and sometimes dysaesthetic face and is sensible enough to protect an anaesthetized cornea, there are several possible surgical approaches:
- alcohol injection, section or avulsion of the relevant branches of the trigeminal nerve in the face provides temporary relief
- percutaneous phenol, glycerol or alcohol injection of the trigeminal sensory root ganglion
- percutaneous thermo- or electro-coagulation of the sensory root ganglion
- root section at craniotomy (probably obsolete because of operative risk)
- decompression of the sensory root, usually from a small artery crossing the nerve, does not cause any anaesthesia or analgesia of the face but does require a posterior fossa operation

Glossopharyngeal neuralgia

This is much less common than trigeminal neuralgia. The pain is similar in character but felt in the tonsillar region and ear and is precipitated by coughing or swallowing due to a 'trigger point' in the throat. Rarely it is due to compression of the glossopharyngeal nerve by tumours, etc., or multiple sclerosis. Occasionally bradycardia and syncope occur, perhaps as a vasovagal response to the pain, although in some cases the pain is mild.

Atypical facial pain

This is a vague condition, usually in women, in which there is a constant ache or pain in one cheek or frontal region. Antidepressants may help.

Pain in and around the eye

Any cause of headache (p. 134) may cause pain around the eye. Additional or particular causes are:
- refractive errors causing 'eye strain'
- glaucoma
- iritis
- optic neuritis (p. 343)
- cavernous sinus, superior orbital fissure (p. 184) and orbital (p. 174) lesions
- distal carotid or posterior communicating artery aneurysm (p. 232)
- dissection of the internal carotid artery (p. 210)
- diabetic third nerve palsy (p. 454)
- post-herpetic neuralgia (p. 523)
- migrainous neuralgia (p. 141)
- osteitis or tumour of the petrous apex, often with sixth nerve palsy (Gradenigo's syndrome, p. 188)
- nasopharyngeal tumours
- ophthalmoplegic migraine (p. 138)
- Tolosa-Hunt syndrome (p. 189)

Carotodynia

This rare syndrome consists of bouts of pain and tenderness superimposed on a background ache over the carotid artery in the neck and is occasionally due to arterial inflammation (e.g. giant cell arteritis, p. 450) or dissection (p. 210). In the majority no cause is found. It may respond to indomethacin, lithium or methysergide (doses, see pp. 140 and 142). In a very few cases it appears to be part of a migrainous syndrome.

6   Disorders of memory and intellect

Cognitive defects encompass impairments of verbal and non-verbal memory, reasoning, learning and focal cortical functions such as language and visuo-spatial ability.

Dementia

Dementia is a syndrome not a diagnosis. It is defined as decline in previously normal memory and/or intellect (i.e. cognitive function) in an alert patient. A gradual decline is inevitable with normal ageing, particularly in memory for names, so there is a quantitative, and perhaps qualitative, difference between this normal age-related decline and the abnormal decline called dementia. About 5% of the population over the age of 65 are said to be demented and 20% over the age of 80.

There are many causes of dementia, not all of which are progressive. Only about 5% of patients presenting to medical attention primarily with dementia have a treatable underlying disorder and even fewer are curable; the majority have Alzheimer's disease (p. 160) and/or multi-infarct dementia (p. 161).

The *aims of management* are to:
- ensure that the patient definitely has dementia, not something else (p. 154)
- diagnose the cause of the dementia, particularly if it is treatable, at an early stage (p. 156). Although more effort is usually made in younger patients, there are still many treatable causes of dementia in the very elderly (e.g. hypothyroidism, p. 457). Subdivision into 'pre-senile' and 'senile' categories is unhelpful; it is better to subdivide into 'treatable' and 'not-treatable' dementias
- control the symptoms and behaviour as far as possible and care for the patient and family (p. 159)

Causes of dementia

Neurological disorders

Almost any disorder of the brain can cause dementia but it may be a more or less prominent part of the following conditions:
- Alzheimer's disease (p. 160)
- Pick's disease (p. 160)
- multi-infarct (vascular or arteriosclerotic) dementia (p. 161)
- head injury:
    post-severe head injury
    chronic subdural haematoma (p. 235)
    repetitive moderate head injuries (boxing, steeple chasers, etc.)

- intracranial tumours (p. 266) and malignant meningitis (p. 267)
- intracranial infection:
  syphilis (general paresis of the insane, p. 516)
  post-severe encephalitis (p. 498)
  post-severe bacterial (p. 491), tuberculous (p. 512) or fungal (p. 531) meningitis (p. 532)
  post-cerebral abscess (p. 503)
  AIDS (p. 526)
  Creutzfeldt–Jakob disease (p. 531)
  subacute sclerosing panencephalitis (p. 525)
  chronic rubella encephalitis (p. 526)
  progressive multifocal leucoencephalopathy (p. 530)
  Whipple's disease (p. 463)
- 'normal' pressure hydrocephalus (p. 262)
- degenerative disorders such as:
  Huntington's disease (p. 298)
  Parkinson's disease (p. 154)
  Steele–Richardson–Olszewski syndrome (p. 290)
  multiple sclerosis (p. 345)
  tuberous sclerosis (p. 487)
  dominant and idiopathic cerebellar ataxia (p. 201)
  ataxia telangiectasia (p. 202)
  xeroderma pigmentosum (p. 203)
- biochemical disorders such as:
  lysosomal storage diseases (p. 477)
  inborn errors of amino and organic acid metabolism (p. 480)
  progressive myoclonic epilepsies (p. 75)
  adrenoleucodystrophy (p. 456)
- limbic encephalomyelitis (p. 475)

General medical disorders

Dementia can occur as a consequence of many general medical disorders and sometimes these present to a neurologist before the underlying disorder has been diagnosed. The same disorders may also present with coma (p. 122) and confusional states (p. 161), depending on their severity, speed of onset and the circumstances.
- metabolic:
  renal failure (p. 465)
  dialysis dementia (p. 467)
  hepatic encephalopathy (p. 467)
  hyper- and hypo-calcaemia (p. 457)
  hyponatraemia (p. 464)
  hypoglycaemia (p. 108)

anoxia (chronic anoxia, post-severe acute anoxia, p. 292, carbon monoxide poisoning, p. 549)

hypercapnia and respiratory failure

Wilson's disease (p. 310)

mitochondrial cytopathy (p. 429)

- endocrine:

hypothyroidism (p. 456)

Addison's disease (p. 455)

hypopituitarism (p. 273)

Cushing's syndrome (p. 455)

- nutritional deficiencies:

vitamin B_1 (beri-beri, p. 468)

vitamin B_{12} (p. 470)

folic acid (p. 470)

nicotinic acid (pellagra, p. 471)

- toxins:

chronic alcoholism (p. 544)

organic solvents (p. 546)

metals (p. 547)

- drugs which cause confusional states (p. 162)

Clinical features

Although the rate of progression, and to some extent the type of cognitive deficit, depends on the nature of the underlying disease, some generalizations are possible.

Patients may or may not have insight into their own progressive decline of memory or intellect. If they have insight they may be able to adjust to it (by making lists, etc.). Without insight they are likely to be brought to medical attention by family, friends, workmates, neighbours or the police (and in children by teachers) from whom the history is best taken:

- Decline in verbal and non-verbal recent memory, e.g. forgetting where things are put, plans for the day, events of yesterday, names and faces, how to get to places, recent events. Distant memory is usually less affected. Losing the thread in conversation and perhaps confabulating. Unfamiliar routines cannot be coped with. Often there is mild nominal aphasia (p. 23) and eventually disorientation in time and place, and inability to recognize familiar friends and relatives.
- Decline in reasoning, e.g. poor comprehension of conversations, TV, newspapers; difficulty with ordinary tasks around the house and handling money; loss of initiative; perseveration (p. 156).
- Decline in interest in work, hobbies, friends, TV, newspapers.
- Errors of judgement and reasoning which are difficult for the patient to appreciate and correct. The patients may appear bewildered and upset by their all too obvious mistakes.

- Behavioural changes. Some patients become apathetic and depressed, particularly if insight is preserved. Others become irritable and agitated with violent outbursts and disinhibition. Behaviour is irrational with nocturnal wanderings, delusions, illusions, hallucinations and paranoia. The patients begin to neglect their appearance and personal hygiene. However, in public and in the clinic they may appear socially well preserved, at least in the early stages.
- Urine and faecal incontinence are usually late features.

At first there are usually no *prominent* focal neurological features (e.g. partial seizures, hemiparesis, marked aphasia, etc.) unless there is an underlying focal neurological disorder such as an intracranial tumour. Later, more obvious dominant hemisphere (asphasia, etc.) and non-dominant hemisphere cognitive features develop (e.g. dressing and constructional apraxia). Generalized epileptic seizures are common in some degenerative brain disorders (e.g. the progressive myoclonic epilepsies, p. 75) and myoclonus is a feature of Creutzfeldt–Jakob disease (p. 531) and occasionally of Alzheimer's disease (p. 160).

It follows, therefore, that a demented patient may present to medical attention in several ways:
- their own concern about failing memory
- other people being concerned about their failing memory
- depression or anxiety secondary to failing memory
- acute confusional state (p. 161) precipitated by fever, hospital admission, bereavement, etc.
- during the follow-up of an already diagnosed disease (e.g. Parkinson's disease, p. 282, Huntington's disease, p. 298, etc.)

Differential diagnosis

Various conditions may be mistaken for dementia:

Deafness

This should be obvious but is sometimes missed. If present, it certainly makes the assessment of any dementia more difficult.

Depression

Depression may lead to apathy, poor concentration, slowed mental and physical responses, loss of interest and delusions (so-called pseudodementia) but, if tested properly, memory and intellect are more or less normal and there are certainly no abnormal neurological signs. The patients tend to fail even to try cognitive tasks, unlike demented patients who usually try and then fail. Of course, patients may become depressed as a consequence of dementia which makes the underlying dementia more difficult to diagnose.

Parkinson's disease

This can, in the late stages, be associated with dementia (p. 282) and any of the anti-parkinsonian drugs can cause confusion and hallucinations. Parkinsonian patients, because they are slow to do things and look rather depressed, may be incorrectly thought to be demented. In any advanced dementia some rigidity and poverty of movement may develop but without other major parkinsonian features.

Aphasia (p. 23)

Aphasia can be mistaken for dementia or confusion.

Non-convulsive status epilepticus (p. 97)

This is more likely to be mistaken for an acute confusional state than dementia.

Confusional states (or delirium)

These are distinguished from dementia by the acute or subacute onset and associated impairment of consciousness (p. 161).

Hypotension

Hypotension chronically induced by drugs or cardiac failure, or intermittently by cardiac arrhythmias, tends to cause intermittent confusional states rather than dementia.

Excessive day-time sleepiness (p. 114)

The diagnosis of dementia

The first step is to ensure that the patient is demented and the second is to find the cause, particularly if it is treatable. Although rarely found, the treatable dementias are not very difficult, dangerous or expensive to diagnose.

Dementia versus non-dementia

When assessing cognitive function (i.e. memory and intellect) it is important to first test conscious level (p. 122), language function (spontaneous speech, object naming, repetition, reading, writing, comprehension, p. 23) and hearing before necessarily concluding that a patient is demented. Anxiety and depression may also interfere with mental state testing.

The *mini-mental state* examination is a simple bedside procedure which, although crude and inapplicable in dysphasic patients because it is weighted in favour of verbal skills, has the great advantage of being standardized:

- *Orientation* (1 point for each correct answer)

  what is the: time

                   date

                   day

                   month

                   year   5 points

  what is the name of this: ward

                              hospital

                              district

                              town

                              country   5 points

- *Registration*: name three objects, (e.g. pencil, cow, house), score 1–3 points according to how many are correctly repeated. Resubmit list until patient is word perfect in order to use it for a later test of recall. Score only first attempt.

                                             3 points

- *Attention and calculation*: ask the patient to subtract 7 from 100 and then from the result a total of five times down to 65. Score 1 point for each correct subtraction.

                                           5 points

- *Recall*: ask for the three objects used in the registration test, 1 point being awarded for each correct answer.

                                           3 points

- *Language*: 1 point each for two objects correctly named (e.g. pencil and watch).

                                           2 points

1 point for correct repetition of 'No ifs, ands or buts'   1 point

3 points if three stage command correctly obeyed, e.g. 'Take this piece of paper in your right hand, fold it in half, and place it on the table'.   3 points

1 point for correct response to a written command such as 'close your eyes'.

                                         1 point

ask the patient to write a sentence. Award 1 point if the sentence is meaningful, has a verb and a subject.

                                         1 point

● *Visuospatial*: test the patient's ability to copy a complex diagram of two intersecting pentagons.

1 point

Total score = 30

Score
<20 probably demented (provided not aphasic)
21–25 equivocal
>25 probably normal, but may miss a non-dominant hemisphere disorder

Other informal bedside tests of cognitive function include:
● ask patient to describe recent events from newspapers, TV, etc.
● digit span with immediate recall; normally individuals can remember at least 6 digits forwards
● orientation in the ward for toilet, bed, etc.
● further drawing tasks, e.g. bicycle, house
● reasoning can be tested by asking the patient to explain a proverb
The interpretation of cognitive tests depends on assessment of the patient's premorbid ability (from education, job, vocabulary). Formal neuro-psychological evaluation may be needed in cases of doubt or if an objective baseline is required. Performance IQ is usually more depressed than verbal IQ. Both verbal and non-verbal memory can be quantified to determine if both are affected equally, and to what extent.

In addition, it is important to look for focal cognitive defects (such as aphasia, dressing apraxia, etc.) and focal neurological deficits (such as hemiparesis).

Note: Perseveration is the phenomenon of repetition of the response to one command when it is countermanded by a second command. It has no local-izing value and is found in demented, confused and dysphasic patients but not to any extent in depression.

Determining the cause of the dementia

History
It is crucial to have an account from relatives, friends, etc. and important to consider alcohol consumption, drug history, past head injury, speed of progression, etc.

Neurological examination
This is often normal, apart from impaired cognitive function, but there may be non-specific signs of no particular localizing value which would not be

expected in depression (e.g. prominent grasp, palmomental and pout reflexes). Focal signs or seizures early in the course, drowsiness and raised intracranial pressure should prompt a search for a structural intracranial lesion. Dysarthria and nystagmus suggest intoxication with alcohol (p. 544) or drugs; chorea suggests Huntington's disease (p. 298); and myoclonus, Creutzfeldt–Jakob disease (p. 531).

General examination

This also is often normal but it is important to consider such disorders as hypothyroidism (p. 456), chronic liver disease (p. 467), etc.

Routine investigations

These must include:
- full blood count and ESR
- urea and electrolytes
- liver function
- plasma glucose
- plasma calcium
- thyroid function
- serum B_{12} and folate
- syphilis serology
- chest X-ray
- skull X-ray if no CT scan planned

Other investigations depend on the clinical situation, e.g. blood lead, blood alcohol, drug screen, blood and urine amino acids, HIV antibody, leucocyte enzymes, etc. Four merit special discussion:

CT scan. CT scan will detect intracranial mass lesions, hydrocephalus, focal hypodensities presumed to be infarctions, and severe white matter disorders (e.g. leucodystrophies, Binswanger's disease, p. 161). It is *not* particularly helpful in distinguishing dementia from non-dementia, nor for assessing the severity of dementia on the basis of the amount of cortical atrophy. Nonetheless, *marked* cortical atrophy provides some confirmation of dementia in doubtful cases but does not indicate any particular cause. In a severely symptomatic patient, a *completely* normal scan might resurrect the possibility of depression, Creutzfeldt–Jakob disease, or some other diagnosis (p. 154).

CT is used mainly to exclude treatable intracranial pathology and is particularly indicated if the following conditions prevail:
- recent onset of dementia (weeks)
- recent head injury (weeks)
- focal neurological features (e.g. aphasia, hemiparesis)

- evidence of raised intracranial pressure
- seizures
- clinical picture of normal pressure hydrocephalus (p. 262)
- no general medical cause and the patient is reasonably well preserved
- age less than about 70, but older if CT available

provided no other definite cause has been discovered earlier, particularly if treatment then reverses the dementia (e.g. alcoholism, hypothyroidism, etc.).

CSF examination. This may sometimes be helpful:
- obscure dementia in young patients
- positive blood serology for syphilis (p. 516)
- possible chronic infective meningitis (p. 497)
- possible malignant meningitis (p. 277)
- possible multiple sclerosis (oligoclonal bands) (p. 345)
- possible progressive multifocal leucoencephalopathy (p. 530)
- subacute sclerosing panencephalitis (p. 525)

EEG. This can occasionally be helpful:
- diagnosis of Creutzfeldt–Jakob disease (p. 531), subacute sclerosing panencephalitis (p. 525)
- perhaps to help distinguish dementia, when the EEG may be abnormal, from depression when it is normal
- non-convulsive status epilepticus (p. 97)
- in metabolic encephalopathies (p. 124) there is usually marked generalized slowing of the EEG even when clinical symptoms are relatively slight

Brain biopsy. Brain biopsy is unhelpful except in rare situations:
- possibility of cerebral vasculitis (p. 444)
- possibility of chronic meningeal infection (p. 497)
- need for definite diagnosis to aid genetic counselling

Amnesia (memory impairment)

Pure amnesia without any focal cortical deficits such as aphasia, dyscalculia, visuospatial problems, etc., normal personality and consciousness, and with no other neurological signs, is a restricted form of 'dementia'. Dominant and non-dominant cerebral hemisphere lesions may lead to verbal and non-verbal memory impairment respectively. *Bilateral* temporal lobe, hippocampal and medial thalamic lesions produce a global amnesia (verbal and non-verbal) and the causes include:
- trauma (including neurosurgery)
- bilateral ischaemia (via posterior cerebral circulation)
- Korsakoff's syndrome (p. 468)
- transient global amnesia (p. 159)

- encephalitis (p. 498)
- limbic encephalomyelitis (p. 475)
- cerebral anoxia (p. 292)

Transient global amnesia (TGA)

TGA is a very characteristic syndrome which occurs in middle-aged and elderly people. Quite suddenly the patient is unable to remember any new material for more than a minute or so (anterograde amnesia) and also fairly recent material stretching back a few weeks or sometimes longer (retrograde amnesia). There is no disturbance of consciousness or any other feature except perhaps a mild headache. There is no loss of personal identity although the patients are often confused in the sense that they do not know what they have just done, can be agitated, and they tend to ask the same questions repetitively. The amnesia lasts a few hours and the patient is left with a more or less dense amnesic gap for the period of the attack.

Most patients are medically and neurologically well and the prognosis is good. Just occasionally there is an explanation such as complex partial seizures (the attacks tend to be shorter and recurrent, p. 71), vertebrobasilar ischaemia affecting the thalamus and temporal lobes bilaterally (usually there are additional features such as weakness, diplopia, etc., p. 220), or the use of benzodiazepines.

The attacks may recur but usually not very frequently unless they are actually epileptic. In otherwise clinically well patients no particular investigations or treatments are required.

Treatment of dementia

Any underlying treatable cause for dementia should be managed on its merits. Important general points are:
- Discussion of diagnosis and prognosis with the patient, if possible and appropriate, and the relatives or carers.
- Advice on retirement, driving, financial responsibility, etc.
- Support in the home for the patient and carer; homehelp, meals on wheels, district nurse, laundry service, benefits, etc.
- Relief of burden on carer; day centre attendance, holiday and respite admissions, long-term care in nursing home or psychogeriatric unit.
- Treatment of any complicating depression or intercurrent deafness, cataracts, etc.
- Maintenance of a normal and familiar routine. Admission to hospital or bereavement can cause major exacerbations of dementia and precipitate an acute confusional state. Patients are best kept in familiar surroundings without too many different people being involved with their care. They should not be moved from bed to bed or ward to ward.

• Attention to adequate fluid intake and if necessary the use of a fluid chart.
• Withdrawal and avoidance of all except necessary medications, particularly sedative, psychotropic and other drugs which may cause confusion (p. 162).
• Night-time, and sometimes day-time, sedative is required for very restless and confused patients, but not as a routine. Useful drugs are: haloperidol (1 mg), thioridazine (10 mg), promazine (25 mg). The dosage should be increased slowly as appropriate to the patients' needs as well as bearing in mind any effect their confused behaviour may be having on other people or patients. Larger parenteral doses may be needed for very disturbed behaviour.

Alzheimer's disease

This is the most common cause of patients presenting to medical attention with dementia. The brain shows what may be the exaggerated changes of ageing: widespread neurofibrillary tangles, argyrophilic senile plaques, neuronal loss and often amyloid deposition in small blood vessel walls (i.e., congophilic angiopathy, p. 474). It can be familial.

It seldom presents under the age of 40 (except in Down's syndrome) and is much more common in the elderly. Memory decline is insidious over several years to death and there are seldom any other prominent neurological features until late in the course. Eventually cortical deficits become obvious (verbal and non-verbal difficulties such as aphasia, dressing apraxia, sensory inattention, etc.) and there may be muscular rigidity and corticospinal tract signs in the late stages. In a few patients there is a rather focal 'cortical' onset with prominent aphasia or visuospatial defects. Some patients develop myoclonic jerks and occasionally seizures. The EEG is either normal or shows generalized slow wave activity. The CT scan is normal or shows cortical atrophy and corresponding ventricular dilatation. During life, the diagnosis is largely one of exclusion of other causes of progressive dementia.

Useful address

Alzheimer's Disease Society
158/160 Balham High Road
London SW12 9BN
Tel: 081-675-6557

Pick's disease

There is brain atrophy, particularly of the frontal and temporal lobes, with neuronal loss, gliosis, and neuronal argentophilic inclusion bodies. It is much rarer than Alzheimer's disease; the clinical picture is the same, but the diagnosis may be suspected during life from the pattern of atrophy on CT.

Multi-infarct dementia (vascular or arteriosclerotic dementia)

Clearly patients may become demented after one or more strokes of any cause, particularly if the infarct or haemorrhage involves the cerebral cortex or medial thalamus (Chapter 8). In some patients episodes of ischaemia (and possibly even haemorrhage) may be rather insidious, unrecognized or truly subclinical so that there is a slowly progressive dementia, usually in the context of obvious vascular risk factors (old age, hypertension, cervical arterial bruits, ischaemic heart disease, etc.).

A progressively dementing patient is more likely to have multi-infarct dementia than Alzheimer's disease if:
- focal neurological symptoms and signs
- past history of stroke/TIA
- focal hypodense lesions on CT
- good evidence of generalized vascular disease, e.g. arterial bruits, absent pulses, claudication, angina, hypertension

However, these features are far from specific; many patients have Alzheimer's disease as well. It is important to remember that some vascular disorders are treatable and *may* present with multi-infarct dementia (e.g. giant cell arteritis, p. 450).

Binswanger's disease (subcortical arteriosclerotic encephalopathy) has no good operational definition. Some progressively dementing elderly patients, with or without stroke-like episodes, have very marked lucency of the periventricular white matter on CT. This syndrome has been ascribed to vascular disease. However, the same CT pattern can be found in some normal elderly. There are no treatment possibilities and the cause is often said to be hypertension but in reality is unknown.

Confusional states

Many demented patients are confused, but the term 'confusional states' (or delirium) is restricted to episodes of acute and subacute confusion with failure of recent memory, clouding of consciousness, disorientation in time and place, often with marked behavioural disturbances (hyperactivity, aggression, fear, visual hallucinations, etc.). The severity tends to fluctuate. The patients are disturbed, incoherent, irrational and can be difficult to control.

Clearly there are innumerable possible causes, many of which are the same as the causes of dementia (p. 150) and coma (p. 122). Indeed, many demented patients may become acutely confused as a result of infection, bereavement or hospitalization. Therefore, the distinction between confusion and dementia is rather more quantitative than qualitative.

Causes of confusional states

- infections:
  intracranial (meningitis, encephalitis, Chapter 18)
  extracranial (urine infection, pneumonia, etc.)
  generalized (septicaemia, typhoid, p. 509, malaria, p. 534, etc.)
  non-specific effect of high fever
- intracranial tumours (p. 266)
- stroke (p. 161)
- ischaemic/anoxic brain damage (p. 123)
- metabolic encephalopathies (p. 124)
- non-convulsive status epilepticus (p. 97)
- toxins (see also Chapter 19):
  alcohols and glycols (p. 542)
  organic solvents (p. 546)
  metals (lead, p. 547, mercury, p. 547, tin, p. 547, bismuth, p. 548, etc.)
  organophosphorus compounds (p. 548)
  carbon monoxide (p. 549)
  mushrooms (p. 553)
  plants (p. 552)
- drugs:
  amphetamines
  anticholinergics
  anticonvulsants (p. 88)
  alpha interferon
  antidepressants
  antituberculous drugs (isoniazid, PAS, cycloserine)
  barbiturates
  benzodiazepines
  bromide
  bromocriptine
  cannabis
  clioquinol (p. 550)
  cimetidine
  cyclosporin
  cytarabine
  digoxin
  diuretics
  hypnotics
  hypoglycaemic drugs
  hypotensive drugs
  ifosfamide/mesna
  indomethacin
  lithium

ʟ-dopa
lysergic acid diethylamide (LSD)
mexiletine
neuroleptics
opiates
procainamide
quinine
ranitidine
sedatives
sympathomimetic drugs (p. 294)
tocainide
tranquillizers
vidarabine

Differential diagnosis

Hysterical fugue

In an hysterical fugue the patient claims loss of all memories including personal identity but is alert and there are no general or neurological abnormalities. This state may last hours, days or sometimes weeks and is the usual explanation for the disappearance of a patient and their reappearance in some distant place without having had any difficulty getting on and off numerous buses and trains.

Transient global amnesia (see p. 159)

Schizophrenia

This is manifest more by thought disorder in a fully conscious patient than by confusion; auditory (rather than visual) hallucinations, paranoid ideas and behavioural disturbances are common.

Mania

Mania is distinguished by normal consciousness and there is no real confusion of thought.

Mental retardation

Unlike dementia, in mental retardation the patient has impaired memory and/or intellect from birth or early neonatal life and, depending on the cause, there may or may not be progression. There are numerous causes including:

- genetic abnormality:
  Down's syndrome
  lysosomal storage diseases (p. 477)
  amino and organic acid inborn errors of metabolism (p. 480)
  Lesch–Nyhan syndrome (p. 482)
  Menkes' kinky hair syndrome (p. 482)
  Cockayne syndrome (p. 482)
  Rett's syndrome (p. 483)
  tuberous sclerosis (p. 487)
- intrauterine brain damage:
  anoxia
  trauma
  infection (rubella, p. 526, cytomegalovirus, p. 525, AIDS, p. 526, toxoplas-
    mosis, p. 536, etc.)
  drugs
  cretinism
  kernicterus (p. 300)
  hydrocephalus (p. 259)
- perinatal brain damage:
  trauma
  anoxia
  intraventricular haemorrhage
  meningitis (p. 491)

Such early brain damage may cause not just mental retardation but also seizures; physical neurological disability (so-called cerebral palsy) such as hemiplegia, paraplegia, dystonia, chorea, etc., or perhaps only delayed motor milestones and clumsiness; and behavioural disturbance.

7 Disorders of the cranial nerves, vision, cerebellum and brainstem

Smell

Unilateral loss of smell sensation is seldom if ever noticed by the patient and even bilateral loss may be unnoticed or merely described as impaired taste. Smell should be tested with an aromatic odour (such as an orange or cordial bottle top from the patient's locker) and not with an acrid odour such as ammonia.

Impaired smell sensation may be due to:
- nasal obstruction or inflammation, which is by far the most common
- head injury, not necessarily severe
- meningitis (p. 491)
- inferior frontal tumour compressing the olfactory tract(s) (p. 22)
- Parkinson's disease (p. 280)
- Refsum's disease (p. 397)
- sarcoidosis (p. 472)
- idiopathic, usually bilateral but can be unilateral
- congenital

It is only worth testing smell in patients who may have a frontal tumour (i.e. with dementia or progressive visual failure) and in those complaining of altered taste or smell.

Disturbance of smell sensation can occur in depression and schizophrenia, and transiently in complex partial seziures (p. 71).

Vision

Visual acuity should be 6/6 in each eye, or better. If with distance spectacles or a pinhole it is less, then there *must* be a reason in the eye itself (usually visible with an ophthalmoscope, e.g. cataract, retinal lesion, etc.), optic nerve, or optic chiasm. Lesions of the optic tract, radiation and the visual cortex in the occipital lobe are much less likely to impair visual acuity. Unilateral amblyopia (i.e. impaired visual acuity) may also be due to a congenital squint.

Visual failure is monocular or binocular, sudden or gradual in onset, transient or persistent. The localization of the causative lesion requires detailed examination of the visual fields, pupils and the first six cranial nerves along with the assessment of any optic atrophy, exophthalmos, papilloedema, the eye itself and any general medical or neurological disorders. Depending on the exact site, and likely nature of the lesion, imaging may include X-rays of the skull, pituitary fossa, orbits and sinuses; CT and MRI of the same regions; and carotid angiography. The CSF may also be informative.

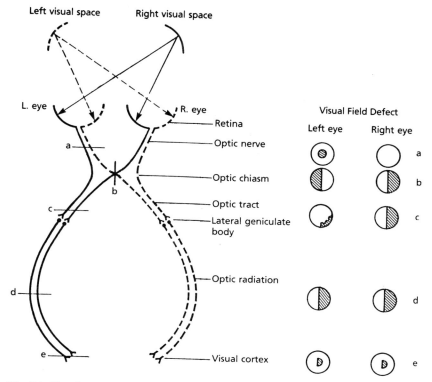

Fig. 7.1 The characteristic visual field defects resulting from lesions at various points in the visual pathway.

No patient must be allowed to go progressively blind without a confirmed and accurate diagnosis, and perhaps a trial of corticosteroids if no cause is apparent. Even if no diagnosis can at first be made, follow-up must be thorough in case clues appear later.

The visual fields

Lesions of the optic nerve (Fig. 7.1a)

These cause a monocular field defect which is usually a central scotoma or sometimes centrocaecal (embracing the blindspot), occasionally a scotoma elsewhere in the visual field, or complete monocular blindness. Visual acuity is reduced and usually the patient notices this early. Retro-orbital optic nerve lesions may involve some of the nasal crossing fibres from the other eye to produce an upper temporal field defect in that eye as well.

Note: Macular lesions also cause a central scotoma but are usually visible with an ophthalmoscope (e.g. senile macular degeneration, etc.).

Lesions of the optic chiasm (Fig. 7.1b)

These almost always affect the crossing fibres first. Pressure on, or lesions in, the lower chiasm (e.g. pituitary adenoma, p. 273) first cause an upper bitemporal hemianopia, whilst upper chiasmal lesions (e.g. craniopharyngioma, p. 274) first cause a lower bitemporal hemianopia. In either situation the visual field defect expands to a complete bitemporal hemianopia. This may be unnoticed by the patient or any symptoms may be vague such as double vision, vertical splitting of the image and difficulty with close work. Eventually the uncrossed temporal fibres become involved and the visual field defect crosses the midline when acuity is reduced and noticed by the patient, perhaps abruptly. A bitemporal hemianopia can be very asymmetrical, incongruous, or spare the peripheral field (i.e. scotomatous bitemporal hemianopia); however, the important feature is that there is a midline vertical division between the normal and abnormal field although this can be subtle and only detectable with a red target.

Chiasmal compression may be due to:
- pituitary adenoma (p. 273)
- craniopharyngioma (p. 274)
- meningioma of tuberculum sellae, olfactory groove or sphenoid wing (p. 271)
- epidermoid/dermoid tumour (p. 274)
- carotid siphon or ophthalmic artery aneurysm (p. 232)
- hydrocephalus and dilatation of the 3rd ventricle (p. 259)
- nasopharyngeal carcinoma
- chordoma of the clivus (p. 275)
- sarcoid granulomas (p. 472)
- subacute and chronic meningitis (p. 497)
- secondary carcinoma (rare)
- primary hypothyroidism (p. 456)

The chiasm may be invaded by retrograde spread of an optic nerve astrocytoma (p. 176) and compressed by retrograde spread of an optic sheath meningioma (p. 176). It is not affected by ischaemia because of its very extensive blood supply from many small arteries but haemorrhage in the chiasm can result from a ruptured vascular malformation.

Lateral compression of the chiasm (e.g. from carotid aneurysm) very occasionally causes an ipsilateral nasal field defect.

Lesions of the optic tract and lateral geniculate body (Fig. 7.1c)

These are rare, usually tumours in the middle cranial fossa. They cause a homonymous hemianopia which tends to be incongruous.

Lesions of the optic radiation (Fig. 7.1d)

These lesions cause a homonymous field defect which tends to be congruous and involve central vision. Temporal lobe lesions affect the lower fibres to cause an upper temporal homonymous quadrantanopia; parietal lobe lesions affect the upper fibres to cause a lower temporal homonymous quadrantanopia. If the whole radiation is involved (proximally by a small lesion near its origin or distally by a large lesion such as a tumour or infarct) then a homonymous hemianopia results.

Lesions of the occipital cortex

These can also cause a homonymous hemianopia which may or may not spare the macula. Lesions of the very tip of the occipital lobe cause a scotomatous homonymous hemianopia (Fig. 7.1e).

In any form of homonymous field defect the central visual acuity is normal. The patient has difficulty reading, bumps into objects on the blind side, or loses sight of approaching traffic, etc. If the macula is 'split' the patient may complain of seeing 'half of things'.

Bilateral occipital lobe lesions

Such lesions (usually due to anoxia or vertebrobasilar ischaemia, p. 220) cause an upper or lower altitudinal defect in both eyes, or bilateral cortical blindness which is sometimes strangely ignored or denied by the patient, particularly if there are additional cognitive deficits (amnesia, sensory inattention, etc.). If the occipital pole is spared, there is bilateral macular sparing which leaves tubular vision. On the other hand, if *only* the occipital poles are involved, there is a bilateral central scotoma.

Note: Pupil responses are normal in lesions posterior to the lateral geniculate body even if the patient is blind, since the visual afferents destined for the midbrain leave the optic tract just before the lateral geniculate body.

The causes of visual failure

Transient monocular visual failure (or amaurosis fugax)

This lasts seconds, minutes or hours. The causes are:
- retinal (or occasionally optic nerve) ischaemia (p. 222)
- papilloedema due to raised intracranial or intraorbital pressure (p. 172)
- glaucoma
- retinal lesions (e.g. haemorrhage, macular degeneration) — should be visible

- Uhthoff's phenomenon in multiple sclerosis (p. 345)
- orbital tumour (p. 174)
- retinal migraine (p. 222)
- hysteria and malingering

Sudden and persistent monocular visual failure

This may be caused by:
- retinal infarction (p. 175)
- ischaemic optic neuropathy (p. 175)
- retinal venous infarction, central or branch vein
- retinal or vitreous haemorrhage and other visible retinal lesions
- papilloedema due to raised intracranial pressure (p. 172)
- cavernous sinus thrombosis (p. 188)
- carotico-cavernous fistula (p. 189)

Transient binocular visual failure

This may be caused by:
- vertebrobasilar transient ischaemic attacks (p. 220)
- vertebral angiography (p. 243)
- systemic hypotension (p. 216)
- head injury
- migraine (p. 137)
- bilateral papilloedema due to raised intracranial pressure (p. 256)
- benign in adolescence (p. 220)

Sudden and persistent binocular failure

This may be due to:
- pituitary apoplexy (p. 273)
- bilateral ischaemic optic neuropathy (p. 175)
- profound hypotension and parieto-occipital infarction (normal pupil response to light) (p. 216)
- bilateral occipital infarction due to vertebrobasilar thromboembolism (normal pupil response to light) (p. 239)
- vertebral angiography causing cortical blindness (normal pupil response to light) (p. 243)
- head injury

Progressive monocular visual failure

This is due to progressive lesions in one eye or optic nerve such as:
- visible ocular lesions (cataract, senile macular degeneration, glaucoma, etc.)
- optic neuritis (p. 173)

- orbital tumour (p. 174)
- lesions which compress the optic chiasm but which, if they are anterior or the chiasm is more posterior than usual, compress only one optic nerve retro-orbitally (p. 168)
- Paget's disease of the skull (p. 483)
- anterior communicating artery aneurysm (p. 232)
- irradiation (p. 486)
- meningovascular syphilis (p. 515)
- dysthyroid eye disease (p. 456)
- Tolosa–Hunt syndrome (p. 189)
- subacute and chronic meningitis (p. 497)
- orbital or paranasal suppuration, fungal infection (p. 531)

Progressive binocular visual failure

This is due to lesions behind the orbit, or a systemic ocular/optic nerve disorder:

- optic chiasm compression (p. 168)
- bilateral optic neuritis (p. 173)
- toxins:
  alcohols and glycols (p. 545)
  heavy tobacco consumption (p. 545)
  mercury (p. 547)
  clioquinol (p. 550)
  chronic cyanide poisoning (p. 549)
- drugs:
  chloramphenicol
  chloroquine
  desferrioxamine
  ethambutol (p. 514)
- glaucoma
- irradiation (p. 486)
- systemic disorders:
  dysthyroid eye disease (p. 437)
  diabetic retinopathy (p. 453)
  sarcoidosis (p. 472)
  lysosomal storage diseases (p. 477)
  adrenoleucodystrophy (p. 456)
- subacute and chronic meningitis (e.g. tuberculosis, syphilis, fungal) (p. 497)
- malignant meningitis (p. 277)
- bilateral severe papilloedema (p. 172)
- nutritional deficiency (vitamin B_{12}, E, etc.) (p. 468)
- Leber's hereditary optic atrophy (p. 174)
- hysteria/malingering (normal pupil response to light)

Note: Toxins and drugs tend to produce a bilateral centrocaecal scotoma.

Papilloedema (or a swollen optic disc)

Oedema of the optic nerve head is called papilloedema and has several causes:
- raised intracranial pressure (p. 256)
- orbital tumour (p. 174)
- cavernous sinus thrombosis (p. 188)
- carotico-cavernous fistula (p. 189)
- malignant hypertension (p. 214)
- retinal venous occlusion
- optic neuritis (p. 173)
- ischaemic optic neuropathy (p. 175)

The normal cup of the optic nerve head fills in and the optic disc becomes swollen, the disc margin is blurred, the disc itself looks pink, the retinal veins become engorged and non-pulsatile, and retinal haemorrhages appear around the disc. Fluorescein angiography usually shows leakage of dye from the disc. Occasionally drusen in the optic nerve head resemble papilloedema, but they show auto-fluorescence, and infiltration of the optic disc may simulate papilloedema (e.g. by sarcoidosis, leukaemia, astrocytoma). The visual acuity is at first normal if the papilloedema is due to raised intracranial or intraorbital pressure whereas in most other cases it is reduced.

In raised pressure cases there may be brief monocular or binocular visual obscurations (lasting seconds), most obvious on standing, bending quickly or exercise; such blurring or complete blindness occurs because raised intracranial and intraorbital pressure causes obstruction to venous outflow and reduces optic nerve perfusion which becomes critical when lowered further by even a small drop in systemic blood pressure. Also, the blindspot is enlarged and sometimes the visual field is constricted, particularly inferonasally. Persistent impaired visual acuity occurs later as raised pressure papilloedema increases and spreads towards the macula, or because of macular haemorrhage. In severe cases, optic atrophy follows and the optic disc becomes grey or pale.

Note: The nasal side of the normal optic disc often looks a little blurred.

Note: Retinal venous pulsation is absent in about 25% of normal individuals.

Optic atrophy

Pallor of the optic disc is called optic atrophy. The disc appears more distinct than usual. Mild degrees of disc pallor, particularly on the temporal side, should be ignored. *Significant* optic atrophy is always accompanied by some

defect of visual acuity, visual fields or pupil response to light, unless it is a sequel to optic neuritis in which case the only abnormality may be an alteration in the visual evoked potential (p. 55). It may be due to:
- damage to retina, optic nerve or chiasm with subsequent loss of optic nerve myelin
- chronic papilloedema (p. 172)
- glaucoma
- severe myopia

The Foster–Kennedy syndrome. This rare combination of optic atrophy in one eye is due to optic nerve compression by a frontal tumour which is large enough to cause raised intracranial pressure and thus papilloedema in the other eye. The same combination can be found with acute anterior optic neuritis in one eye and optic atrophy in the other due to previous optic neuritis; however, in this situation visual acuity is impaired in *both* eyes, not just the eye with optic atrophy.

Proptosis (or exophthalmos)

This is protrusion of one or both eyeballs and must be distinguished from lid retraction, traumatic displacement of the globe and buphthalmos (enlargement of the eyeball). The causes are:
- orbital tumour (p. 174) or inflammation (e.g. bacterial, mucormycosis, p. 533)
- dysthyroid eye disease (p. 456)
- cavernous sinus thrombosis (p. 188)
- carotico-cavernous fistula (p. 189)
- arteriovenous malformation in cavernous sinus region (p. 233)
- craniofacial congenital anomalies
- Paget's disease of the skull (p. 483)
- orbital haematoma (usually traumatic)

Miscellaneous ocular and orbital conditions

Optic neuritis

Optic neuritis (inflammatory or demyelinating) is discussed with multiple sclerosis (Chapter 12) which is its most common cause. Others include:
- Leber's hereditary optic atrophy (p. 174)
- postviral infection (p. 502) (usually bilateral), e.g. chicken pox (p. 523), measles (p. 525), Epstein–Barr virus (p. 524)
- syphilis (p. 515)
- Devic's disease (p. 346)
- sarcoidosis (p. 472)
- orbital cellulitis

Leber's hereditary optic atrophy

This condition is very rare, variably inherited, and males are more often affected than females. In the second or third decade there is subacute bilateral (simultaneous or sequential) painless visual failure progressing over weeks or months and stopping short of complete blindness. Optic atrophy develops, there are central scotomas and recovery does not occur. Occasionally, dementia, ataxia and spastic paraplegia are present.

Orbital tumours

These are rare but often treatable. They may cause:
• progressive monocular visual failure due to optic nerve compression with a monocular visual field defect, usually a central scotoma
• optic atrophy
• sometimes papilloedema
• proptosis or some other deviation of the globe if the tumour is large
• pain in and around the orbit depending on the nature and size of the tumour
• involvement of the intra-orbital cranial nerves: 3rd, 4th, 6th and first division of the 5th cranial nerve
• very rarely, transient monocular blindness on eye movement
    Orbital tumours include:
• optic nerve astrocytoma (usually children with neurofibromatosis, p. 277)
• optic sheath meningioma (p. 176)
• arteriovenous malformation (p. 233)
• haemangioma and lymphangioma
• dermoid and epidermoid tumours (p. 275)
• secondary tumours*
• local spread from nasopharyngeal carcinoma, lacrimal gland carcinoma, rhabdomyosarcoma, retinoblastoma
• lymphoma* (p. 275) and leukaemia* (p. 459)
• myeloma* (p. 460)
• Wegener's granulomatosis* (p. 447)
• sarcoid granuloma (p. 472)
• orbital pseudotumour (p. 174)

Note: Small tumours at the back of the orbit can be extremely difficult to detect with X-rays of the skull and optic foramina and even with CT and MRI of the orbits.

Note: Occasionally a chronic granulomatous mass is found in the orbit. This may be due to sarcoidosis or is idiopathic when it is then referred to as a

* Can be bilateral.

pseudotumour (this may be either diffuse, or localized to an extraocular muscle, the optic nerve sheath, lacrimal gland or epibulbar connective tissue). These conditions may respond to corticosteroids in high dosage.

Retinal infarction

This has the same causes as cerebral infarction (p. 208). It may also be preceded by transient ischaemia, i.e. transient monocular blindness, one cause of amaurosis fugax (p. 222). Occlusion of the central retinal artery causes sudden and painless monocular blindness due to infarction of the retina which becomes pale and swollen. The choroid vascular supply remains normal, so at the macula, where the retina is thin, it stands out as a cherry-red spot against the pale surrounding retina. The retinal arterioles are attenuated and sometimes there is segmentation or 'cattle-trucking' in the retinal veins. In a few weeks the oedema subsides, the macular cherry-red spot disappears and the optic disc becomes pale. Vision seldom recovers. Occlusion of a retinal branch artery causes more restricted infarction with a symptomatic upper or lower altitudinal field defect, or a smaller scotoma which is often not noticed by the patient.

In transient or permanent ischaemia emboli may be observed within the retinal circulation:

• Cholesterol emboli from proximal atheromatous arteries are golden glittering particles which usually do not obstruct the circulation although they appear wider than the arterioles. They are often multiple and scattered throughout the retina. Many such emboli are asymptomatic.

• Calcific emboli from calcified aortic or mitral valves are white and tend to occlude an arteriole at the edge of the optic disc.

• Fibrin-platelet emboli are seldom seen since they move through the retinal circulation as white bodies.

Any type of embolus may become organized, so leading to 'sheathing' of occluded blood vessels which appear white on ophthalmoscopy.

Ischaemic optic neuropathy

This is acute ischaemic infarction of the optic nerve head due to occlusion of the posterior ciliary arteries by hypertensive vascular disease, giant cell arteritis (p. 450), other collagen vascular disorders (p. 444), emboli from proximal arterial or cardiac sources (p. 217), and other rare causes of cerebral infarction (p. 207). There may be preceding amaurosis fugax. Monocular blindness is painless, sudden and involves the whole visual field or the upper or more often lower part with papilloedema and eventually atrophy affecting the corresponding part of the optic disc. It usually does not recover (cf. optic neuritis in multiple sclerosis, p. 343).

In unilateral cases the other eye may become affected, particularly in giant cell arteritis. Bilateral ischaemic optic neuropathy can complicate sudden profound hypotension (p. 216).

Ischaemic oculopathy

This is the condition of ischaemia and infarction of the retina *and* other parts of the globe. It is due to severe carotid artery disease, usually involving not just the internal carotid artery but the external carotid artery as well so that there is restriction of collateral blood supply to the eye (p. 211). The eye is blind with retinal haemorrhages, ocular pain and low pressure glaucoma.

Optic sheath meningioma

Optic sheath meningioma is notoriously difficult to diagnose since it may present with only progressive, painless and monocular loss of vision with optic atrophy and be very difficult to image (CT and MRI of the orbits being the most effective methods). It may spread intracranially to compress the chiasm and other optic nerve, and into the cavernous sinus.

Optic nerve astrocytoma

This presents as an orbital mass or with progressive monocular blindness in children. It can be difficult to image. It may infiltrate back into the chiasm, hypothalamus and third ventricle to cause hydrocephalus and endocrine disturbance. Many patients have neurofibromatosis (p. 277).

Pupils

The normal pupils are regular, equal, react to light directly and consensually and react to accommodation as the eyes converge. Convergence and pupil constriction depend on adequate close vision and therefore reading glasses may need to be worn or the patients simply asked to look at the tip of their nose. Unequal pupils (anisocoria) are of no pathological significance if there are no other pupillary or neurological abnormalities.

A small pupil (meiosis) is due to:
- Horner's syndrome (p. 178)
- pontine lesion (p. 28)
- Argyll Robertson pupil (p. 177)
- pilocarpine and other constricting eyedrops
- organophosphorus poisoning (p. 548)
- opiates (bilateral)

- autonomic neuropathy (p. 403)
- trauma to the iris (usually irregular)
- normal in old age, but usually bilateral
- congenital

A large pupil (mydriasis) is due to:
- parasympathetic lesion, i.e. 3rd cranial nerve lesion (p. 179)
- Holmes–Adie syndrome (p. 178)
- Parinaud's syndrome (high midbrain lesion, p. 179)
- autonomic neuropathy (p. 403)
- anxiety (bilateral and symmetrical)
- atropine and other dilating eyedrops
- amphetamines (bilateral)
- brain death (p. 131)
- trauma to the iris (usually irregular)
- normal in infants (bilateral)

Impaired pupil response to light is found in:
- 3rd cranial nerve lesion (p. 179)
- optic nerve lesion (an early feature as well as late) (p. 167)
- chiasmal lesion (but slight and inconstant until late) (p. 168)
- Argyll Robertson pupil (p. 177)
- Parinaud's syndrome (high midbrain lesion, p. 179)
- ocular disease causing severe impairment of visual acuity
- very small pupils
- trauma to the iris
   The response is normal with lesions of the lateral geniculate body and behind (p. 168).

Argyll Robertson pupils

These are almost pathognomonic of meningovascular syphilis, tabes dorsalis and general paresis of the insane (p. 516).
   Similiar but fragmentary features can be found in:
- diabetic autonomic neuropathy (p. 453)
- late Holmes–Adie pupil (p. 178)
- Parinaud's syndrome (p. 179)
- trauma to the iris
- amyloid neuropathy (p. 473)
- hypertrophic polyneuropathy (p. 396)
   The pupils are unequal, small, irregular and do not constrict to light but they do constrict to accommodation. There may be iris atrophy. The lesion is in the periaqueductal grey matter or ciliary ganglia.

Horner's syndrome

This is due to a lesion anywhere in the ipsilateral sympathetic pathway to the pupil. This starts in the hypothalamus, runs down through the brainstem and cervical spinal cord, emerges with the T1 anterior nerve root close to the apex of the lung, and then ascends in close proximity to the internal carotid artery through the base of the skull and cavernous sinus, and then through the superior orbital fissure to the dilator muscles of the pupil.

Lesions anywhere along this pathway can cause a Horner's syndrome and the position can be deduced from associated features (e.g. brainstem signs, high cervical cord signs, carcinoma of the apex of the lung, neck trauma, thyroidectomy scar, etc.). Lesions in the cavernous sinus and orbit also usually damage parasympathetic nerves to the constrictor muscles of the pupil running with the 3rd cranial nerve; the pupil is then fixed and dilated, or semidilated. A Horner's syndrome can appear with no detectable underlying cause. It can also appear transiently or permanently in migrainous neuralgia (p. 141).

The features are:
- small pupil which constricts to light and accommodation
- mild incomplete ptosis (because of damaged sympathetic nerve supply to eyelid elevators)
- impaired ipsilateral facial sweating is inconstant

Note: Horner's syndrome developing *in utero* or infancy interferes with pigmentation of the iris so that the eyes are of different colours.

Note: Bilateral Horner's syndrome from a brainstem or cervical cord lesion is easily missed since the pupils although small do react, they are equal, and ptosis is symmetrical.

Note: There are usually no symptoms although the patient and others may notice the small pupil and ptosis.

Holmes–Adie syndrome

This is the combination of a Holmes–Adie pupil with absent or depressed tendon reflexes. This is asymptomatic apart perhaps from some photosensitivity in bright light. Usually only one (occasionally both) pupil is dilated; it is regular and first appears in adolescence or young adults, women more often than men. The pupil hardly reacts at all to light but there is reasonable constriction with convergence. Dilatation after constriction is very slow, hence the alternative name of 'myotonic pupil'. The pupil usually constricts with 2.5% methacholine drops because of denervation hypersensitivity, whereas normal and Argyll Robertson pupils do not. Eventually the pupil may become small and irregular, very like an Argyll Robertson pupil (p. 177).

Parinaud's syndrome

This is the combination of failure of upward gaze, bilateral pupil dilatation with a poor response to light and often to accommodation as well, sometimes accompanied by convergence-retraction nystagmus on attempted up-gaze. This is due to a dorsal upper midbrain lesion, usually a tumour in the pineal region (p. 274).

Third, fourth and sixth cranial nerves

The 3rd (oculomotor), 4th (trochlear) and 6th (abducens) cranial nerves carry lower motor neurone fibres from the midbrain and pons, forward through the cavernous sinus and supraorbital fissure into the orbit to supply the extraocular muscles and elevator of the upper eyelid. Lesions of these nerves, or of the extraocular muscles they innervate, cause dysconjugate eye movements and diplopia which is binocular (i.e. abolished by closing either eye).

The upper motor neurone pathway to these cranial nerve nuclei arises in the cerebral cortex and projects to midbrain and pontine centres. Upper motor neurone lesions cause defective conjugate gaze but usually no diplopia.

Voluntary lateral gaze

This is mediated by the frontal (mostly saccadic movements) and occipital (mostly following or pursuit movements) lobes and by the pons. Frontal lesions impair saccadic gaze to the opposite side (p. 20) and lateral pontine lesions impair gaze to the ipsilateral side (p. 28). Occipital lesions tend to impair pursuit to the same side (p. 23). In cerebral lesions the eyes can be made to move involuntarily by having the patient look ahead and then passively rotating the head (doll's eye manoeuvre) and by irrigating the external ear with ice-cold water (oculovestibular reflex); however, these reflexes are impaired in pontine lesions, if there is a lower motor neurone lesion of the 3rd, 4th or 6th cranial nerves, and if the extraocular muscles are affected by myasthenia (Chapter 15) or a myopathy (p. 416).

Voluntary up- and down-gaze

This is mediated largely via the upper midbrain and is therefore impaired by tumours in that region (usually pineal, p. 274) or by pressure from downward herniation of the temporal lobes in raised supratentorial pressure (p. 257). Up-gaze is usually more affected than down-gaze. In normal people both can be produced reflexly by vertical doll's eye manoeuvres.

Note: Impaired conjugate gaze can be found in:
- elderly normal people, particularly up-gaze and convergence
- in Parkinson's disease (p. 280) and some of the parkinsonian syndromes (e.g. progressive supranuclear palsy, p. 290)
- Miller Fisher syndrome (p. 399)
- hexosaminidase deficiency (p. 479)
- Whipple's disease (p. 463)
- vitamin E deficiency (p. 471)
- dominant and idiopathic cerebral ataxia (p. 201)
- Wernicke's encephalopathy (p. 468)

Internuclear ophthalmoplegia

An internuclear ophthalmoplegia is caused by a lesion of the medial longitudinal fasciculus which connects the 3rd with the ipsilateral 6th cranial nerve nucleus. Lesions can be bilateral or unilateral, most commonly due to multiple sclerosis (p. 345). With a unilateral lesion there is incomplete or slow adduction of the ipsilateral eye but normal abduction of the contralateral eye when looking away from the lesion. Usually there is nystagmus in the abducting eye (so-called ataxic nystagmus). Impaired adduction of the ipsilateral eye can be shown not to be due to a medial lateral rectus palsy since convergence and monocular movements are reasonably normal.

One-and-a-half syndrome

This is due to a unilateral lesion (usually ischaemic or multiple sclerosis) of the pons, with paralysis of conjugate deviation of the eyes to the same side and an internuclear ophthalmoplegia; the eye ipsilateral to the lesion does not abduct or adduct and the contralateral eye can only abduct, often with associated ataxic nystagmus.

Note: In ocular myopathies (p. 416) and myasthenia gravis (Chapter 15) there is often weakness of extraocular muscles which can sometimes masquerade as a gaze palsy or internuclear ophthalmoplegia; of course, the pupils are normal and reflex oculocephalic and oculovestibular movements are impaired because of the extraocular muscle weakness.

Note: In a *congenital squint* there is visual suppression and amblyopia in one eye so that although gaze is dysconjugate there is no diplopia. A latent squint may break down in adult life often as a result of intercurrent illness. When this occurs there may be intermittent diplopia. This can be distinguished from acquired extra-ocular muscle weakness by normal monocular eye movements and the cover test: one eye is covered and an object is fixated and, when the cover is removed, there is a quick fixating movement of the previously covered eye.

Congenital oculomotor apraxia

This is seen in children who have difficulty with horizontal eye movements and need to blink to produce them.

Hysterical convergence spasm

This may mimic bilateral sixth nerve palsies but the convergence varies and the pupils are small and constrict on attempted lateral gaze because of the functional convergence and accommodation.

Ocular bobbing

Ocular bobbing is spontaneous and repeated fast downward movements of both eyes, a pause, and then a slow drift back to the resting position. It is seen in large pontine lesions causing coma and horizontal gaze paresis, and in severe generalized encephalopathies.

Ocular dipping

Ocular dipping is spontaneous and repeated slow downward movements of both eyes, a pause and then a rapid return. It is seen in anoxic coma.

Various other forms of conjugate and dysconjugate roving or more apparently directed disorders of eye movement are seen in anoxic, toxic and metabolic coma.

Diplopia

This may be binocular or uniocular, the latter due to refractive errors, vitreous lesions, retinal lesions in the affected eye, and hysteria. Binocular diplopia is due to any lesion which prevents the eyes moving conjugately, such as a dislocated eye ball (trauma, orbital tumour), myasthenia gravis (Chapter 15), ocular myopathy (p. 416) rarely, or a lesion of the 3rd, 4th or 6th cranial nerves. To determine which cranial nerve is involved (or which muscle) it is necessary to determine in what direction of gaze diplopia is maximal (Fig. 7.2) by asking the patient to:
- Look to each side. Abduction of one eye (lateral rectus) should be conjugate with adduction of the other eye (medial rectus).
- Look to each side and then down. The downward movement of the abducting eye is mediated by the inferior rectus and the downward movement of the adducting eye by the superior oblique.
- Look to each side and then up. The upward movement of the abducting eye is mediated by the superior rectus and the upward movement of the adducting eye by the inferior oblique.

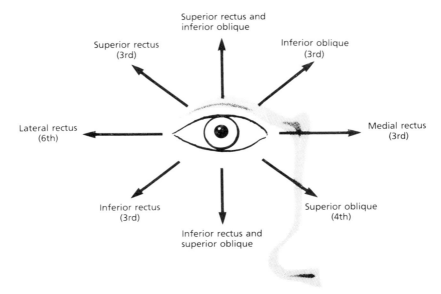

Fig. 7.2 Actions of the extraocular muscles. The arrows indicate the position of the right eye, viewed from in front, where the action of each muscle is most effective, i.e. oblique muscles are most effective elevating and depressing the *adducted* eye, and the superior and inferior rectus muscles are most effective when the eye is *abducted*.

With these six movements it is possible to determine which pair of extraocular muscles is at fault (diplopia being maximal in the appropriate direction of gaze) and then by looking at the eyes to determine which muscle of the pair is the one affected. If the dysconjugate gaze is not obvious in the direction of maximal diplopia then each eye should be covered in turn; the false image arises from the paralysed eye and is the more peripheral and usually less distinct of the two and it disappears when that eye is covered.

Clinical features of third, fourth and sixth cranial nerve palsies

Third nerve lesion

- weakness of all extraocular muscles except lateral rectus and superior oblique. At rest the eye is deviated downwards and outward
- ptosis which can be complete and thus abolish diplopia
- pupil dilated with impaired or no response to light or accommodation due to involvement of parasympathetic nerves running with the third nerve

However, the pupil is usually spared in diabetic and 'ischaemic' third nerve palsies. It is almost always affected if there is pressure on the nerve (i.e. a 'surgical' lesion), unless the extraocular muscle weakness is mild in which case the pupil usually becomes involved a few days after the onset of diplopia as any pressure increases. In cavernous sinus lesions the pupil may not be fully dilated because of an additional Horner's syndrome (p. 178), but it is usually fixed.

An intact fourth nerve is shown by attempted down-gaze when the eye will show some rotation.

Fourth nerve lesion

• weakness of the superior oblique with diplopia and oblique separation of the images looking ahead (abolished by head tilt) and worse on looking down and inwards

Sixth nerve lesions

• weakness of lateral rectus with diplopia and lateral separation of the images on looking to the affected side
  Pseudo sixth nerve palsy may be due to:
• hysterical convergence spasm but the pupils are constricted, particularly on attempted abduction of the eye(s) with apparent weakness of the lateral rectus muscle
• Duane's syndrome is a congenital anomaly due to fibrous replacement of the lateral rectus muscle causing impaired abduction of the eye; however, on attempted adduction there is retraction of the eyeball and narrowing of the palpebral fissure.
  Extraocular muscle weakness may also be due to:
• myasthenia gravis (usually but not always bilateral) (Chapter 15)
• ocular myopathies (bilateral) (p. 416)
• orbital tumour (unilateral) (p. 174)
• dysthyroid eye disease (usually but not always bilateral) (p. 456)
• giant cell arteritis (p. 450)

Causes of third, fourth and sixth cranial nerve lesions

Within the midbrain and pons (see also p. 203):
• tumour (p. 266)
• stroke (p. 239)
• multiple sclerosis (p. 345)
• encephalitis (p. 498)
• Wernicke's encephalopathy (p. 468)

Around the brainstem:
• acute and chronic meningitis (p. 497)
• malignant meningitis (p. 277)

- meningovascular syphilis (p. 515)
- basilar artery aneurysm or ectasia (p. 232)
- posterior communicating artery aneurysm (3rd nerve only) (p. 232)
- tumour (e.g. chordoma, p. 275, nasopharyngeal carcinoma)
- diabetes (p. 454)
- sarcoidosis (p. 472)
- Guillain–Barré syndrome and other neuropathies (p. 393)

Petrous bone apex (6th cranial nerve only):
- raised intracranial pressure (p. 257)
- infection from middle ear
- nasopharyngeal carcinoma

Cavernous sinus:
- pituitary adenoma/apoplexy (p. 273)
- meningioma sphenoid wing (p. 271)
- nasopharyngeal carcinoma
- metastasis
- carotid siphon aneurysm rupture or expansion (p. 232)
- cavernous sinus thrombosis (p. 188)
- carotico-cavernous fistula (p. 189)

Superior orbital fissure:
- sphenoid wing meningioma (p. 271)
- optic sheath meningioma (p. 176)
- metastasis
- pseudotumour (p. 175)
- Tolosa–Hunt syndrome (p. 189)

Orbit:
- tumours (p. 174)
- cellulitis

Others:
- trauma to head or orbit
- giant cell arteritis (p. 450)
- ophthalmoplegic migraine (3rd nerve only, p. 138)
- infections, e.g. herpes zoster (p. 523), AIDS (p. 526), borrelia (p. 517)
- 'ischaemic' although exact site uncertain in brainstem or peripheral nerve

It follows, therefore, that important features to look for include:
- uniocular or binocular visual failure (p. 169)
- visual fields (p. 167)
- papilloedema (p. 172)

- optic atrophy (p. 172)
- proptosis (p. 173)
- anosmia (p. 166)
- pain around the eye/face/head (p. 147)
- fifth cranial nerve (and others) involvement (p. 186)
- excessive fatiguability (myasthenia gravis) (Chapter 15)

Note: An acute, isolated but complete lesion of one nerve in late middle age and the elderly is quite common and usually 'ischaemic' (or perhaps traumatic). There may or may not be pain around the ipsilateral eye. If there are no other neurological symptoms or signs, then, apart from checking for diabetes, syphilis and vascular risk factors, there is nothing more to do if recovery starts in 2–4 weeks, particularly if the pupil is spared in a third nerve lesion. Recovery is usually complete. If the pupil is dilated, there is pain, other neurological signs appear, the patient is known to have or has had cancer, or recovery does not occur, then it is important to look for compressive lesions (skull and sinus X-ray, CT scan and carotid angiography, examination of nasopharynx) and meningeal inflammation, infection or malignancy (CSF examination).

Treatment

Treatment of diplopia is symptomatic by covering one eye and if it becomes permanent and static then prisms can be incorporated into spectacles or the appropriate extraocular muscles weakened or shortened.

Causes of ptosis

- third nerve lesion (can be complete ptosis) (p. 182)
- Horner's syndrome (partial ptosis only) (p. 178)
- myasthenia gravis/Lambert–Eaton myasthenic syndrome (Chapter 15)
- midbrain lesion (p. 27)
- tabes dorsalis (p. 515)
- myopathies, e.g. myotonic dystrophy (p. 424), ocular dystrophies (p. 424), mitochondrial cytopathy (p. 429)
- congenital
- senile (usually bilateral)
- orbital trauma

Fifth cranial (trigeminal) nerve

The motor nucleus of the 5th cranial nerve is in the pons and the efferent nerve fibres leave the base of the skull through the foramen ovale to supply the muscles of mastication. A unilateral lesion can be difficult to detect; the open jaw deviates to the same side due to pterygoid muscle weakness and there may be wasting of the masseter and temporalis muscles ipsilaterally. Bilateral lesions are more obvious with the jaw hanging open and clearly weak.

The complicated central connections of the sensory fibres have been described (p. 15). There are three peripheral sensory branches. The 1st (ophthalmic) division passes in relation to the cavernous sinus through the superior orbital fissure into the orbit and supplies the forehead and scalp (Fig. 7.3); the 2nd (maxillary) division passes inferior to the cavernous sinus through the foramen rotundum, while the 3rd (mandibular) division runs with the motor fibres through the foramen ovale. The oral cavity, anterior tongue and gums are supplied by the lower two sensory divisions. The distribution of any sensory loss indicates where the lesion is: proximal lesions in or near the brainstem cause numbness in all three divisions; lesions near the cavernous sinus spare the 3rd division; lesions in the orbit affect only the 1st division; and lesions at the foramen ovale or within the mandible affect the 3rd division, perhaps merely with unilateral numbness of the chin. Sometimes the sensory loss can be a very restricted patch when only a few fibres of a division are affected by a skull base tumour, for example. The afferent pathway for the corneal response is carried mostly by the 1st division, with perhaps some contribution from the 2nd for the lower half of the cornea.

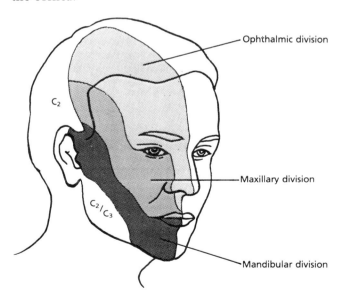

Fig. 7.3 The cutaneous distribution of the 5th cranial (trigeminal) nerve. *Note:* hysterical sensory loss often extends to the hairline and angle of the jaw and the corneal response is normal.

The nerve may be damaged in:
- the medulla (pain loss only, see p. 15), e.g. syringobulbia (p. 334), tumour (p. 266)
- pons (pain and touch loss, see p. 15, with or without motor loss), e.g. multiple sclerosis (p. 343), tumour (p. 266), stroke (p. 239)
- cerebello-pontine angle (p. 194), including trigeminal neuroma
- base of skull (sensory and/or motor loss):
  meningitis (p. 495)
  malignant meningitis (p. 277)
  sarcoidosis
  meningovascular syphilis (p. 515)
  carcinoma nasopharynx
  chordoma (p. 275)
  metastasis
- petrous temporal bone apex (Gradenigo's syndrome, p. 188)
- cavernous sinus lesions (usually only 1st but sometimes also 2nd sensory division affected, p. 188)
- superior orbital fissure (1st sensory division only, p. 188)
- orbital tumours (p. 147) or cellulitis (1st division only)
- mandible, e.g. tumour, infection (3rd sensory division only)
- Guillain–Barré syndrome and other peripheral neuropathies (p. 389), motor more obvious than sensory loss
- herpes zoster (usually 1st sensory division, p. 523)
- polio (p. 522) (motor division only)
- skull trauma
- isolated trigeminal sensory neuropathy (p. 187)
- trichloroethylene toxicity (p. 546)
- organic mercury poisoning (p. 547)

The jaw muscles may also be weak as a result of a myopathy (Chapter 16), myasthenia gravis (Chapter 15), or motor neurone disease (Chapter 13).

Isolated trigeminal sensory neuropathy

This condition is rare. A small numb patch may appear on the face and spread throughout the whole division of the nerve and then to the adjacent divisions as a result of a skull base tumour. Sometimes, however, no cause can be found for such a sensory disturbance even when the whole face becomes numb, and often uncomfortable, first on one side and sometimes then on the other with depression of the corneal response if the 1st division is involved. Severe loss of pain sensation may lead to ulcerative lesions around the nose and of the cornea. Taste sensation may be impaired. Some patients have systemic sclerosis (p. 447), mixed connective tissue disease (p. 447) or other collagen vascular disorders (p. 444). Recovery sometimes occurs after weeks or months. Skull base tumours must be excluded by appropriate imaging and

CSF examination, both of which may need to be repeated and the patient kept under review.

Gradenigo's syndrome

This syndrome is the combination of a 6th nerve palsy with ipsilateral facial and/or ear pain and trigeminal sensory loss due to an inflammatory or neoplastic lesion at the apex of the petrous temporal bone.

Lesions in the region of the cavernous sinus and superior orbital fissure

These cause 3rd, 4th and 6th nerve palsies; impairment of sensation in the 1st division of the trigeminal nerve and occasionally the 2nd if the lesion is posterior and inferior; and pressure on the optic chiasm (p. 168) or optic nerve (p. 170):

- tumours:
  pituitary adenoma/apoplexy (p. 273)
  sphenoid wing meningioma (p. 271)
  nasopharyngeal carcinoma
  metastasis
  malignant meningitis (p. 277)
- vascular:
  aneurysm of carotid siphon or ophthalmic artery (p. 231)
  carotico-cavernous fistula (p. 189)
  cavernous sinus thrombosis (p. 188)
- inflammation:
  acute and chronic meningitis (p. 497)
  sarcoidosis (p. 472)
  Tolosa–Hunt syndrome (p. 189)

Several of the above lesions can cause pain above and within the orbit. If there is venous obstruction, then proptosis, episcleral vasodilatation, and often papilloedema follow. Accurate diagnosis in this area requires high quality plain X-rays, narrow collimated i.v. contrast enhanced CT, MRI, carotid angiography and CSF examination.

Cavernous sinus thrombosis

This condition is rare and usually due to suppuration spreading from the paranasal sinuses, face or orbit (staphylococcal, p. 508, streptococcal, p. 507, mucormycosis, p. 533) and results in:

- pain around the eye and face
- conjuctival and eyelid oedema, episcleral reddening
- proptosis
- 3rd, 4th, 6th with 1st and perhaps 2nd sensory divisions of 5th nerve involvement

- papilloedema, decreased visual acuity and blindness

Thrombosis may spread to the contralateral cavernous and other dural sinuses, and suppuration may spread to cause bacterial meningitis (p. 491) or subdural empyema (p. 503). The patients are generally ill with clinical evidence of infection.

Carotico-cavernous fistula

This occurs as the result of:
- ruptured dural arteriovenous malformation (p. 233)
- ruptured intracavernous carotid aneurysm (p. 232)
- closed head injury, penetrating injury
- spontaneous in the elderly
- Ehlers–Danlos syndrome (p. 484)
- pseudoxanthoma elasticum (p. 484)

There is sudden onset of unilateral pulsating exophthalmos with an orbital bruit often audible to the patient. There may also be ipsilateral orbital pain, papilloedema, chemosis, monocular visual loss and involvement of the 3rd, 4th, 6th and 1st and perhaps 2nd sensory division of the 5th cranial nerves. It can often be obliterated successfully by a balloon introduced on the end of an arterial catheter.

Tolosa–Hunt syndrome

This syndrome is extremely rare. The main features are subacute onset of severe unilateral orbital pain which may be accompanied by 3rd, 4th, 6th and 1st and perhaps 2nd sensory division of the 5th cranial nerve impairment, monocular visual loss and sometimes a raised ESR. Other painful inflammatory and neoplastic causes of the same syndrome (see lesions of the superior orbital fissure) (p. 188) *must* be excluded by CT or MR imaging of the region of the cavernous sinus and orbit, carotid angiography and CSF examination before starting prednisolone (80 mg daily) which normally suppresses the symptoms in a few days. Maintenance treatment in a lower dose may be needed for some years and the patient may need to be closely followed in case another cause of the syndrome eventually declares itself. Some cases turn out to be due to chronic inflammation behind and/or within the orbit (p. 174).

Seventh cranial (facial) nerve

The facial nerve is entirely motor and the nucleus is in the pons. It leaves the brainstem to pass across the cerebello-pontine angle into the internal auditory canal along with the 8th cranial nerve. It then lies close to the inner and middle ear in the temporal bone, and leaves the skull through the stylomastoid foramen to supply the muscles of facial expression and platysma. Lower motor neurone facial weakness includes the forehead as well as the other facial muscles and, if the lesion is proximal, there may be ipsilateral hyperacusis due to involvement of the small branch to the stapedius muscle.

In the temporal bone the facial nerve is joined by the chorda tympani nerve carrying taste from the anterior two thirds of the tongue and efferent autonomic fibres to the salivary glands. This nerve is only variably affected in proximal facial nerve lesions. Of more consequence is that after recovery of a proximal lesion there may be aberrant reinnervation not just to the wrong muscles (synkinesia, so that a blink may be accompanied by ipsilateral movement of the lips) but between autonomic nerves so that lacrimation may accompany salivation during eating (crocodile tears).

Causes of facial nerve lesions

- idiopathic acute (or Bell's) palsy (p. 191)
- pontine lesion (stroke, multiple sclerosis, etc.) (p. 203)
- cerebello-pontine angle mass (p. 194)
- subacute and chronic meningitis (p. 497)
- infections:
  herpes zoster (p. 523)
  syphilis (p. 515)
  leprosy (p. 514)
  borrelia (p. 517)
  polio (p. 522)
  Epstein–Barr virus (p. 524)
  AIDS (p. 526)
- middle or inner ear suppuration
- malignant meningitis (p. 277)
- sarcoidosis (p. 472)
- diabetes (p. 454)
- Guillain–Barré syndrome and other severe neuropathies (p. 389)
- head injury/neurosurgery
- parotid tumour, inflammation, injury
- Melkersson's syndrome (p. 191)
- Mobius' syndrome (p. 191)

Note:
- Facial nerve lesions must be distinguished from myopathic weakness (p. 416) which is usually bilateral and myasthenia gravis (Chapter 15) which is much more often bilateral than unilateral.
- Facial asymmetry is universal and can sometimes be surprisingly prominent, giving the false impression of unilateral facial weakness.

• Squeezing the eyes shut should cause elevation of the eyeballs (Bell's phenomenon). If the facial muscles appear weak but the eyes look straight ahead during this manoeuvre then the patient may not be trying.
• Congenital and unilateral absence of the muscle to the lower lip (depressor anguli oris) can be confused with a facial palsy.

Bell's palsy

Bell's palsy is an idiopathic, isolated unilateral facial nerve palsy which can occur at any age. Around the onset there may be pain around the ear and discomfort or subjective numbness over the affected side of the face. Weakness comes on rather acutely and is usually complete within 24 hours. Sometimes there is ipsilateral hyperacusis and loss of, or impaired, taste. There are *no* other neurological signs and no objective facial sensory disturbance. About 80% of patients recover spontaneously and completely in a few weeks. Residual *severe* paralysis is very unusual.

The cause may be 'viral' with inflammation of the nerve in the temporal bone and giving steroids within a day or so of the onset may hasten recovery: prednisolone, oral, 60 mg daily, tailing off in 2–3 weeks.

Apart from checking for diabetes, AIDS and syphilis, no investigation is necessary unless there are other cranial nerve lesions, or the weakness is bilateral (p. 198) or recurrent (p. 199) when appropriate imaging and CSF examination must be carried out.

If there is severe residual weakness, a tarsorrhaphy may be required to protect the cornea and plastic surgical procedures may help straighten the face.

Melkersson's syndrome

This is the curious association of recurrent unilateral facial palsy, recurrent inflammatory swelling of the face, with a congenitally and deeply fissured 'geographical' tongue. Obviously sarcoidosis and other causes of recurrent facial palsy must be excluded (p. 199).

Mobius' syndrome

This is congenital absence of the facial and 6th cranial nerve nuclei, occasionally others as well, and the muscles they innervate.

Hemifacial spasm

Hemifacial spasm is not uncommon and starts insidiously with involuntary muscle twitching around one eye which is accentuated by forced eye closure. This may gradually spread to involve the ipsilateral corner of the mouth and the rest of the ipsilateral facial muscles along with the platysma. Although painless, the movements may become so severe that irritation and social embarrassment are major problems. There is usually a little weakness around the corner of the mouth ipsilaterally, but no other signs. It tends to vary in severity over the years, being worse at times of stress. The cause is unknown, although very occasionally a cerebello-pontine angle mass (p. 194) is found but seldom until other signs develop (e.g. absent ipsilateral corneal reflex, sensorineural deafness) or the patient is investigated with an enhanced CT scan at an early stage.

For severe cases carbamazepine occasionally helps (p. 90) and repeated intramuscular injection of botulinum toxin around the eye can be effective (see blepharospasm, p. 304). In rare cases a posterior fossa operation is required to 'decompress' the proximal facial nerve from a small vascular loop and to wrap it in non-absorbable sponge, but why this works is unknown.

Facial myokymia

This is rapid and flickering movement of the facial muscles (usually unilateral but it can be bilateral). It is usually asymptomatic and is observed only by looking carefully at the face. There may or may not be associated lower motor neurone facial weakness. The EMG of myokymia is characteristic. The causes are:
- multiple sclerosis (p. 345)
- brainstem tumour (p. 203)
- Guillain–Barré syndrome (p. 398)
- idiopathic

Eighth cranial nerve

Isolated unilateral or bilateral deafness does not usually present directly to a neurologist although it can sometimes be due to a 'neurological' lesion, particularly if there is evidence of involvement of the lower cranial nerves or brainstem. Deafness is most unusual in cortical lesion and fairly unusual with intrinsic brainstem lesions but is common in:
- cerebello-pontine angle lesions (p. 194)
- acute or chronic meningitis (p. 491)
- malignant meningitis (p. 277)

Tinnitus

Tinnitus can accompany any form or cause of hearing loss, including 'neurological' ones such as a cerebello-pontine angle tumour (p. 194). It is scarcely ever an isolated symptom of neurological disease unless it is pulsatile in which case it is often audible to the examiner:

• dural arteriovenous malformation, usually involving the transverse sinus (p. 233)
• other arteriovenous malformations in the neck or head, less often
• arterial bruit from stenosis of the distal internal carotid artery, or intracranial arterial stenosis but seldom due to a bruit from the carotid bifurcation (p. 240)
• carotico-cavernous fistula (p. 189)
• giant intracranial aneurysm (p. 231)
• glomus jugulare tumour (p. 198)
• high cardiac output

Nystagmus

Nystagmus is a to-and-fro oscillation of the eyes which may be present in the primary position and is usually accentuated (or appears) on horizontal and/or vertical gaze. The movements may be horizontal, vertical or rotatory. It is best to describe nystagmus in terms of the direction of gaze in which it is observed, and the direction of the abnormal movements. The nystagmus itself is seldom symptomatic (although patients may complain of vertigo, p. 105) but a few patients do notice the to-and-fro movements as jerkiness of their visual field which is called oscillopsia. The causes of nystagmus include those of vertigo (p. 105), brainstem (p. 203) and cerebellar lesions (p. 199). There is a rare pendular horizontal nystagmus equal in amplitude in both eyes and in all directions of gaze (including up and down) which is congenital, particularly if vision has been poor since childhood; similar movements can be seen in albinos and miners who have spent years in dim light. Also note opsoclonus-myoclonus-ataxia paraneoplastic syndrome (p. 476).

Some general rules are helpful:

• Nystagmus without the symptom of vertigo is generally due to a brainstem or cerebellar lesion.
• Ataxic nystagmus (p. 180) is always due to a brainstem lesion.
• Nystagmus due to a labyrinthine or a vestibular nerve lesion tends to be fairly transient and not to outlast any vertigo, but that due to a brainstem lesion does.
• Symmetrical horizontal nystagmus on lateral gaze to the left and to the right is usually due to drugs (e.g. alcohol, barbiturates, phenytoin, carbamazepine).
• Vertical nystagmus is always due to a brainstem lesion (usually medullary) which can be a consequence of drugs (e.g. anticonvulsants) as well as structural lesions.
• Rotatory nystagmus has no localizing value.
• Positional nystagmus (and vertigo) which fatigues in seconds is due to

benign positional vertigo (p. 107); if positional nystagmus persists for longer, then it is more likely to be due to a brainstem or cerebellar lesion.

• Unilateral labyrinthine and peripheral vestibular nerve nystagmus tends to be more prominent when looking away from the affected side, and the fast phase of the nystagmus is also away from the side of the lesion.

• Caloric testing by placing warm and then cold water in the outer ear often produces confusing results but an abnormality does at least indicate an organic lesion. Most helpful is a 'canal paresis' when both warm and cold water in one ear cause a reduced duration of nystagmus when compared with irrigating the normal ear; this indicates a lesion of the labyrinth or vestibular nerve.

In most cases the exact characterization of nystagmus and vertigo is less helpful in localizing the site of any lesion than other associated neurological or auditory symptoms and signs.

Note: Nystagmus may appear in normals, usually just transiently, if the direction of gaze is more than 30° from the midline or if the eyes are convergent.

Note: Latent nystagmus is congenital and benign. It occurs when one eye is covered, so frequently is first noticed when looking into the patient's fundus with an ophthalmoscope. It can also occur in patients who are actually viewing with only one eye even when both are open (as a result of amblyopia, squint, etc.)

Cerebello-pontine angle

This is the space between the pons, cerebellum and petrous temporal ridge. It is important because it is a common place for tumours and the 5th, 7th and 8th cranial nerves pass across it. This space may be involved in acute or chronic meningitis (p. 491) and in malignant meningitis (p. 277) and the main mass lesions are:

• acoustic 'neuroma' (p. 272)
• meningioma (p. 271)
• 5th nerve 'neuroma' (p. 272)
• 9th nerve 'neuroma' (p. 195)
• epidermoid/dermoid tumour (p. 274)
• brainstem astrocytoma (children or adolescents) (p. 271)
• chordoma (p. 275)
• metastasis
• carcinoma nasopharynx
• basilar artery ectasia or aneurysm (p. 232)
• arteriovenous malformation (p. 233)

The first symptom of a mass lesion is usually progressive unilateral sensorineural deafness, often with ipsilateral tinnitus. Next the 5th cranial nerve is involved, particularly manifest by an absent corneal reflex and facial numbness, and then the 7th, although weakness is mild and taste seldom affected. Hemifacial spasm (p. 191) and trigeminal neuralgia (p. 145) are both extremely unusual. Pain in the ipsilateral face is rare. Vertigo is unusual but a feeling of imbalance is common. With increasing pressure on the brainstem and cerebellum, pyramidal signs (contra, ipsi, or bilateral) appear along with nystagmus and ipsilateral ataxia. Eventually, as with any posterior fossa mass, there may be raised intracranial pressure due to obstructive hydrocephalus.

Imaging of this region includes a skull X-ray with tomograms of the internal auditory meatus (eventually enlarged by an acoustic neuroma) but CT scanning with i.v. contrast enhancement is more sensitive. Plain X-rays are now hardly necessary since a normal result in clinically suggestive circumstances does not rule out the need for a CT scan. If the CT is negative, it may need to be repeated after contrast or air has been introduced into the subarachnoid space by lumbar puncture, or an MRI performed. The brainstem auditory evoked potential is almost always abnormal (prolonged interpeak latency) with acoustic 'neuromas' (even if very small) but false positive results are a problem. Canal paresis on caloric testing is less sensitive, so may give false negative results.

Ninth to twelfth cranial nerves

Ninth cranial nerve (glossopharyngeal)

This nerve carries sensation from the soft palate and pharynx to the brainstem. An isolated lesion of the 9th nerve with unilateral sensory loss is most unusual (e.g. a 'neuroma'). Bilateral sensory loss with an impaired gag reflex is really only seen when other lower cranial nerves (particularly the 10th) are also involved (p. 195) or in a lower brainstem lesion (e.g. syringobulbia, p. 334, Arnold–Chiari malformation, p. 202, etc.).

Note: The gag reflex is absent in some normal individuals.

Tenth cranial nerve (vagus)

Motor nerves arise in the medullary nuclei of the vagus and leave the brainstem to pass through the jugular foramen to supply the pharynx, larynx and, via the recurrent laryngeal nerve, the vocal cords. Unilateral upper or even lower motor neurone vagal lesions seldom cause more than mild symptoms (dysarthria or dysphonia mostly). Contralateral palatal weakness is very transient with upper motor neurone lesions because of bilateral upper motor neurone palatal control (p. 27). Bilateral upper motor neurone lesions cause a pseudobulbar palsy (p. 29) and bilateral lower motor neurone lesions cause a bulbar palsy (p. 29) with nasal dysarthric speech and nasal regurgitation due to bilateral palatal weakness, dysphagia, choking and aspiration into the lungs. The gag reflex is absent. Paralysis of the vocal cord(s) causes hoarseness with a weak cough and sometimes stridor, particularly during sleep; isolated vocal cord paresis is not usually due to a vagal lesion but a recurrent laryngeal nerve lesion in the neck.

Lesions of the vagal nerve motor nuclei or proximal part of the nerve within, and as it leaves, the skull are due to:

• brainstem lesions (stroke, p. 239, Arnold–Chiari malformation, p. 202, polio, p. 522, motor neurone disease, Chapter 13, Shy–Drager syndrome, p. 291, etc.)
• subacute and chronic meningitis (p. 497)
• malignant meningitis (p. 277)
• jugular foramen syndrome (p. 197)
• Guillain–Barré syndrome and other severe neuropathies (p. 389)
• diabetes (p. 454)
• trauma

Bilateral vagal nerve lesions must be distinguished from a bulbar palsy due to myasthenia gravis (p. 408) or myopathies (e.g. polymyositis, p. 435).

Note: Some children and adults occasionally present with dysphagia or hoarseness due to palatal or vocal cord paralysis respectively (usually unilateral rather than bilateral); no cause is found, and recovery occurs within weeks.

Eleventh cranial nerve (spinal accessory)

The motor fibres arise in and leave the upper cervical cord, pass up through the foramen magnum and then leave the skull through the jugular foramen. This nerve is involved in multiple cranial nerve palsies (p. 198), in the jugular foramen syndrome (p. 197), by trauma and by malignancy in the neck. A unilateral lower motor neurone lesion causes weakness of the ipsilateral sternomastoid and upper part of the trapezius muscles. In an acute upper motor neurone lesion (e.g. stroke) there is weakness of the contralateral trapezius, but *ipsilateral* sternomastoid, so that the patient cannot elevate the shoulder of the paralysed arm nor turn his head towards the paralysed side.

Note: Bilateral weakness of the sternomastoids and neck flexors is characteristic of certain muscle disorders and motor neurone disease (p. 417).

Twelfth cranial nerve (hypoglossal)

The motor nucleus is in the medulla and the nerve leaves the base of the skull through the hypoglossal canal to supply the muscles of the ipsilateral side of the tongue. Mild dysarthria and tongue weakness contralateral to the side of an upper motor neurone lesion may occur transiently (e.g. after stroke) while bilateral upper motor neurone lesions cause spasticity of the tongue and severe dysarthria as part of a pseudobulbar palsy (p. 29). Lower motor neurone lesions cause weakness and wasting with dysarthria and difficulty manipulating food in the mouth, particularly if the lesion is bilateral. The causes are the same as those for a 10th cranial nerve lesion (see above).

Dysphagia

Difficulty in swallowing is most often due to obstruction and/or inflammation of the pharynx or oesophagus and the patient can usually point to the site of the trouble; solids are more troublesome than liquids. Neurological disorders may affect the upper and/or lower motor neurone control of the swallowing muscles: tongue, palate, pharynx and larynx. Facial weakness, oral sensory loss (5th cranial nerve) and difficulty chewing may also make swallowing difficult.

Bilateral lower or upper motor neurone lesions are far more likely to be severely symptomatic than unilateral lesions, e.g.:

- bulbar palsy (p. 27)
- pseudobulbar palsy (p. 27)
- myopathies (Chapter 16)
- myasthenia gravis (Chapter 15)
- Guillain–Barré syndrome and other severe neuropathies (p. 389)
  Swallowing may also be impaired in:
- Parkinson's disease and other parkinsonian syndromes (p. 280)
- myotonic disorders (p. 424)
- cranial dystonia (p. 303)
- hysteria with a feeling of a lump in, or constriction of, the throat (globus hystericus)

Jugular foramen syndrome

The jugular foramen transmits the 9th, 10th and 11th cranial nerves along with the sigmoid sinus. It is adjacent to the hypoglossal canal which transmits the 12th cranial nerve. Anteriorly lies the internal carotid artery with the associated sympathetic nerves which enter the skull through the foramen lacerum.

Lesions in or near the jugular foramen may cause:

- hoarseness, nasal speech, dysphagia (10th cranial nerve palsy)
- wasting and weakness of ipsilateral sternomastoid and trapezius (11th cranial nerve palsy)
- diminished ipsilateral palatal sensation (9th cranial nerve involvement)
- pain in and around the ear if bone erosion or inflammation occur

- brainstem signs if lesion is within the skull
- ipsilateral Horner's syndrome if lesion is outside the skull
- ipsilateral hypoglossal palsy with tongue weakness (12th cranial nerve)
  The usual causes are:
- subacute and chronic meningitis (p. 497)
- malignant meningitis (p. 277)
- neuroma of 9th, 10th or 12th cranial nerves
- meningioma (p. 271)
- epidermoid/dermoid tumour (p. 274)
- glomus tumour (p. 198)
- chordoma (p. 275)
- extension of cerebello-pontine angle mass (p. 194)
- metastasis
- nasopharyngeal carcinoma
- malignant lymph nodes in the neck
- skull base fracture

Investigation requires imaging of the skull base and posterior fossa (skull X-ray, CT often with intrathecal contrast), CSF examination and possibly carotid angiography to display a glomus tumour (below).

Glomus tumours are highly vascular and erosive tumours of ectopic chemoectodermal tissue which are found in the inner ear and jugular foramen. They erode bone and present with the jugular foramen syndrome and/ or a mass in the external auditory meatus.

Multiple cranial nerve lesions

A patient may present with a lesion of one cranial nerve and then later an adjacent (or more distant) cranial nerve is affected, followed by others. If the affected nerves are all on the same side the cause is usually a mass lesion. Possibilities include:

- brainstem lesion (usually with additional brainstem signs):
  polio (p. 522)
  motor neurone disease (Chapter 13)
  syringobulbia (p. 334)
- malignant meningitis (p. 277)
- subacute and chronic meningitis (p. 497)
- sarcoidosis (p. 472)
- collagen vascular disorders (p. 444)
- herpes zoster (p. 523)
- Guillain–Barré/Miller Fisher syndrome (p. 398)
- diabetes (p. 454)
- basilar artery ectasia (p. 212)
- tumours:
  carcinoma nasopharynx

chordoma (p. 275)
lymphoma (p. 275)
metastasis in skull base
* trauma
* idiopathic, presumed 'ischaemic'
* idiopathic familial

Recurrent cranial nerve palsies

The causes to consider are:
* diabetes (p. 454)
* ischaemia
* sarcoidosis (p. 472)
* idiopathic (and sometimes familial)
* intermittent compression from an aneurysm (p. 232)
* Melkersson's syndrome (p. 191)
* collagen vascular disorders (p. 444)
* ophthalmoplegic migraine (p. 138)

The cerebellum

A lesion in one cerebellar hemisphere tends to cause ipsilateral limb ataxia, imbalance, dysarthria and horizontal nystagmus (see also p. 14). If large, it compresses the brainstem to cause brainstem or cranial nerve signs, obstructive hydrocephalus and raised intracranial pressure by blocking the outflow of CSF from the 4th ventricle. Compression of the cerebellar hemisphere by a cerebello-pontine angle mass (p. 194) does much the same. Midline cerebellar mass lesions cause less limb ataxia but more general imbalance with truncal, sitting and gait ataxia and rather little dysarthria and nystagmus. Diffuse cerebellar lesions cause general imbalance and truncal ataxia, any limb ataxia is symmetrical, and dysarthria and nystagmus are inconstant.

Causes of cerebellar lesions

Focal and structural abnormalities:
* tumour:
  cystic astrocytoma in hemisphere (children) (p. 271)
  medulloblastoma in midline (children) (p. 273)
  haemangioblastoma in hemisphere (adults, von Hippel–Lindau syndrome, p. 202)
  ependymoma (children) (p. 272)
  secondary carcinoma (hemisphere or midline)
* haemorrhage (p. 223)

- infarct (p. 223)
- abscess (p. 503)
- multiple sclerosis (Chapter 12)
- developmental:
  Arnold–Chiari malformation (p. 202)
  Dandy–Walker syndrome (p. 202)
- Paget's disease of skull (p. 483)

Generalized disorders:

- hereditary:
  autosomal dominant cerebellar ataxia of late onset (p. 201)
  ataxia telangiectasia (p. 202)
  Friedreich's ataxia (p. 336)
  xeroderma pigmentosum (p. 203)
  Cockayne's syndrome (p. 482)
- toxins:
  alcohol (acute intoxication, chronic consumption, Wernicke's encephalo-
    pathy) (p. 542)
  organic solvents (p. 546)
  bismuth (p. 548)
  mercury poisoning (p. 547)
  lead poisoning (p. 547)
  acrylamide (p. 549)
- drugs:
  aminoglycosides
  amiodarone
  barbiturates (p. 92)
  carbamazepine (p. 90)
  cytarabine
  fluorouracil
  lithium
  phenytoin (p. 88)
  piperazine
- metabolic:
  hypothyroidism (p. 456)
  abetalipoproteinaemia (p. 479)
  Hartnup disease (p. 481)
  argininosuccinic aciduria (p. 481)
  ornithine transcarbamylase deficiency (p. 480)
  Leigh's disease (p. 482)
  mitochondrial cytopathy (p. 430)
  adrenoleucodystrophy (p. 456)
  Refsum's disease (p. 397)
  metachromatic leucodystrophy (p. 478)
  hexosaminidase deficiency (p. 479)

Wilson's disease (p. 310)
vitamin E deficiency (p. 471)
neuronal ceroid lipofuscinosis (p. 480)
• infections:
typhoid fever (p. 509)
brucellosis (p. 510)
legionnaire's disease (p. 510)
enteroviral infections (p. 522)
chicken pox (p. 523)
Epstein–Barr virus (p. 524)
mumps
progressive chronic rubella encephalitis (p. 526)
Creutzfeldt–Jakob disease (p. 531)
kuru (p. 531)
Miller Fisher syndrome (p. 399)
Whipple's disease (p. 463)
• others:
idiopathic sporadic late-onset cerebellar ataxia (p. 201)
paraneoplastic syndrome (p. 475)
progressive myoclonic epilepsies (p. 75)
post cerebral anoxia
radiotherapy (p. 486)
heat stroke (p. 485)
Fahr's syndrome (p. 293)

Autosomal dominant cerebellar ataxia of late onset

This usually starts in middle age with progressive cerebellar ataxia and imbalance along with dysarthria. There can be a variety of other features including supranuclear ophthalmoplegia, dementia, pigmentary retinal degeneration, optic atrophy, rigidity, chorea, sensorineural deafness, pyramidal signs, absent tendon reflexes, muscle wasting (amyotrophy) and impaired position and vibration sense in the feet. Death occurs in a few years. There is considerable variation even within families and the neuropathology is variable, only some cases being due to olivo-ponto-cerebellar atrophy. It must be distinguished from Huntington's disease (p. 298) and vitamin E deficiency (p. 471). On CT the cerebellum and sometimes brainstem are atrophied; the CSF is normal.

Idiopathic sporadic late-onset cerebellar ataxia

This starts in middle age and is similar to the dominant late onset ataxia above except that the additional neurological features are less common. The pathology may be not just olivo-ponto-cerebellar atrophy but also cortical cerebellar atrophy and other patterns of neuronal degeneration. Drugs, toxins, vitamin E deficiency and metabolic causes must be excluded (p. 200).

Arnold–Chiari malformation

This is a developmental anomaly with prolapse of the cerebellar tonsils and sometimes more of the cerebellum and the lower brainstem through the foramen magnum. It can be associated with syringomyelia and syringobulbia (p. 334), spinal dysraphism (p. 329) and fused cervical vertebrae (Klippel–Feil syndrome). It presents at any age, in neonates and children usually with raised intracranial pressure, hydrocephalus and midline cerebellar and low brainstem signs. At older ages the onset can also be with syringomyelia, pain in the neck, down the arms or in the occiput, characteristically aggravated by coughing.

Plain X-rays may show basilar impression (platybasia), widened cervical canal and fusion of cervical vertebrae. Myelography must be done with the patient supine and contrast passed up through the foramen magnum with CT, but MRI is the most sensitive imaging procedure.

Dandy–Walker syndrome

This is a developmental anomaly with cystic dilatation of, or near, the 4th ventricle. It causes obstructive hydrocephalus, cerebellar and/or brainstem signs.

Von Hippel–Lindau syndrome

This is autosomal dominant with variable expression. Features include:
- cerebellar haemangioblastoma (single or often multiple) (p. 272)
- brainstem haemangioblastoma (p. 272)
- retinal angioma
- spinal canal haemangioblastoma
- renal angioma, carcinoma, cysts
- phaeochromocytoma
- pancreatic adenoma or cysts
- cysts of epididymis

Patients presenting with one of the features, and asymptomatic close relatives, should be screened at least once by general physical examination, CT of head and upper abdomen, microscopic haematuria and renal function, ophthalmoscopy and fluoroscein angiography and urine vanilylmandelic acid. Affected families should be kept under regular review.

Ataxia telangiectasia

This is an uncommon autosomal recessive disorder which starts in infancy with cerebellar ataxia. This progresses with dysarthria, titubation of the head, absent tendon reflexes, choreoathetosis, dystonia, disordered eye movements and eventually distal weakness, muscle atrophy and sensory loss due to a peripheral neuropathy. Mental retardation and myoclonus may occur. Conjunctival and skin telangiectases develop after the onset of the neurological symptoms. There is severe immune deficiency (particularly of serum IgA and IgG), raised serum alphafetoprotein, recurrent infections, the children are small and lack secondary sexual characteristics, and often lymphoma or other malignancies develop. Death occurs at about the age of 20.

Xeroderma pigmentosum

This is autosomal recessive and primarily a skin disease with abnormal sensitivity to sunlight. However, it can be complicated by neurological disorders, particularly cerebellar ataxia, chorea, seizures, mental retardation or dementia, deafness, spasticity and peripheral neuropathy.

The brainstem

The clinical features of brainstem lesions have been described (p. 27). The most common causes are:

- stroke (p. 239)
- external pressure:
  transtentorial herniation and tonsillar coning (p. 257)
  cerebello-pontine angle mass (p. 194)
  cerebellar mass (p. 199)
  basilar aneurysm or ectasia (p. 212)
  nasopharyngeal carcinoma
  Arnold–Chiari malformation (p. 202)
  Dandy–Walker syndrome (p. 202)
- multiple sclerosis (Chapter 12)
- motor neurone disease (Chapter 13)
- vascular malformation (p. 233)
- tumours, e.g. pontine astrocytoma (p. 271) in children and young adults, ependymoma (p. 272) of 4th ventricle in children
- syringobulbia (p. 334)
- infections:
  polio (p. 522)
  listeria encephalitis (p. 511)
  abscess (p. 503)
- Wernicke's encephalopathy (p. 468)
- central pontine myelinolysis (p. 465)
- Leigh's disease (p. 482)
  Some patients have a chronic progressive pseudobulbar palsy with no cause becoming obvious; perhaps this is one form of motor neurone disease (Chapter 13).

8 Cerebrovascular disease

Cerebrovascular disease includes spontaneous disorders which cause ischaemia, infarction or haemorrhage within or over the brain. There are three main categories:

Stroke

Stroke (cerebrovascular accident) is a rapidly developing episode of focal and at times global (applied to patients in deep coma or after subarachnoid haemorrhage) loss of cerebral function with *symptoms* lasting more than 24 hours, or leading to death, and with no apparent cause other than that of vascular origin. It may be due to:
- cerebral infarction (approximately 80% of cases) (p. 207)
- primary intracerebral haemorrhage (approximately 15% of cases) (p. 227)
- subarachnoid haemorrhage (approximately 5% of cases) (p. 228)

Transient ischaemic attack (TIA)

TIA is an acute loss of focal cerebral or monocular function with *symptoms* lasting less than 24 hours and which, after adequate investigation, is presumed to be due to embolic or thrombotic vascular disease.

Multi-infarct (vascular or arteriosclerotic) dementia (p. 161)

Note: The difference between *ischaemic* stroke and TIA based on the 24-hour time criterion is arbitrary but widely accepted. In practice, a more useful distinction for management and planning services is between patients who recover in minutes, days, or weeks (i.e. a *reversible ischaemic attack*) and those who do not.

In developed countries, stroke is the third most common cause of death after ischaemic heart disease and cancer and is the most common cause of serious physical disability. In some countries the incidence is declining.
In the UK:
- the incidence of first ever stroke is approx. 2 per 1000 population per annum
- the incidence of TIA is approx. 0.4 per 1000 population per annum
- the prevalence of stroke survivors is approx. 8 per 1000 population
- after first ever stroke about 20% of patients are dead at 1 month and 35% of survivors are dependent at 6 months

Note: The exact figures depend on the age structure of the population because cerebrovascular disease is strongly associated with increasing age; only 25% of strokes occur below the age of 65.

Cerebral ischaemia and infarction

Thrombotic or embolic occlusion of an artery (for any reason) causes a reduction in blood flow and ischaemia in its territory of supply. In the brain this results in impaired neuronal function, causing a clinical deficit which may be anything from mild and localized (e.g. clumsiness of one hand) to severe and widespread (e.g. hemiplegia with aphasia). The *pattern* of the deficit depends on which part of the brain is ischaemic. If the reduction in blood flow is severe and/or prolonged (which is more likely if the collateral blood supply is poorly developed or affected by arterial disease), then some or all of the ischaemic brain will infarct.

Recovery of function following cerebral infarction depends on:
- the size of the infarct
- revascularization of ischaemic areas by collateral blood supply (p. 211) or reflow through previously occluded arteries
- resolution of any cerebral oedema associated with ischaemia or infarction
- ability of other parts of the brain to take over lost functions; this is greatest in children and least in the elderly
- adaptation to the clinical deficit (i.e. impairment, p. 59), so reducing its functional significance (i.e. handicap, p. 60).

Therefore, the clinical manifestations of cerebral ischaemia and infarction range from none at all if the involved area of brain is small or of apparently little functional importance, to a transient ischaemic attack, to a stroke which may or may not recover, to death due to stroke and its complications. However, the underlying causes (p. 208) and risks of subsequent serious vascular events (stroke, myocardial infarction, sudden death, p. 251) are much the same whatever the severity of the initial ischaemic event.

Note: Emboli to the brain consist of any combination of:
- fibrin (from left atrial or left ventricular thrombus, thrombus on atheromatous plaque)
- platelet aggregates (from thickened aortic valve, thrombus on atheromatous plaque)
- cholesterol (from ruptured atheromatous plaque)
- calcium (from calcified heart valve)
- tumour (e.g. myxoma)
- bacterial vegetations (infective endocarditis)
- fat (p. 487)
- air (e.g. cardiac surgery, p. 219)

Cerebral blood flow

Cerebral blood flow (CBF) is more or less constant (about 50 ml/100 g brain/minute) if the systolic blood pressure remains between a mean of about 60 and 160 mmHg (this is cerebral autoregulation). Blood pressure above this increases CBF and causes hyperaemia of the brain, breakdown of the blood brain barrier, cerebral oedema and raised intracranial pressure (and the clinical features of hypertensive encephalopathy, p. 214). If the blood pressure falls below the range for autoregulation, then ischaemia and eventually infarction occur. Autoregulation is set higher in chronic hypertension so that the patients are more likely than usual to develop symptoms with low blood pressure and are more resistant to developing cerebral oedema with very high blood pressure. Autoregulation is impaired in and around ischaemic and haemorrhagic brain lesions; also, it gradually tends to become less effective with increasing age.

CBF is strongly influenced by $PaCO_2$; an acute rise of $PaCO_2$ by 1 mmHg increases CBF by about 5%. However, in chronic hypercapnia the CBF is normal. CBF is less influenced by blood oxygen tension but rises when the PaO_2 is low enough to reduce oxygen saturation. CBF falls with increasing haematocrit which is largely due to the increased oxygen-carrying capacity of the blood rather than its greater viscosity.

The causes of cerebral ischaemia and infarction

Artheroma and its complications (p. 211) are the most common causes of TIA and cerebral infarction (at least 50% of cases). Small vessel disease within the brain (so-called lipohyalinosis, p. 213) causes about 25% of symptomatic cerebral infarcts, and embolism from the heart another 10% (p. 217). The rest are caused by rarer arterial disorders (p. 214) and blood disorders (p. 210).

Definite risk factors for stroke due to cerebral infarction

- those which increase the risk of degenerative arterial disease in general:
  increasing age
  increasing blood pressure (p. 213)
  diabetes mellitus (p. 453)
  cigarette smoking
  increasing plasma cholesterol
  increasing plasma fibrinogen
  excessive alcohol consumption (probably by causing hypertension)
  males slightly more than females
- markers for arterial disease:
  ischaemic heart disease (angina, previous myocardial infarction)
  peripheral vascular disease
  TIA
  cervical arterial bruit
- cardiac embolic source (p. 217), e.g. atrial fibrillation, recent myocardial infarction

Hypertension is the most important risk factor, not only because it is so common in the general population but also because it is very common in cerebral infarction and TIA patients (about 50% have a prior BP of >160/90 mmHg twice).

Note: More strokes occur as a result of mild to moderate hypertension in large numbers of people than as a result of severe hypertension in a few individuals.

Causes of occlusive arterial disease

- atheroma in large vessels (p. 211)
- lipohyalinosis in small vessels (p. 213)
- inflammatory arterial disease:
  giant cell arteritis (p. 450)
  systemic lupus erythematosus (p. 444) and Sneddon's syndrome (p. 446)
  systemic vasculitis (p. 447)
  rheumatoid disease (p. 448)
  Sjögren's syndrome (p. 449)
  relapsing polychondritis (p. 449)
  Behçet's syndrome (p. 449)
  malignant atrophic papulosis (p. 450)
  isolated granulomatous angiitis of the nervous system (p. 450)
  Takayasu's disease (p. 453)
  necrotizing angiitis due to drug abuse (cocaine, heroin, amphetamines, etc., p. 551)
  sarcoid angiitis (p. 472)
  rheumatic fever
- infections causing inflammation of the vessel wall:
  tonsillitis, pharyngitis and cervical lymphadenitis causing carotid artery inflammation
  herpes zoster (p. 523)
  mucormycosis (p. 533) and other fungi (p. 531)
  arteritis due to TB (p. 512), syphilis (p. 515) and other causes of meningitis (p. 491)
- trauma (p. 214):
  penetrating neck injury
  blow to neck
  cervical manipulation
  yoga
  cervical rib
  'whiplash' injury
  tonsillectomy
  attempted strangulation

atlanto-axial dislocation
fractured clavicle
cervical rib
fractured base of skull
cerebral angiography (p. 243)
- dissection:
trauma (see above)
atheroma (p. 211)
fibromuscular dysplasia (p. 215)
cystic medial necrosis
inflammatory arterial disease (see above)
Ehlers–Danlos syndrome (p. 484)
pseudoxanthoma elasticum (p. 484)
Marfan's syndrome (p. 484)
Menkes' kinky hair syndrome (p. 482)
- congenital:
aneurysms (p. 231)
loops and coils
fibromuscular dysplasia (p. 215)
- miscellaneous:
migraine (p. 215)
oral contraceptives (p. 216)
pregnancy (p. 215)
homocystinaemia (p. 481)
malignant angioendotheliosis (p. 276)
neoplastic invasion of arterial wall
irradiation of arteries (p. 486)
Fabry's disease (p. 397)
mitochondrial cytopathy (p. 429)
inflammatory bowel disease (p. 463)

Haematological causes of cerebral ischaemia and infarction

- sickle cell disease/trait (p. 460)
- polycythaemia (p. 458)
- essential thrombocythaemia (p. 459)
- leukaemia (p. 459)
- thrombotic thrombocytopenic purpura (p. 462)
- paroxysmal nocturnal haemoglobinuria (p. 462)
- disseminated intravascular coagulation (p. 462)
- hyperviscosity syndrome (multiple myeloma, p. 460, Waldenstrom's macroglobulinaemia, p. 461)
- anaemia (transient ischaemia only, p. 460)
- 'hypercoagulability' (p. 462)

If cerebral ischaemia or infarction occurs at a young age *in families* then consider:

- familial hypercholesterolaemia
- sickle cell disease/trait (p. 460)
- familial causes of 'hypercoagulability' (e.g. antithrombin III, protein C, protein S deficiencies, p. 462)
- pseudoxanthoma elasticum (p. 484)
- Ehlers–Danlos syndrome (p. 484)
- Marfan's syndrome (p. 484)
- homocystinaemia (p. 481)
- Fabry's disease (p. 397)
- mitochondrial cytopathy (p. 429)
- migraine (p. 215)

Atheroma

Most cerebral infarcts and TIAs are due to the thrombotic and embolic complications of atheroma affecting the extracranial neck arteries and the medium sized arteries at the base of the brain. Atheroma tends to occur at points of arterial branching (e.g. carotid bifurcation), tortuosity (e.g. carotid syphon) and confluence (e.g. basilar artery) (Fig. 8.1).

Occlusion of a neck artery may not cause cerebral infarction in its territory of supply if the distal collateral blood supply is adequate (see below). On the other hand, embolism to the origin of, or branches of, the intracranial arteries is likely to cause cerebral infarction since more distally there is less potential for collateral blood supply.

Collateral channels include:
- circle of Willis (Fig. 8.2) but parts of it are often absent or hypoplastic even in normal individuals. Also, it is often affected by atheroma
- anastomoses between branches of the internal carotid artery and ipsilateral external carotid artery around and within the orbit
- leptomeningeal anastomoses between cortical branches of the middle, posterior and anterior cerebral arteries
- meningeal anastomoses between branches of the internal carotid artery, external carotid artery and vertebral artery
- anastomoses in the neck between branches of the occipital and ascending pharyngeal branches of the external carotid artery, muscular branches of the vertebral artery, and branches of the deep and ascending cervical arteries.

Note: Atheroma is a multi-arterial disease. Patients with clinical manifestations of atherothromboembolism affecting one organ (e.g. the brain) almost always have atheroma affecting the blood supply to other organs (e.g. heart, legs) with or without symptoms (e.g. angina, claudication, etc.).

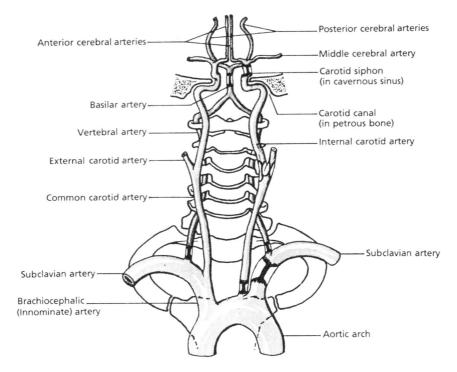

Fig. 8.1 The arterial blood supply to the brain. Sites most often affected by atheroma are shown as white indentations into the arterial wall.

Note: Occasionally atheroma is complicated by dilatation (ectasia) which can become aneurysmal. These dilatations are usually asymptomatic but can cause pressure on adjacent structures (e.g. an ectatic basilar artery or aneurysm can compress the brainstem and lower cranial nerves).

Note: Dissection of an atheromatous aortic arch may cause occlusion of the major vessels arising from it with subsequent ischaemia of the arm, brain or eye. Usually there is chest pain and reduced or absent arterial pulsation in the arm(s) and neck.

Cholesterol embolization syndrome

This is a rare disorder in which there is deposition of cholesterol and atheromatous debris in the microcirculation of many organs, particularly the kidneys and skin. It occurs after instrumentation or surgery of large atheromatous arteries such as the aorta. The clinical picture can be easily confused with systemic vasculitis (p. 447):

• proteinuria, renal failure

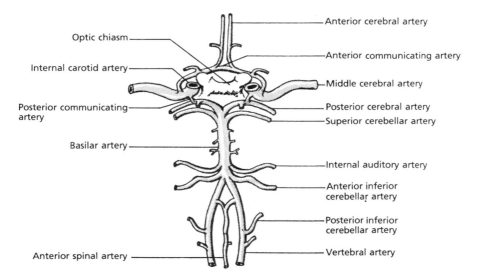

Fig. 8.2 The circle of Willis at the base of the brain.

- skin petechiae, livedo reticularis
- drowsiness and occasionally TIA and stroke-like episodes
- raised ESR and neutrophil leucocytosis
- eosinophilia
  The diagnosis is made by finding cholesterol debris in the microcirculation of biopsy material (skin, kidney, etc.).

Intracerebral small vessel disease (lipohyalinosis)

The small arteries which penetrate the base of the brain (e.g. lenticulostriate arteries arising from the proximal middle cerebral artery) can become tortuous with thickened, hyalinized and lipid-rich (so-called lipohyalinosis). How this pathological change relates to atheroma is unclear but it may be a separate and distinct disorder. Certainly occlusion of these arteries leads to the clinically recognizable lacunar syndromes which have a good prognosis (p. 237). It is not inconceivable that the same small vessel disease is complicated by microaneurysms (Charcot–Bouchard aneurysms) which may rupture to cause intracerebral haemorrhage, typically in the basal ganglia region. Patients with this small vessel disorder may be hypertensive, but not always.

Hypertension

Hypertension is the most important risk factor for cerebral infarction, primary intracerebral haemorrhage and subarachnoid haemorrhage; an increase in diastolic BP by about 7.5 mmHg doubles the risk of subsequent stroke. Hypertension accelerates the formation and distal spread of atheroma in the arterial system and probably is partly the cause of lipohyalinosis. Hypertension itself seldom causes symptoms, with the possible exception of headache when the diastolic blood pressure is over at least 120 mmHg.

Malignant hypertension with hypertensive encephalopathy is now rare. It seldom occurs in chronic hypertensives because autoregulation has been set higher (p. 208); it is more likely in acute hypertension when the upper limit of autoregulation is normal and can therefore be more easily exceeded (e.g. eclampsia, acute nephritis). There is widespread cerebral oedema, ischaemia and occasionally intracerebral haemorrhage(s) which cause:
- headache, nausea and vomiting
- drowsiness, confusion, leading to coma
- bilateral papilloedema and blurring of vision
- partial and generalized seizures
- stroke and TIA-like episodes due to focal cerebral ischaemia, or less often intracerebral haemorrhage

Rare arterial disorders

Trauma

Trauma to arteries in the neck, penetrating or indirectly and not necessarily very severe (p. 209), may cause the following:
- Dissection of the carotid or vertebral arterial wall. Blood or haematoma in the false lumen in the arterial wall may occlude the true lumen which, if there is an adequate distal collateral blood supply, is of no particular consequence. However, if thrombus forms on the damaged intima (usually where the dissection communicates with the true lumen), it may embolize distally to cause cerebral infarction within minutes, hours, or even days of injury, but seldom later since by then most dissections resolve to leave a normal artery with no further likelihood of thromboembolism. Carotid dissection may cause pain in the ipsilateral face, eye and neck along with a Horner's syndrome (p. 178). The angiographic picture is characteristic with a smooth tapering stenosis ('string sign') or occlusion, perhaps with a double lumen, and sometimes with aneurysm formation. Duplex ultrasound can be diagnostic. Anticoagulation may reduce the risk of thrombosis and embolism in the acute stage, but this is uncertain.
- Disruption of an atheromatous plaque with immediate or delayed distal embolization to the brain.
- Rupture of the arterial wall.
- Traumatic aneurysm. This may enlarge and the thrombus within it may embolize distally, even months or years after the injury. However, the usual presentation is with a pulsatile mass in the neck some months or years after trauma.

Note: Arterial aneurysms in the neck may also be congenital or due to local irradiation (p. 486), fibromuscular dysplasia (see below) and infections (e.g. tonsillitis).

Fibromuscular dysplasia

Fibromuscular dysplasia of the carotid, and less often the vertebral arteries, is rare and seldom causes any problems except by dissection (clinical features, see above). It can be associated with intracranial saccular aneurysms (p. 231) and vascular malformations (p. 233) as well as with fibromuscular dysplasia of other arteries (e.g. the renal arteries to cause hypertension).

Moyamoya syndrome

This is a radiological diagnosis of a characteristic pattern of abnormal arterial anatomy. There is obstruction of the terminal internal carotid artery, non-filling of portions of the Circle of Willis, and collateral formation taking the form of a mesh of fine vessels throughout the basal ganglia region with the appearance of a haze-like puff of smoke on angiography (moyamoya in Japanese). This condition tends to occur only in Asians and usually no cause is found; it is sometimes the result of meningeal infection.

Symptoms usually arise in infants and children (rather than in adults) and are due to primary intracerebral haemorrhage, subarachnoid haemorrhage and recurrent cerebral infarction.

Migrainous stroke

Occasionally, during the aura of a previously experienced and otherwise unremarkable attack of classical migraine (p. 137), the neurological deficit persists for days or longer. For example, a homonymous hemianopia persists in a patient whose auras were of a homonymous visual field disturbance, or a sensory-motor stroke occurs when previous auras were tingling down the same side of the body. CT is normal or shows infarction. The cause is presumably arterial occlusion, perhaps due to vasospasm. Recurrence is unusual.

Pregnancy

Stroke complicates the last trimester of pregnancy and the puerperium in no more than 5 per 10 000 deliveries in the UK. It is often due to middle cerebral artery occlusion, perhaps as a consequence of paradoxical embolism from the venous system of the legs or pelvis. Occasionally it is due to intracranial haemorrhage during eclampsia, but in this condition widespread cerebral oedema with hypertensive encephalopathy (p. 214) is more likely. Intracranial venous thrombosis occurs more often in developing countries. Arteriovenous malformations (p. 233) have a tendency to bleed during pregnancy and labour.

Oestrogens

Oral contraceptive users have about three times the usual risk of stroke, and an even higher risk if they are smokers; however, the *absolute* risk remains extremely small. This excess risk appears to apply to both cerebral infarction and intracranial haemorrhage and the underlying mechanism is unknown. Some years after stopping oral contraceptives the risk declines to the normal background level.

Men taking oestrogens (e.g. for prostatic carcinoma) also have an excess risk of stroke.

There is no excess risk of stroke in women taking hormone replacement therapy; there may even be a modest protective effect.

Hypotension and cerebral infarction

Systemic hypotension, from whatever cause, usually causes non-focal neurological symptoms (e.g. faintness, muzzy head, dimming of vision bilaterally, loss of consciousness, p. 100) and, if more severe and prolonged, persistent coma, the vegetative state (p. 126) and death. These are no *focal* symptoms unless there is *also* severe stenosis or occlusion of a major artery in the neck or at the base of the brain, a previous stroke has impaired autoregulation in a focal area of brain, or boundary zone infarction occurs (see below). A fall in blood pressure as the cause for a transient ischaemic attack or stroke is suspected if:

● focal symptoms occur when a fall in blood pressure is likely to have occurred:

    standing up quickly
    after a heavy meal
    after a hot bath
    after exercise
    shortly after starting hypotensive drugs (e.g. nifedipine)
    shortly after taking vasodilators (e.g. glyceryl trinitrate)
    during general anaesthesia
    during cardiac arrhythmias
    during circulatory arrest

● measured blood pressure is low at the onset of the attack (but seldom practical to record at that moment)
● the eye and ipsilateral cerebrum are affected simultaneously
● chest pain and/or palpitations at the onset of attack suggesting a cardiac arrhythmia
● boundary zone infarction (see below)
● early loss of consciousness along with the focal signs

Boundary zone (watershed) infarction

This is infarction *between* rather than within the territories of supply of the cerebral arteries, e.g. in the fronto-parietal lobe between the anterior and middle cerebral artery territories, and in the parieto-occipital area between the anterior, middle and posterior cerebral artery territories. This tends to occur under two sets of circumstances:

- low blood flow due to severe arterial disease in the neck or at the base of the brain, usually in the presence of a poor collateral blood supply
- profound and prolonged hypotension (e.g. as a result of cardiac arrest)

Embolism from the heart

The consequences of embolism to the brain and eye are the same whether the embolus arises from a proximal arterial site or from the heart. In an individual patient it is extremely difficult to be sure of the cause of an ischaemic stroke or TIA when there is evidence of both a potential cardiac source of embolism (e.g. atrial fibrillation) and proximal arterial disease (e.g. a cervical bruit, p. 240) which is commonly the case in the elderly. A *potential* cardiac source of embolism is present in about 30% of cerebral infarction/ TIA patients but is often a coincidence or an association of atheromatous arterial disease affecting the brain (to cause ischaemic stroke/TIA) and the heart (to cause atrial fibrillation, left ventricular aneurysm, etc.). Probably no more than 10% of ischaemic stroke/TIA cases are *actually* due to embolism from the heart (non-rheumatic atrial fibrillation being the most common cause).

Cardiac sources of embolism to the brain and elsewhere (in anatomical sequence):

- paradoxical embolism from the venous system:
  atrial septal defect
  patent foramen ovale
  pulmonary arteriovenous malformation (p. 234)
- left atrium:
  thrombus, particularly with atrial fibrillation or sinoatrial disease
  myxoma
- mitral valve:
  infective endocarditis
  rheumatic endocarditis
  marantic (non-infectious or non-bacterial thrombotic) endocarditis associated with cancer or cachexia (p. 477)
  prosthetic valve
  Libman-Sacks endocarditis (p. 445)

mitral annulus calcification*
mitral leaflet prolapse*
- left ventricular mural thrombus:
myocardial infarction
left ventricular aneurysm
cardiomyopathy
- aortic valve:
infective endocarditis
rheumatic endocarditis
marantic endocarditis (p. 477)
prosthetic valve
syphilis
sclerosis/calcification*
- congenital cardiac disorders (usually with right to left shunts)
- cardiac surgery (p. 219), cardiac catheterization, coronary angioplasty

Evidence for embolism from the heart to the brain in an individual patient

- A *major* potential cardiac embolic source is present, e.g. echocardiographically definite mural thrombus complicating recent myocardial infarction, atrial fibrillation with rheumatic valvular heart disease, infective endocarditis or prosthetic valve. Atrial fibrillation is present in about 15% of ischaemic stroke/TIA patients but is not usually associated with the above cardiac disorders, making it uncertain whether embolism from the left atrium to the brain has occurred or not in these circumstances.
- No other likely causes of cerebral ischaemia or infarction, i.e. no evidence of vascular disease such as angina, cervical bruit, peripheral vascular disease, or on duplex imaging of the neck arteries and no hypertension.
- Infarction in separate parts of the brain, or in other organs as well as the brain.
- Calcific emboli visible in the retina (from calcified aortic or mitral valves).
- Patient under the age of about 50.
- Lacunar infarcts are rarely embolic (p. 238).

Note
- Atrial thrombus is difficult if not impossible to image with conventional echocardiography (a transoesophageal approach is more sensitive).
- Left ventricular mural thrombus is easier to image and is particularly likely after a large anterior myocardial infarction and in a left ventricular aneurysm.
- The mere diagnosis of intracardiac thrombus by echocardiography does not necessarily mean that parts of it have embolized to the brain, or will do so

---

* Uncertain causes.

in the future. Such thrombus may be a coincidence in a patient who has both coronary atheroma and atheroma affecting the arteries to the brain. Stroke complicates less than 5% of all acute myocardial infarcts and yet left ventricular thrombus is present in at least 20%.

• Lack of demonstrable intracardiac thrombus does not exclude embolism to the brain; there may be no thrombus left, or what is left may be too small to be imaged.

Cardiac surgery

Cardiac surgery causes perioperative stroke and symptomatic retinal infarction in 1–5% of cases. More common is postoperative confusion and drowsiness for a few days and subtle cognitive defects, most, but not all, of which resolve in a few weeks. These complications are more likely with increasing age, longer operation times, and in patients with widespread atheromatous disease. The possible causes are:

• macro- and micro-embolization of atheromatous and cholesterol debris from the aorta
• platelet aggregates, fibrin fragments and non-organic debris from the tubing used for cardiac bypass
• hypotension with cerebral hypoperfusion during cardiac bypass
• hypoxia during and after surgery
• aortic dissection during surgery
• air embolization during surgery
• intracranial haemorrhage due to anticoagulation

Clinical features and differential diagnosis

Transient ischaemic attacks

Transient ischaemic attacks (TIAs) start suddenly. All the symptoms start more or less together and are maximal within seconds; there is no gradual build-up or spread of symptoms as occurs during the aura of migraine (cf. transient migrainous accompaniments, p. 138). Headache at the onset is uncommon and never severe; not surprisingly, tension-type headaches are frequent. Most attacks gradually resolve in a few minutes or an hour or so but, by definition, some last up to 24 hours. After symptomatic recovery, a few non-functionally significant signs may be found (e.g. reflex asymmetry, extensor plantar responses) and even evidence of focal infarction on CT.

The attacks may be single or repetitive up to many times in a day. Sometimes they are remarkably stereotyped. In most cases no clear precipitant can be identified. Rarely attacks occur as a result of sudden hypotension (p. 216) or compression of the vertebral arteries during neck turning in the presence of cervical spondylosis (p. 328); however, in both cases atheromatous stenosis or occlusion is usually present in the sympto-matic artery and/or the collateral supply to the brain.

The pattern of symptoms depends on which part of the brain or eye is affected by ischaemia, and that depends on which arteries are occluded.

The *internal carotid artery* (Fig. 8.1) arises at the common carotid bifurcation in the neck and supplies the eye (via the ophthalmic artery), the anterior two thirds of the cerebral hemispheres (via the anterior and middle cerebral arteries) and the anterior part of the basal ganglia region (via the lenticulostriate penetrating arteries and the anterior choroidal artery). Ischae-mic symptoms therefore include:

• transient ipsilateral monocular visual loss (amaurosis fugax, p. 222)
• language disturbance (dysphasia, dysgraphia, dyslexia, p. 23) if dominant hemisphere
• contralateral motor and/or sensory loss involving some or all parts of the face, upper and lower limbs. Any dysarthria is in proportion to facial weakness

The *two vertebral arteries* (Fig. 8.1) arise from the subclavian arteries, unite to form the basilar artery (whose branches supply the brainstem and cerebellum), which divides into the two posterior cerebral arteries which supply the posterior part of the cerebral hemispheres and posterior part of the basal ganglia and thalamus region. Ischaemic symptoms therefore include:

• unilateral or bilateral motor and/or sensory loss involving some or all parts of the face, upper and lower limbs. Crossed sensory disturbance of one side of the face and the opposite limbs due to medullary ischaemia is very unusual
• homonymous hemianopia (p. 169)
• sudden blindness in both eyes *
• cortical blindness (p. 169)
• dysarthria (which must not be confused with dysphasia) (p. 24)
• dysphagia (p. 197)
• diplopia† (p. 181)
• vertigo†, nausea, imbalance

Note: It is not possible to distinguish carotid from vertebrobasilar ischaemia if there are *only* unilateral motor and/or sensory symptoms although such attacks are usually assumed to be 'carotid'.

Note: Ischaemic symptoms are usually 'negative' and reflect *loss* of function (e.g. weakness, numbness, clumsiness, blindness) whereas epileptic and

---

* In adolescence, acute transient bilateral loss of vision is usually benign.
† If these symptoms are *isolated*, then, although the attack may have been a TIA, other causes of diplopia (p. 181) and vertigo (p. 105) must be considered. Non-specific 'dizziness' on its own is *not* diagnostic of a vertebrobasilar TIA.

migrainous symptoms are usually 'positive' and reflect *excessive* function (e.g. jerking of a limb, visual scintillation). A Todd's paresis (p. 70) should be obvious from the history of a preceding seizure. During both focal seizures and ischaemia there can be tingling or even pain but in the former the symptoms spread along a limb and from one body part to another (p. 71), whereas in the latter they come on all at once. Transient speech arrest is usually epileptic (p. 72) rather than ischaemic and dysphasic speech is usually ischaemic.

Note: Impairment or loss of consciousness is *very* unusual in TIAs and if present suggests a non-focal neurological problem such as generalized seizure (p. 70), syncope (p. 100) or metabolic disturbance such as hypoglycaemia (p. 108).

Subclavian steal occurs as a result of occlusion or severe stenosis of the subclavian artery proximal to the origin of the vertebral artery so that vertebral blood flow may be reversed away from the brain, particularly during exercise of the ipsilateral arm which increases its blood flow. Although this haemodynamic situation is quite common, it rarely causes transient vertebrobasilar symptoms (e.g. vertigo, diplopia, bilateral blurring of vision) and probably never causes a brainstem stroke. There is an obvious difference in the radial pulses and the blood pressures between the two arms, and often a supraclavicular bruit over the stenosed subclavian artery.

Transient global amnesia (p. 159), confusional episodes (p. 161) and drop attacks (p. 222) are rarely due to cerebral ischaemia.

Transient focal neurological attacks can also be caused by:
- migraine (p. 137)
- partial seizures (p. 70)
- multiple sclerosis (p. 342), but usually not in the vascular age group
- intracranial mass lesions rarely, e.g. tumour (p. 266), chronic subdural haematoma (p. 235), giant aneurysm (p. 232). In these cases the symptoms often turn out, on reflection, to be due to partial seizures
- cerebral vascular malformations (p. 233) may cause TIA-like episodes, perhaps due to vascular steal or small haemorrhages. On the other hand, many such episodes may in fact be epileptic rather than ischaemic
- metabolic disturbances (e.g. hypoglycaemia, p. 108, hyponatraemia, p. 464) rarely cause focal symptoms. However, focal neurological attacks in treated diabetes should always arouse suspicion, especially if they are present on waking or occur before a meal or after exercise
- hypertensive encephalopathy (p. 214)
- severe anaemia (p. 460)
- peripheral nerve pressure or ischaemia
- psychogenic. Functional overbreathing usually causes bilateral sensory symptoms (p. 110), but occasionally the symptoms are unilateral which

causes diagnostic confusion. The context of the attack may help in the diagnosis. Hysteria and malingering are other possibilities

Transient monocular visual loss (amaurosis fugax) has several causes (p. 169). Retinal ischaemia causes *sudden* visual loss in the whole visual field, or just in the bottom or top half. Often it is described as though a blind or shutter has fallen over the eye. Normally it lasts no more than a few minutes. Attacks due to low flow may last longer; also, such attacks may cause bleaching of vision looking like a photographic negative, particularly when the patient moves from darkness into light.

Note: Unless the patient covers each eye to check, it can be very difficult in retrospect to distinguish between transient homonymous hemianopia and transient monocular visual loss.

Drop attacks

These are episodes which occur while walking and sometimes just standing. Without any warning, there is very sudden collapse to the ground without loss of consciousness. Apart from any injury, the patient is otherwise perfectly well and can stand up immediately and carry on walking. The attacks may be isolated or recurrent on a number of occasions and tend to occur in middle-aged and elderly women.

Retinal migraine

Retinal migraine is an uncertain entity. The diagnosis tends to be made in young adults with episodes of transient monocular visual loss developing over minutes and lasting for up to half an hour. Often blindness is incomplete and there may be 'positive' visual symptoms such as stars, shimmering, etc. If headache occurs subsequently, as in the usual types of migraine (p. 137), the diagnosis of retinal migraine is more secure.

Cerebral infarction

The onset is almost always sudden or the patient wakes with a focal neurological deficit consistent with a lesion somewhere in the brain (the main clinical syndromes are described on p. 237). The deficit is at its maximum in minutes or an hour or so, although occasionally it increases in one or more definite 'steps', so-called 'stroke-in-evolution'. In rare cases stroke onset is slowly progressive over days or weeks; usually this is due to very low focal cerebral blood flow (e.g. as a result of internal carotid artery occlusion and poor collateral flow). Headache at onset is quite common but usually rather modest.

Deterioration in neurological function after the onset may be due to:

Neurological causes:
- propagating thrombosis
- recurrent embolization
- haemorrhagic transformation tends to occur in large infarcts and increases any mass effect though sometimes there are no clinical consequences. This is probably due to blood flowing under systemic pressure back into an area of ischaemic brain with disrupted microvasculature, or due to the use of antihaemostatic drugs. It is said to be a particular consequence of embolic arterial occlusion when the embolus is lysed by the natural fibrinolytic processes in the arterial wall
- cerebral oedema (p. 263) which causes further reduction in local cerebral blood flow, mass effect, brain shift, increasing intracranial pressure and transtentorial herniation. Cerebral oedema begins to develop a day or two after infarction and is maximal on the third to fifth day
- seizures
- obstructive hydrocephalus (cerebellar infarction, below)

General causes:
- hypoxia (pneumonia, inhalation, pulmonary embolism, cardiac failure)
- hypotension (hypotensive drugs, cardiac failure, pulmonary embolism, pneumonia, dehydration, septicaemia)
- cardiac failure (pulmonary embolism, myocardial infarction, cardiac arrhythmias, neurogenic pulmonary oedema)
- septicaemia (pneumonia, urine infection, skin sepsis)
- water and electrolyte imbalance
- hyperglycaemia (usually due to the stress response, p. 246)
- depression
- drugs (sedatives, hypotensives, anticonvulsants, hypnotics)
- admission of elderly patients to hospital, particularly if demented

or, the diagnosis is incorrect and the patient has an expanding intracranial lesion (p. 236).

Commonly, the neurological deficit slightly worsens in the first day or two, usually for no obvious reason. Deciding exactly what has caused deterioration requires both a general medical evaluation (e.g. chest examination and X-ray, blood urea, electrolytes, etc.) *and* a careful consideration of the neurological situation for which CT scanning is usually necessary.

Cerebellar strokes

The clinical features of infarction and haemorrhage in the cerebellum are similar. Although less than 5% of all strokes are cerebellar, it is important to recognize them since surgery can be lifesaving.

The onset is sudden with vertigo, nausea and perhaps vomiting, imbalance and usually quite severe headache (cf. bacterial meningitis, p. 491, subarachnoid haemorrhage, p. 228). Ataxia of gait, ipsilateral limb ataxia, and perhaps dysarthria and nystagmus may be found. However, a lesion of any size rapidly obstructs the flow of CSF from the fourth ventricle to cause acute hydrocephalus, raised intracranial pressure, meningism and coma. At this stage any focal neurological signs reflect compression of the brainstem and are subtle: impaired horizontal gaze towards the side of the lesion, ipsilateral lower motor neurone facial weakness, abnormal breathing pattern, bilateral extensor plantar responses. Limb weakness and sensory loss are usually mild or absent and cerebellar signs cannot be evaluated because of the depressed conscious level. Death may occur in hours or days of the onset but recovery can sometimes be very good. Some patients present with merely vertigo, some imbalance, and no obvious brainstem or cerebellar signs (cf. 'viral' labyrinthitis, p. 106).

Diagnosis is by CT scan to show intracerebellar haemorrhage or infarction. However, early after an infarct there may merely be compression and shift of the fourth ventricle due to oedema along with hydrocephalus, or the scan can be normal and the lesion visible only on MRI. Lumbar puncture is contraindicated for fear of causing tonsillar coning.

In severe or deteriorating cases, the treatment is urgent lateral ventricular drainage and/or removal of the haemorrhage or infarct, often with a good functional outcome.

Intracranial venous thrombosis

Thrombosis of the dural sinuses and/or cerebral and cortical veins is rare. It may be due to the following:

Local conditions affecting the veins and sinuses directly:
- head injury
- intracranial surgery
- local sepsis (sinuses, ears, mastoids, scalp, nasopharynx)
- bacterial meningitis (p. 491)
- subdural empyema (p. 503)
- meningovascular syphilis (p. 515)
- tumour invasion of dural sinuses
- catheterization of jugular veins for parenteral nutrition, etc.

Systemic disorders:
- dehydration, hypernatraemia
- septicaemia
- pregnancy and the puerperium
- oral contraceptives
- blood disorders (p. 210)
- 'hyperviscosity' syndrome (p. 461)

- inflammatory arterial diseases (p. 209)
- diabetes mellitus (p. 453)
- congestive cardiac failure
- inflammatory bowel disease (p. 463)
- androgen therapy
- non-metastatic effect of extracranial malignancy, perhaps due to 'hyper-coagulability'

The clinical syndromes occur in isolation or combination:

Sagittal and/or transverse sinus thrombosis

This is one cause of 'benign' intracranial hypertension (p. 264) and presents with headache along with papilloedema and obscurations of vision. It may be suspected on an unenhanced CT scan if the straight and other sinuses appear prominent and even more so if, after intravenous enhancement, there is an avascular gap at the confluence of the superior sagittal and transverse sinus (empty delta sign). MRI is even more sensitive.

Cortical venous thrombosis

This usually causes a subacute and generalized encephalopathic illness rather than stroke or TIA-like syndromes. There is headache, confusion, drowsiness, partial and generalized seizures, raised intracranial pressure, and coma with or without focal neurological signs. Widespread venous infarcts and haemorrhages are usually visible on CT. The CSF is normal or contains a modest excess of lymphocytes, polymorph neutrophils, red blood cells and protein. The differential diagnosis is encephalitis (p. 498), severe bacterial meningitis (p. 491), subarachnoid haemorrhage (p. 228), subdural empyema (p. 503) and cerebral abscess (p. 503).

Cavernous sinus thrombosis (p. 188)

Treatment

Anticoagulation is worth trying for patients with dural sinus thrombosis and 'benign' intracranial hypertension, and may be helpful for cortical venous thrombosis even in the presence of haemorrhagic infarction. Any underlying cause should be treated if possible.

Intracranial haemorrhage

Spontaneous intracranial haemorrhage may occur mainly into the subarach-noid space over the surface of the brain (subarachnoid haemorrhage, SAH), mainly within the brain (primary intracerebral haemorrhage, PICH), into the ventricles (ventricular haemorrhage) or into the subdural space (subdural haematoma). The clinical, CT, and even pathological distinction is not always easy since a PICH may rupture onto the surface of the brain or into the ventricles, and a saccular aneurysm may rupture into the brain as well as into the subarachnoid space.

Causes of intracranial haemorrhage

- hypertension (the most common cause of PICH, p. 213)
- saccular aneurysm (the most common cause of SAH, p. 231)
- vascular malformation (p. 233)
- atheromatous aneurysm (p. 212)
- congophilic angiopathy (p. 474)
- haemostatic failure (p. 462), e.g. haemophilia, thrombocytopenia, anti-coagulation, aspirin, streptokinase, polycythaemia rubra vera
- disseminated intravascular coagulation (p. 462)
- sickle cell disease/trait (p. 460)
- inflammatory arterial disease (p. 209)
- mycotic aneurysm (p. 232)
- cortical venous thrombosis (p. 225)
- vascular tumours, e.g. malignant astrocytoma (p. 271), oligodendroglioma (p. 272), medulloblastoma (p. 273), haemangioblastoma (p. 272), melanoma, hypernephroma, choriocarcinoma, endometrial carcinoma
- hereditary haemorrhagic telangiectasia (p. 234)
- moyamoya syndrome (p. 215)
- oral contraceptives (p. 216)
- drugs which increase blood pressure, e.g. amphetamines (p. 551), cocaine (p. 551), monoamineoxidase A inhibitors, sympathomimetics (p. 294)
- snake bite (p. 551)
- asparaginase

Note: The CSF may contain red blood cells in encephalitis (p. 498) and anthrax meningitis (p. 511).

A head injury, even without visible scalp trauma, can cause intracranial haemorrhage which may be thought 'spontaneous' if the injury is unwitnessed. Also, there may be diagnostic difficulty if at the onset of a stroke the patient falls, sustains a head injury, and on CT an intracranial haemorrhage is found.

Even after angiography of both carotid and vertebral arteries, no definite cause for bleeding is found in about 15% of SAH cases, and in a large proportion of patients with PICH.

Familial causes of intracranial haemorrhage

- haemophilia and other inherited coagulation and platelet disorders (p. 462)
- sickle cell disease/trait (p. 460)
- saccular aneurysm sometimes (p. 231)
- vascular malformations sometimes (p. 233)
- hereditary haemorrhagic telangiectasia (p. 234)
- congophilic angiopathy (Iceland and Holland) (p. 474)
- von Hippel–Lindau syndrome (p. 202)
- Ehlers–Danlos syndrome (p. 484)
- pseudoxanthoma elasticum (p. 484)

Causes of multiple intracerebral haemorrhages

- congophilic angiopathy (p. 474)
- metastases (p. 276)
- haemostatic defect (p. 462)
- cortical venous thrombosis (p. 225)
- inflammatory arterial disease (p. 209)
- malignant hypertension (p. 214)
- multiple haemorrhagic infarcts (usually embolic) (p. 223)
- head injury

Primary intracerebral haemorrhage

Clinical features

Usually primary intracerebral haemorrhage (PICH) is not distinguishable from stroke due to cerebral infarction on clinical grounds alone. In a patient with a clinically definite stroke, it is best first to delineate the stroke syndrome and site of the lesion on clinical grounds (p. 237), and then do a CT scan which will reliably diagnose PICH (p. 239). PICH *must* be excluded by CT before starting anticoagulants and perhaps even aspirin.

The site of an intracerebral haemorrhage may suggest its cause. Hypertensive PICH tends to occur in the basal ganglia region, thalamus, brainstem and cerebellum. Other disorders cause PICH not just in these areas but also peripherally in the cerebral hemispheres (lobar haemorrhage).

Outcome and treatment

About 50% of patients die within the first month, usually in the first week as a consequence of supratentorial haemorrhage large enough to cause transtentorial herniation, or haemorrhage in the posterior fossa (see cerebellar stroke,

p. 223). About 50% of the survivors remain dependent; small and even medium-sized haemorrhages may cause remarkably little residual disability.

Early deterioration in the first week or so may be due to the same general causes as after cerebral infarction (p. 223) and neurological causes including:

- recurrent haemorrhage
- hydrocephalus if blood has entered the CSF (see SAH, p. 229) or if haematoma in the cerebellum or brainstem obstructs CSF flow down the aqueduct and out of the fourth ventricle
- cerebral oedema causing local cerebral ischaemia, raised intracranial pressure, brain shift and transtentorial herniation
- seizures

The *treatment* is:

- general support for the stroke patient (p. 245)
- stop any antihaemostatic drugs
- ventricular drain if symptomatic hydrocephalus occurs
- operative removal of a superficial haematoma which is causing progressive impairment of consciousness and/or neurological deterioration in a patient who might otherwise recover (e.g. haemorrhage in the frontal lobe, cerebellum, etc.)
- prevention of recurrence which depends on the cause (p. 226), particularly the treatment of saccular aneurysms (p. 231), vascular malformations (p. 231) and hypertension (p. 252)

Spontaneous subarachnoid haemorrhage

Clinical features

Sometimes spontaneous subarachnoid haemorrhage (SAH) is obviously precipitated by activities which raise the blood pressure: heavy exertion, defaecation, lifting, sexual intercourse, etc. Otherwise, onset is spontaneous but rarely during sleep. There is *sudden* headache which is usually, but not always, severe. At first the pain may be localized, often in the occipital area, and later becomes generalized and spreads down the back, or it is generalized from onset. In severe cases coma and death occur within minutes; SAH is the only type of stroke which can cause death within an hour or so (i.e. 'sudden death'). In milder cases there is no loss of consciousness but merely drowsiness, or the patient can be completely alert. Irritability, nausea, vomiting, photophobia, confusion and sometimes seizures may develop in the first few hours. Meningism (p. 492) develops within 6 hours or so but can be absent in deep coma. Subhyaloid haemorrhages may be seen in the eye and are probably due to the sudden increase in intracranial pressure.

Focal neurological signs (e.g. hemiparesis, dysphasia, etc.) occur at onset if there is intracerebral as well as subarachnoid bleeding. Bilateral extensor plantar responses are common. A ruptured (or unruptured) posterior communicating/distal internal carotid artery aneurysm may cause an ipsilateral third cranial nerve palsy. The headache usually resolves within a week or two, occasionally longer.

The *differential diagnosis* is:

- bacterial meningitis (p. 491)
- cerebellar stroke (p. 223)
- benign orgasmic cephalgia (p. 143)
- thunderclap headache (p. 144)
- migraine (p. 137)
- acute painful neck conditions

Subarachnoid haemorrhage may be complicated by:

- Hydrocephalus due to blood clot, and later fibrosis, obstructing CSF flow. This may occur at or near onset or within a few days. It can be asymptomatic or cause increasing intracranial pressure and deteriorating conscious level. Hydrocephalus may develop months or even years after SAH and is one cause of 'normal' pressure hydrocephalus (p. 262).
- Any intracerebral haemorrhage, with or without brain shift, is usually present fairly soon after the onset. This commonly occurs with bleeding from a vascular malformation and may occur after aneurysmal rupture, e.g. a middle cerebral artery aneurysm can rupture into the temproal lobe and an anterior communicating artery aneurysm into the frontal lobe.
- Focal cerebral ischaemia. After severe SAH (usually due to rupture of an aneurysm rather than a vascular malformation) with a large amount of blood in the subarachnoid space, focal ischaemia may occur with narrowing of the cerebral arteries (so-called vasospasm which usually affects the aneurysm-bearing artery but can be more widespread). Increasing drowsiness and focal neurological signs develop 2–10 days after SAH onset. The cerebral oedema and transtentorial herniation can be fatal but recovery may occur in a matter of weeks.
- Rebleeding from an aneurysm is most likely within the first 2 weeks of rupture, perhaps in 20% of cases. In the acute stage rebleeding is far less likely with a vascular malformation.
- Seizures at onset, or later, particularly if there has been intracerebral haemorrhage.
- General complications of stroke (p. 246).

Diagnosis

The sudden onset of headache is characteristic and with the rapid development of meningism the diagnosis is usually obvious. However, to confirm the presence of blood in the CSF around the cerebral hemispheres and brainstem, or in the ventricles, a CT scan must be performed urgently. This will not only confirm SAH but also:

- demonstrate any haematoma in the brain, ventricles or subdural space
- demonstrate any hydrocephalus
- demonstrate cerebral oedema
- suggest from where the bleeding has originated. This is particularly useful if later more than one aneurysm is shown by angiography
- after enhancement with i.v. contrast, large aneurysms or vascular malformations may be shown; this is unnecessary if angiography is going to be required later

However, if the CT scan is negative (usually because the SAH is mild or the scan has been done more than a few days after onset) or not *quickly* available (within an hour or so), a lumbar puncture *must* be performed, mainly to exclude bacterial meningitis but also to confirm blood in the CSF. Xanthochromia (p. 42) usually appears within a few hours of bleeding and persists for a week or two. It is demonstrated in the supernatant after spinning the CSF or allowing it to stand for an hour. If it cannot be seen with the naked eye, then spectrophotometry is more sensitive. The CSF glucose is normal or slightly reduced and there is often a modest increase in lymphocytes and polymorph neutrophils.

Note: Just occasionally blood does not reach the lumbar CSF until a few hours after onset of SAH, or there is even no blood staining at all either because the haemorrhage has been minor or because of impaction of the brain at the foramen magnum.

Note: Three specimens of CSF *must* be taken to differentiate SAH from a 'traumatic tap' (p. 42).

Outcome and treatment

After aneurysmal SAH about 25% of patients die in the first 48 hours and another 25% within the next month. Survivors can recover completely but many are left with focal neurological deficits, seizures, poor memory, behavioural disturbances, anxiety and depression. Early mortality and later morbidity is less with vascular malformations.

The general measures for stroke are required (p. 245). It is important to relieve headache with adequate analgesia (but not with aspirin which may promote bleeding) particularly because the pain may be responsible for restlessness and an increase in blood pressure. Extremely raised blood pressure should be carefully controlled (see p. 249). Normally patients are kept in bed until either the headache resolves or the ruptured blood vessel has been dealt with surgically.

Nimodipine should be given routinely to reduce the risk of 'vasospasm' and cerebral infarction: oral, or by nasogastric tube, 60 mg 4-hourly for up to about 21 days, provided the blood pressure does not fall excessively. Other adverse effects: flushing, headache, nausea.

The main concern is to prevent rebleeding, particularly in the first few weeks (see p. 229), and in the long-term. The approximate risk of long-term rebleeding is about 3% per annum for both ruptured saccular aneurysms and ruptured arteriovenous malformations. After subarachnoid haemorrhage of unknown cause (i.e. cerebral angiography is normal), not only is the early mortality low but the risk of rebleeding is extremely small.

Whether an aneurysm can be clipped, or a vascular malformation removed, is a technical neurosurgical decision. On the whole, the sooner the patient is operated on the better, provided the operative risks are acceptably low. In practice, conscious patients with no focal deficits have a low operative risk and can be operated on within 48 hours of SAH onset, which is usually before any focal ischaemia has developed, to reduce the risk of early, as well as late, rebleeding. Otherwise, surgery is normally delayed until the patient is in a good neurological and general condition, perhaps 1 or 2 weeks after SAH onset.

Surgery may be required to relieve symptomatic hydrocephalus or to remove a localized haematoma if it is causing an increasing focal neurological deficit or progressive decline in conscious level.

Inoperable vascular malformations (usually because they are too large or within very sensitive brain areas) sometimes may be embolized or treated with radiotherapy.

Note: Angiography to demonstrate the source of bleeding need not be performed until just before surgery is planned. It should include intracranial views of both carotid and both vertebral artery systems even if an aneurysm or vascular malformation is found after one vessel is injected, in case there are multiple aneurysms, or a vascular malformation is supplied from more than one arterial source.

Note: Even an unconscious patient *may* have a remedial cause of coma, e.g. acute hydrocephalus, lobar haematoma, hyponatraemia, hypotension.

Intracranial saccular aneurysms

Saccular aneurysms arise at points of arterial branching in the Circle of Willis and proximal parts of the main intracranial arteries at the base of the brain. They vary from a few mm to several cm in diameter. About 35% occur on the anterior communicating artery complex, 30% on the posterior communicating artery or distal internal carotid artery, 30% on the middle cerebral artery, and about 5% in the posterior circulation. Aneurysms are multiple in about 25% of cases. They are an incidental postmortem finding in 2%. Many aneurysms are thought to be congenital but some are acquired as a result of hypertension and atheroma. They are more common in smokers. Clearly some, but not all, enlarge with time.

Clinical features

• Rupture to cause SAH (p. 228), PICH (p. 227) or both is by far the most common presentation. Occasionally they rupture into the subdural space.

• Pressure on cranial nerves, e.g. 3rd from a posterior communicating/distal internal carotid artery aneurysm which usually causes pain behind the eye and involves the pupil (p. 182); optic nerve from anterior communicating artery complex aneurysm; optic chiasm (p. 168) along with 3rd, 4th, 5th, and 6th cranial nerves from a distal internal carotid artery aneurysm (cf. pituitary adenoma, p. 273); brainstem and lower cranial nerves from a basilar aneurysm. The neurological deficit develops over days, weeks or months and relapses and remissions can occur.

• Presentation as a mass lesion with a focal cerebral deficit is unusual.

• Seizures are unusual if the aneurysm is unruptured.

• Hydrocephalus occasionally occurs if an unruptured aneurysm obstructs the flow of CSF (e.g. basilar aneurysm).

• Embolization from thrombus in the aneurysmal sac to cause a TIA or cerebral infarct more distally is very unusual.

• Carotico-cavernous fistula (p. 189) from rupture of a distal internal carotid artery aneurysm within the cavernous sinus.

Note: Saccular aneurysms may be associated with:
• polycystic kidneys*
• fibromuscular dysplasia of the carotid and other arteries (p. 215)
• coarctation of the aorta
• Ehlers–Danlos syndrome* (p. 484)
• pseudoxanthoma elasticum* (p. 484)
• Marfan's syndrome* (p. 484)
• hereditary haemorrhagic telangiectasia* (p. 234)
• moyamoya syndrome (p. 215)
• progeria
• Klinefelter's syndrome

Mycotic aneurysms

These are rare. One or more develop on peripheral as well as proximal branches of cerebral arteries as a result of septic emboli during the course, or within a few weeks, of infective endocarditis; other causes are septicaemia, particularly fungal; and occasionally due to tumour emboli. Many remain asymptomatic and probably disappear but others rupture into the brain, subdural or subarachnoid space.

* Familial cases likely.

Vascular malformations

Arteriovenous malformations (AVM)

These are the most common. They are probably congenital, sometimes familial, and occasionally due to head trauma. They consist of an abnormal fistulous connection between one or more hypertrophied feeding arteries and dilated draining veins. The fistulae may vary from a few mm to several cm in diameter and most probably grow during life; a few shrink or disappear, perhaps as a consequence of haemorrhage. They occur in or on the brain (or spinal cord, p. 336) and in the dura.

Presentation is with some combination of:
- partial or secondary generalized seizures (p. 69)
- primary intracerebral haemorrhage (p. 227)
- spontaneous subarachnoid haemorrhage (10% of SAH cases) (p. 228)
- hydrocephalus (post SAH, or as a result of obstruction to CSF flow)
- as a mass lesion causing a progressive focal neurological deficit is rare, or as an orbital tumour (p. 174)
- intermittent focal symptoms, often with a brainstem AVM, may be mistaken for TIAs or even multiple sclerosis; these symptoms may be due to vascular steal or microhaemorrhage
- audible bruit to the patient (see also p. 193), particularly with a dural AVM
- carotico-cavernous fistula (ruptured dural AVM) (p. 189)
- high output cardiac failure in neonates and infants

Non-specific headaches and migraine are common features but not to the extent that an AVM should be suspected unless there are *additional* features (e.g. cranial bruit, seizures, focal deficit).

AVMs may be suspected clinically if the following conditions prevail:
- cranial (orbits, skull) or carotid bruit in patients presenting with intra-cranial haemorrhage, headache or seizures
- subarachnoid haemorrhage with past history of seizures
- known saccular aneurysm or hereditary haemorrhagic telangiectasia

Venous malformations

These consist of a collection of venous channels of various sizes. They usually present with low pressure haemorrhage into the ventricles or the brain (such haemorrhages are therefore small and carry little morbidity).

Cavernous malformations

These are sharply circumscribed lesions of varying size consisting of collections of thin-walled sinusoidal vessels. They may be familial and are quite often multiple. They usually present with partial or secondary generalized seizures. Low pressure intracerebral haemorrhage is unusual.

Telangiectases

Telangiectases are collections of dilated capillaries which usually have no clinical significance (see hereditary haemorrhagic telangiectasia, below).

Diagnosis

The definitive investigation is intra-arterial cerebral angiography but this may be negative if the vascular malformation is very small (e.g. cavernous malformation), has been destroyed by haemorrhage, or possibly early after rupture when the vascular malformation may be compressed by the haemorrhage. MRI is more sensitive for cavernous malformations. CT may reveal some lesions, particularly with i.v. contrast enhancement to show the dilated and abnormal vessels. Calcification is quite common.

However, all forms of imaging may fail to show small vascular malformations.

Sturge–Weber syndrome

This is a rare, congenital and sporadic condition affecting males and females equally. At birth there is a cutaneous capillary angioma (port wine stain) somewhere on the face. It is usually unilateral but can be asymmetrically bilateral. There may be associated ipsilateral glaucoma, choroidal angioma and hypertrophy of the face. In addition, there is meningeal angiomatosis, usually ipsilateral to the skin lesion, with underlying atrophy and calcification of the cerebral cortex (this is best shown on CT, skull X-ray merely showing 'tramline' calcification).

Apart from the cosmetic issue, the main problem is partial and secondary generalized seizures due to the cortical pathology. Seizures may be easy to control, or intractable with a progressive neurological deficit causing hemiparesis and mental retardation.

Note: Isolated facial port wine stains without neurological complications occur in 1 per 5000 births.

Hereditary haemorrhagic telangiectasia (Osler–Rendu–Weber syndrome)

This is an autosomal dominant condition of multiple cutaneous, mucosal and visceral telangiectases (particularly in the nose, pharynx and gut) causing recurrent bleeding. Neurological complications are unusual.
• Pulmonary arteriovenous malformation usually has a right to left shunt

and so allows parodoxical embolism to the brain and cerebral abscess (p. 503), and can lead to polycythaemia (p. 458) and cerebral hypoxia.

- Intracranial arteriovenous malformation (p. 233).
- Spinal arteriovenous malformation (p. 336).
- Intracranial saccular aneurysm (p. 231).
- Hepatic encephalopathy (p. 467).
- Cerebral and spinal telangiectases are usually asymptomatic.

Chronic subdural haematoma

Immediately after head injury there may be haemorrhage into the subdural space and the cause is obvious. Acute subdural haematoma may also be caused by rupture of a saccular or mycotic aneurysm, vascular tumour and ventricular decompression for hydrocephalus. Of more diagnostic concern is the slow development, over some weeks or months, of a collection of altered blood and fluid in the subdural space, usually supratentorial rather than in the posterior fossa, which causes compression of the underlying brain and increasing intracranial pressure, leading to transtentorial herniation. Chronic subdural haematomas can be bilateral.

Clinical features

About 50% recall a head injury which may however have been mild. Most patients are elderly. The onset is usually gradual over weeks and symptoms tend to fluctuate with headache, mild focal neurological signs (hemiparesis, aphasia, etc.) and eventually raised intracranial pressure which may be manifest merely by drowsiness and confusion rather than by obvious signs such as papilloedema. Seizures are rare. Occasionally there may be only subacute dementia or a confusional state, but usually there is some additional focal feature, drowsiness, or fluctuation of the dementing state.

Diagnosis

Diagnosis is made by CT scan which shows brain shift (unless the haematomas are bilateral) and a thin rim of hyper- or hypodensity over the cerebral hemisphere. On occasion the subdural haematoma is isodense with brain and the only sign may be the brain shift, or effacement of the underlying cortical sulci. Intravenous contrast enhancement, and even carotid angiography with oblique views, may be needed to demonstrate the thin rim of avascular haematoma below the skull.

Treatment

Treatment is usually to drain the subdural collection, although in mild cases the haematoma may disappear spontaneously and only observation is required until it does.

Diagnosis and investigation of stroke

The questions to be answered are:
- Is it a stroke or something else? (p. 236)
- Where is the stroke lesion? (p. 237)
- If it is a stroke, is it due to primary intracerebral haemorrhage, cerebral infarction or subarachnoid haemorrhage? (p. 239)
- If it is a cerebral infarct (or TIA), what is the cause? (p. 208)
- If it is a primary intracerebral haemorrhage, what is the cause? (p. 226)
- If it is a subarachnoid haemorrhage, what is the cause? (p. 226)

How far attempts are made to answer these questions depends on how much the patient's management will be affected, i.e. it depends on the patient's age, previous disability and the severity of the stroke.

Stroke versus not-stroke?

The differentiation of stroke from something else is usually straightforward if a clear history is available. There is almost nothing else which causes a *sudden* disturbance of focal brain dysfunction and which persists for more than a few hours (for *transient* focal neurological attacks, see p. 221). Strokes may occasionally be confused with:
- intracranial tumour (p. 266). A sudden onset is rare but can occur as a result of haemorrhage within the tumour (p. 268). Partial seizures, perhaps with a Todd's paresis (p. 70), are seldom confused with stroke
- chronic subdural haematoma (p. 235). The focal signs are usually rather mild by comparison with depression of consciousness and confusion; a severe focal neurological deficit in an alert patient is most unusual. The signs often fluctuate and may be accompanied by headache
- encephalitis (p. 499) seldom causes a focal neurological deficit, and even when it does the patient is usually drowsy or unconscious, febrile and has a progressive history associated with malaise, meningism and seizures
- occasionally head injury is occult and confused with stroke, particularly when the stroke is due to intracranial haemorrhage (p. 226)
- multiple sclerosis (p. 342) presents in younger patients but sometimes has a fairly abrupt onset and, like stroke, recurs with clinical evidence of several brain lesions which, on both CT and MRI, may appear like infarcts
- hypoglycaemia (p. 108) may cause focal symptoms, even without adrenergic features such as sweating and tachycardia
- cerebral abscess (p. 503) causes more systemic upset than stroke (malaise, fever, neutrophil leucocytosis) and patients seldom present suddenly
- peripheral nerve lesions (Chapter 14) may occasionally be confused with stroke if they start suddenly but the signs are different from those of a cerebral lesion
- hysteria or malingering (p. 38) is only likely to be a diagnostic problem in young 'stroke' patients

Coma soon after onset is most unusual in stroke unless there is:
• subarachnoid haemorrhage
• intracerebral haemorrhage, but only if it is large or in the cerebellum or brainstem
• large cerebral infarct, but coma does not usually occur on the day of onset

Therefore, stroke seldom enters into the differential diagnosis of coma (p. 122), particularly if there are no focal neurological symptoms or signs to suggest a focal brain lesion.

Where is the stroke lesion?

The clinical features of subarachnoid haemorrhage are distinctive and described on p. 228. The site of a cerebral infarct or primary intracerebral haemorrhage is deduced in the normal way for localizing neurological lesions (see Chapter 1) although this can be difficult if there is a residual deficit from a previous stroke. There is a definite advantage in defining the main *clinical syndromes* since their prognoses are certainly different (Table 8.1) and their underlying causes may be. To define the syndromes accurately, it is important to have a clear history and to examine the patient shortly after the stroke before any signs have resolved.

Total anterior circulation syndrome

There is weakness with or without sensory impairment of the whole of one side of the body including the face; homonymous hemianopia; and a focal cognitive deficit (i.e. language disturbance or neglect if the dominant

Table 8.1 Approximate outcome after first ever stroke

	% dead at one month	% dead at 6 months	% dead or dependent at 6 months	% of survivors dependent at 6 months
All cases	20	25	55	40
Cerebral infarction	10	20	50	40
Primary intracerebral haemorrhage	50	60	80	50
Subarachnoid haemorrhage	50	50	65	30
Total anterior circulation infarction (p. 237)	40	50	95	90
Partial anterior circulation infarction (p. 238)	5	10	45	40
Lacunar infarction (p. 238)	2	10	35	30
Posterior circulation infarction (p. 239)	5	15	30	20

hemisphere is affected, and visuospatial disturbance or neglect if the non-dominant hemisphere is). Transient dysarthria and dysphagia are common, usually in proportion to any facial or palatal weakness. Such a large clinical deficit must be due to a large cerebral hemisphere haemorrhage, or occlusion of the internal carotid artery or middle cerebral artery origin to cause a large infarct in the cerebral hemisphere (this is usually the result of thrombosis or embolism complicating atheroma in the large neck arteries, or embolism from the heart). The patient is likely to be drowsy within hours of the onset and it is this clinical type of stroke (whether haemorrhagic or occlusive) which may progress to transtentorial herniation, brainstem compression and death.

Partial anterior circulation syndrome

There are only two of the three main components of the total syndrome present, or an isolated focal cognitive deficit, or an isolated but predominantly proprioceptive sensory deficit. The motor and/or sensory deficit may be restricted to one limb, or even one hand and one or two fingers, depending on the site of the lesion which almost always involves the cerebral cortex but is not large enough to cause the total anterior circulation syndrome. This partial syndrome is due either to a lobar haemorrhage or an infarct caused by occlusion, usually embolic, of a branch of the middle or anterior cerebral artery, or boundary zone infarction (p. 217).

Lacunar syndromes

These reflect small lesions (infarction much more often than haemorrhage) deep in the basal ganglia region, internal capsule, thalamus, cerebral peduncle or pons, usually as a consequence of disease of the small penetrating arteries (p. 213). These arteries do not very often seem to be occluded by embolism from either the heart or extracranial atherothrombosis. In all cases the patient is alert and has neither a hemianopia nor cognitive deficit. There are four main syndromes:

• Pure motor stroke is the most common with weakness of the whole of one side of the body including the face, or the upper and lower limbs, or the face and the upper limb. In addition there may be mild dysarthria and dysphagia with unilateral weakness of the palate.

• Pure sensory stroke. There is cutaneous sensory loss in the same distribution as a pure motor stroke above. Also joint position sense may be impaired but *isolated* joint position sense loss without disturbance of pain or light touch sensation is usually caused by a parietal cortical lesion and is a feature of the partial anterior circulation syndrome.

• Sensory-motor stroke is a combination of pure motor stroke and pure sensory stroke.

• Ataxic hemiparesis is the combination of hemiparesis and ipsilateral ataxia, often with marked clumsiness of the hand, dysarthria and imbalance.

Sudden hemichorea, hemiballismus (both of which may be caused by a lesion in the contralateral subthalamic nucleus) and 'thalamic' pain syndromes (p. 26) are probably all 'lacunar'.

Posterior circulation syndrome

This type is characterized by clearcut brainstem (p. 27) and/or cerebellar signs (p. 14) and/or a homonymous hemianopia or cortical blindness. If there is brainstem *and* occipital cortex involvement, the cause must be thrombotic or embolic occlusion of the basilar and posterior cerebral arteries. If only the brainstem, cerebellum or occipital cortex is involved, then the cause may be occlusive due to lipohyalinosis affecting the small vessels of the brainstem, atherothromboembolism in the basilar or posterior cerebral circulations, embolism from the heart, or due to primary intracerebral haemorrhage.

Is the stroke due to intracerebral haemorrhage or infarction?

The clinical picture of subarachnoid haemorrhage (p. 228) is usually distinct from intracerebral haemorrhage or infarction. However, a sudden lesion *in* the brain causes the same clinical deficit whether it is haemorrhagic or ischaemic. Occasionally one can be reasonably certain that a stroke is due to primary intracerebral haemorrhage if:
- coma occurs at onset or within a few hours
- *severe* headache occurs at or shortly after onset
- meningism, which is due to a large haematoma in the posterior fossa, or blood in the CSF from rupture of a PICH into the ventricles or onto the surface of the brain

A stroke following a series of TIAs is usually due to infarction but it *can* be due to haemorrhage, for example as a result of antithrombotic drugs.

Note: The lumbar CSF becomes blood stained after a PICH in less than 50% of cases.

Therefore, to distinguish PICH from cerebral infarction a CT scan must be performed within a week or two of onset (p. 242). MRI does not distinguish the two except days or weeks after onset. The differentiation of intracerebral haemorrhage from infarction is only required if this is likely to alter the management of the patient, e.g. if anticoagulants, aspirin, carotid endarterectomy, etc. are contemplated.

Once the main pathological type of stroke is known (i.e. PICH or cerebral infarction), the clinically defined stroke *syndromes* (p. 237) can be refined to 'total anterior circulation *infarction*' (or haemorrhage), 'partial anterior circulation *infarction*' (or haemorrhage), 'lacunar *infarction*' (or haemorrhage) and 'posterior circulation *infarction*' (or haemorrhage).

What is the cause of the stroke or transient ischaemic attack?

It is unusual for a stroke or TIA to occur in patients who do not already have known vascular risk factors (particularly hypertension or clinically evident ischaemic heart disease), a cardiac source of embolism, or a rare but quite easily diagnosable disorder (e.g. giant cell arteritis).

The nature of the onset and the clinical deficit does not normally give any more information than the fact that a stroke has occurred. Eliciting the cause depends on:

History

- past history of vascular disease (e.g. myocardial infarction, angina claudication, etc.) makes atheroma a likely cause
- recent history of neck trauma (p. 214)
- hypertension (p. 213)
- past history of epilepsy (vascular malformation)
- antihaemostatic drugs or a known coagulation defect
- malaise, loss of weight, etc. (inflammatory arterial disease)
- migraine (p. 215)
- pregnancy and oral contraceptives (p. 215)
- family history of stroke (pp. 211 and 227)

Examination

- Horner's syndrome due to carotid dissection is ipsilateral to a cerebral hemisphere lesion. It also occurs in a brainstem stroke (p. 178).
- Orbital or cranial bruit may be heard with a vascular malformation (p. 233).
- Cervical bruit (Fig. 8.3). The presence of a carotid arterial bruit more or less doubles the probability of greater than 50% stenosis of the origin of that artery. However, very tight carotid stenosis, or occlusion, may not be associated with a bruit and ulcerating non-stenotic (but still embologenic) lesions may have no associated bruit either. Therefore, the decision to angiogram a patient to show proximal internal carotid artery stenosis, which might be suitable for carotid endarterectomy (p. 253), depends less on the presence or absence of a bruit than on the symptoms (i.e. carotid ischaemia) and, if available, duplex ultrasound imaging (p. 244). Very few patients can hear their own carotid bifurcation bruit (see pulsatile tinnitus, p. 193).
- Extracranial pulses. An absent carotid pulse in the neck indicates common carotid occlusion, and an absent or delayed superficial temporal pulse indicates external carotid artery stenosis or occlusion.
- Atrial fibrillation, but this may occur coincidentally in primary intra-cerebral haemorrhage and in cerebral infarction due to atheroma of the neck or cerebral arteries; it does not necessarily indicate the cause of the stroke.
- Cardiac valvular disease or congenital heart disease.

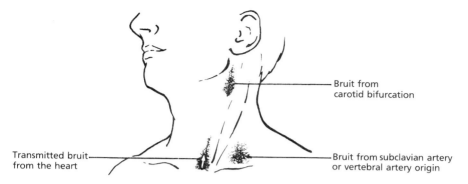

Fig. 8.3 Diagram to show the sites of maximal intensity of localized arterial bruits in the neck and diffuse bruits transmitted from the arch of aorta or the heart (e.g. from aortic stenosis). Diffuse neck bruits may also be due to increased blood flow, e.g. anaemia, hyperthyroidism, intracranial vascular malformation, occlusion of contralateral internal carotid artery, goitre and fever. Venous hums are low pitched and continuous roaring sounds heard in the supraclavicular fossa; they are abolished by light pressure over the jugular vein. In young adults bruits in the supraclavicular fossa are seldom of any significance.

- Blood pressure in both arms, unequal wrist pulses (subclavian stenosis or occlusion) and postural hypotension.
- Aortic aneurysm associated with ischaemic cerebrovascular disease.
- Peripheral vascular disease associated with ischaemic cerebrovascular disease.
- Retinal emboli (cholesterol, calcific, etc., p. 175).
- Skin (telangiectases, p. 234, pseudoxanthoma, p. 484, malignant atrophic papulosis, p. 450, Sneddon's syndrome, p. 446, etc.).

Note: There is no reliable clinical or angiographic way to differentiate infarction due to arterial thrombosis, embolism from the heart, or embolism from proximal arterial sites. The distinction is based on the balance of probabilities (see p. 218 for cardiac embolism). However, on balance, most infarcts causing a partial anterior circulation syndrome (p. 238) are embolic from the heart or proximal arteries rather than due to thrombus of intracranial arteries. Few lacunar infarcts are due to embolism from the heart or, probably, from atheromatous disease of the extracranial arteries.

Investigation

All stroke patients should have the following investigations:
- haemoglobin and haematocrit (? polycythaemia, anaemia, etc.)
- white blood cell count (? infective endocarditis, septicaemia, leukaemia)
- platelet count (? thrombocythaemia or thrombocytopenia)
- ESR (? inflammatory arterial disease, infective endocarditis, myeloma myxoma)

- blood glucose (? diabetes, hypoglycaemia)
- ECG (arrhythmia, recent myocardial infarction, left ventricular hypertrophy as a consequence of hypertension, etc.)
- urine examination (glycosuria, proteinuria, red blood cells, etc.)

The following investigations may also be indicated:
- urea and electrolytes in severe strokes (for fluid balance), if hypertensive, or on diuretics
- cardiac enzymes (? recent myocardial infarction)
- syphilis serology
- blood cholesterol
- coagulation screen (? haemostatic defect, lupus anticoagulant (p. 446), protein C or protein S deficiencies, etc.)
- platelet function tests
- anticardiolipin antibodies, anti-nuclear factor, DNA binding (? SLE)
- chest X-ray (cardiac source of embolism, ? hypertension, ? pulmonary arteriovenous malformation, baseline in severe stroke)
- skull X-ray gives no more information than the CT scan, usually a lot less
- sickle cell screen (in negroes only)
- liver function (? alcohol, ? inflammatory arterial disease)
- thyroid function (if in atrial fibrillation)
- protein electrophoresis (? myeloma)
- plasma and urine amino acids (? homocysteinaemia)
- temporal artery biopsy (? giant cell arteritis)
- muscle biopsy (? systemic vasculitis, mitochondrial cytopathy)
- blood culture (? infective endocarditis)
- venogram (? paradoxical embolism)

CT scan is particularly indicated:
- to exclude non-stroke intracranial pathology if the history is unclear or not characteristic for stroke, particularly if the patient continues to worsen (p. 223)
- to exclude primary intracerebral haemorrhage if:
  patient is on antihaemostatic drugs (e.g. warfarin, aspirin)
  patient may need to start antihaemostatic drugs (p. 253)
  mild carotid distribution stroke possibly suitable for carotid endarterectomy (p. 253)
- in cerebellar and brainstem strokes (in case surgery indicated, p. 223)
- in subarachnoid haemorrhage (p. 228)
- in carotid TIA patients to exclude a mass lesion (present in less than 5% of cases)
  Ideally all stroke and carotid TIA patients should have a CT scan.

After cerebral infarction the CT is normal for the first few hours and maybe even for a day or two. A vague low density area then appears in the infarcted area and gradually becomes more distinct over a few weeks. This hypodense area may disappear temporarily about 2–4 weeks after stroke onset (the 'fogging' effect), but usually at this stage enhancement with intravenous contrast is obvious. With a large oedematous infarct, the CT may show brain shift, haemorrhagic cerebral infarction, and later dilatation of the ipsilateral lateral ventricle due to loss of brain substance.

Note: i.v. contrast should *not* be routine and is seldom needed. It is said to make cerebral infarction worse. Contrast enhancement occurs from a few days to 3 or 4 weeks post-stroke.

Immediately after primary intracerebral haemorrhage the CT shows a high density area, usually well demarcated, sometimes surrounded by a low density halo. If large, there is mass effect with brain shift and perhaps obstructive hydrocephalus. Also there may be blood in the ventricles and over the surface of the brain. The hyperdensity gradually fades and the scan becomes normal, or a low density area appears where the haematoma was and this may be indistinguishable from an old cerebral infarct. As the haematoma disappears it may take on a ring-like appearance, particularly after intravenous contrast enhancement, so mimicking an intracerebral tumour. The distinction between one and the other is usually based on the history or, if necessary, by rescanning in a few weeks; tumours grow while haemorrhages (and infarcts) shrink.

Note: A PICH may disappear completely in a week or two and therefore a scan later than this does not exclude it.

Depending on the quality of the scanner, a *normal* CT after a clinically definite stroke occurs in about 50% of cases and may be due to:
- early scan after infarction before low density appears
- a small infarct or haemorrhage, less than about 0.5 cm diameter
- lesion in the posterior fossa
- 'fogging' stage after cerebral infarction
- late after primary intracerebral haemorrhage when it has become isodense with brain

Note: A focal hypodense lesion on CT may be due to:
- a primary intracerebral haemorrhage more than one or two weeks old
- a cerebral infarct more than a day or two old
- non-stroke pathology, e.g. multiple sclerosis, head injury, etc.

Cerebral angiography should only be carried out if it is likely to influence management. It may, therefore, be required:
- after a carotid TIA or mild carotid ischaemic stroke to image the carotid

bifurcation if carotid endarterectomy is indicated (p. 253) once the patient is neurologically stable. *Selective* intra-arterial injections must be given to show the intracranial as well as extracranial circulation on the symptomatic side. Biplanar or triplanar views of the carotid bifurcation are needed. The main risk of angiography is TIA or stroke in about 4% of examinations, and disabling stroke in 1%. Therefore, the patients should be selected for angiography by prior ultrasound imaging and doppler sonography of the carotid artery (*duplex scanning*). About 50% of patients do *not* have internal carotid artery origin stenosis, usually because they have a cardiac embolic source, atheroma elsewhere in the arterial supply to the brain, or small vessel disease within the brain.

• to image dural sinus thrombosis (p. 224).

• in a patient whose cerebral infarct might have been due to neck trauma and carotid or vertebral artery dissection. Angiography is helpful in the acute phase, before the artery becomes normal, if there is any question of litigation.

• vertebral angiography is seldom required except for the occasional patient with very frequent vertebrobasilar TIAs, or with subclavian steal, whose symptoms may respond to surgery (p. 221).

• after intracerebral haemorrhage, angiography may show
saccular aneurysm (p. 231)
vascular malformation (p. 233)
mycotic aneurysm (p. 232)
but should only be performed if surgery would be considered if a lesion were found.

Note: The diagnosis of TIA and stroke is *clinical* and does not depend on ultrasound or angiography which are only carried out to define the site, size and nature of the underlying arterial pathology.

Lumbar puncture (p. 39) is required only in the following instances:

• subarachnoid haemorrhage cannot be demonstrated by CT (p. 229)

• after 'stroke' if multiple sclerosis (p. 348) or encephalitis (p. 498) are possibilities

• if blood serology for syphilis is positive

Note: For a few days after cerebral infarction the CSF may contain a slight excess of lymphocytes (usually less than 50 per cm^3) and protein (usually less than 1.0 g/l) and occasionally transient oligoclonal bands.

Electroencephalography is rarely needed unless:

• encephalitis (p. 498) is a diagnostic possibility (bilateral slowing of the EEG)

• uncertainty exists between transient ischaemic attack and partial seizure (p. 220)

• seizures occur after stroke (p. 246)

Magnetic resonance imaging is more sensitive than CT in defining small infarcts and haemorrhages, particularly in the posterior fossa, but does not influence management very much. It is not as good as CT in differentiating primary intracerebral haemorrhage from cerebral infarction in the acute stage.

Echocardiography to help delineate a potential cardiac source of embolism is required only if one is likely, i.e. if there is clinical, ECG or chest X-ray evidence of a relevant cardiac abnormality. It is also indicated in patients under the age of 50 if there is no good reason for a cerebral infarct or TIA, or if there is evidence of multiple emboli (see also p. 218).

24–hour ECG monitoring is occasionally required if there is difficulty distinguishing TIA from syncope (which is seldom a problem, p. 220), or if there is concern about intermittent atrial fibrillation as a cause for embolic cerebral infarction and TIA.

Outcome, treatment and secondary prevention of stroke

Stroke patients require:
- general management in the acute stage (p. 245)
- specific early treatment (cerebral infarction, p. 248, primary intracerebral haemorrhage, p. 228, subarachnoid haemorrhage, p. 230)
- rehabilitation (p. 250)
- secondary prevention (p. 251)

and their questions and concerns answered:
- have I had a stroke? (p. 236)
- why have I had a stroke? (pp. 208 and 226)
- will I die? (p. 248)
- will I recover? (p. 250)
- how long will recovery take? (p. 250)
- what treatment is there? (p. 248)
- will I have another stroke and can it be prevented? (p. 251)

General measures in the treatment of acute stroke from any cause

Admission to hospital is required if the diagnosis is in doubt, if complicated treatment is needed (e.g. neurosurgery) and if the patient cannot be nursed, rehabilitated and adequately looked after at home by carers and the domiciliary services (which is the most common reason). Most of the early general management is concerned with preventing the complications of stroke.

The complications of stroke

For a few days after a severe stroke there is a stress response which subsides spontaneously: raised blood pressure, mild fever, neutrophil leucocytosis, hyperglycaemia and perhaps glycosuria, hyponatraemia and ischaemic changes on the ECG. Of more concern are the general complications which often cannot only be treated, but prevented. They are therefore important to recognize:

● Pneumonia is particularly likely if swallowing, the cough reflex or consciousness is impaired, so leading to reduced pulmonary ventilation and inhalation.

● Deep venous thrombosis occurs in about 50% of paralysed legs and, although usually asymptomatic, can cause the leg to become painful and swollen. Pulmonary embolism is present in about 50% of patients who die but is seldom the cause of death; however, presumably it impairs respiratory function in many who survive, at least for a while.

● Urinary infection is particularly likely if bladder function is affected (e.g. incontinence) or if catheterization is needed and can lead on to renal failure and septicaemia.

● Skin pressure sores, particularly if the skin is soaked in urine.

● Constipation is common and is due to immobility, poor diet and dehydration and is perhaps exacerbated by medications. Faecal incontinence is less common than urinary incontinence.

● Septicaemia may be due to urine infection, pneumonia or infected pressure sores.

● Dehydration, water and electrolyte imbalance may be due to impaired swallowing, salt 'wasting', inappropriate intravenous treatment, renal failure and diuretics.

● Cardiac failure is common and may be due to coincidental ischaemic heart disease and myocardial infarction; neurogenic pulmonary oedema following an acute intracranial lesion; arrhythmia; pneumonia.

● Epileptic seizures, partial or secondary generalized, occur in the acute phase in about 2%. The risk of a seizure in the first year is about 5%.

● 'Mechanical' problems are frequent and distressing:
    spasticity and, in the legs, muscle spasms
    dependent oedema in the legs due to impaired muscle pumps or deep
        venous thrombosis
    joint contractures due to spasticity and immobility
    subluxation of the shoulder of the paralysed arm
    frozen shoulder on the paralysed side, stiffness of other immobile joints
    falls and fractures
    osteoporosis of bones in paralysed limbs

● Pressure palsies of peripheral nerves (p. 368).

● Central 'thalamic' pain (p. 26).

- Gastric 'stress' ulceration.
- Concern, anxiety, boredom, frustration, depression and apathy. Excessive emotionalism (affecting crying more often than laughing) tends to be precipitated by stimuli which have an emotional content (e.g. mention of close family, Royal Family, etc.). This phenomenon is also seen in motor neurone disease (Chapter 13) and after head injury.

Therefore, in all stroke patients the following should be attended to:
- Care of the airway, particularly if the patient is drowsy or has difficulty swallowing. Nurse semiprone, use pharyngeal airway if necessary, and oxygen administration if hypoxic. Mechanical ventilation is rarely needed except in the occasional patient with a brainstem stroke who is conscious and expected to recover. Chest physiotherapy is important.
- Position the limbs correctly, turning and skin care every 2 hours (Fig. 8.4).
- Bladder care; if possible, avoid catheterization by toileting frequently. A urinary appliance may be helpful in males. Treat any urine infection with appropriate antibiotics.
- Bowel care; adequate diet and hydration, laxatives and enemas as necessary.
- Fluids must be given, even in the first 24 hours, by mouth or nasogastric tube (about 1500 ml per day). Avoid dehydration and monitor fluid balance.
- Intravenous fluids are seldom necessary and make nursing and rehabilitation more difficult. Oral feeding can start on the first day if feasible but this depends on conscious level and swallowing; if still not feasible by the second

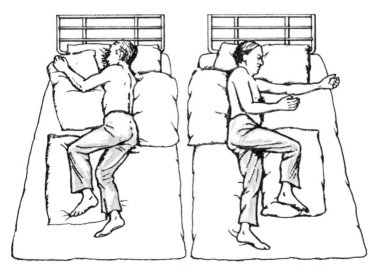

Fig. 8.4 The correct positioning of a hemiplegic patient; in the illustration the hemiplegia is on the left.

day, then a nasogastric tube must be used. Treat nausea and vomiting with appropriate antiemetics.

• Explanation of diagnosis and management to patient and carers.
• Sit the patient out of bed when conscious, headache free and feeling reasonably well.
• Seizures should be treated on their merits (p. 82).
• Deep venous thrombosis and/or pulmonary embolism should be treated with full anticoagulation for a few months *provided* intracranial haemorrhage has been excluded by CT scan.
• In patients with a paralysed leg it is reasonable to attempt to prevent venous thromboembolism with heparin (subcutaneous 5000 units twice daily) until the patient is walking, or for about a month if not already walking within that time; exclude primary intracerebral haemorrhage first by CT scan.
• Attend to other medical disorders, e.g. cardiac failure, diabetes and angina.

The following should be monitored:

Vital signs
• respiratory rate and rhythm (blood gases if necessary)
• heart rate and rhythm
• blood pressure (non-stroke arm)
• temperature (non-stroke axilla since it may be spuriously low under the affected one)
Neurological
• conscious level (Glasgow coma score, p. 122)
• pupils
• limb weakness
• seizures
General
• fluid balance
• electrolytes and urea
• blood glucose
• haematocrit

Early treatment of stroke

About 20% of patients die within a month of a first ever stroke (Table 8.1). This average risk is greater in the following cases:
• intracranial haemorrhage rather than cerebral infarction
• increasing age
• patient already handicapped before the stroke
• reduced conscious level in the first 24 hours
• infarction in the whole of the middle cerebral artery territory (i.e. total anterior circulation syndrome, p. 237)

- the stroke is recurrent
- atrial fibrillation
- hyperglycaemia
- large rather than small intracerebral haemorrhages, particularly if there is blood in the ventricles

In the first week, the cause of death is usually 'neurological' as a consequence of a large infarct or haemorrhage with associated cerebral oedema, haemorrhagic infarction and brain shift causing transtentorial herniation (p. 257), or of direct disruption of the brainstem. Later deaths are more likely to be due to the complications of immobility (pneumonia, pulmonary embolism, renal failure, etc.).

There is no definitely helpful and routine treatment for cerebral infarction (unless in the cerebellum, p. 223), but there may be surgical possibilities in PICH (p. 228) and SAH (p. 230). In cerebral infarction the aim of any treatment is to restore blood supply to the ischaemic area (and certainly not to make it worse), to salvage ischaemic and dying neurones, and to limit the size of the infarct. At the moment there are few if any pharmacological possibilities:

Blood pressure may temporarily rise for a few days after a stroke, although in very severe strokes it can be low. However, many patients are chronically hypertensive and have a raised blood pressure on admission for that reason.

Raising the blood pressure may, in theory, improve cerebral blood flow in ischaemic or haemorrhagic areas of the brain where autoregulation is defective. However, this strategy may increase local blood volume and cause hyperaemia, precipitate cerebral oedema, and therefore make local cerebral blood flow even worse.

Reducing the blood pressure may reduce cerebral oedema but, because of defective autoregulation, local cerebral blood flow may fall, so increasing the ischaemia. In previously hypertensive patients autoregulation is 'set' higher (p. 208), so that reducing the blood pressure is even more likely to reduce local cerebral blood flow; if not documented, previously raised blood pressure can be inferred from evidence of left ventricular hypertrophy, retinopathy, etc.

On balance, it is sensible to leave the blood pressure to stabilize spontaneously unless it is extremely high (greater than 120 mmHg diastolic phase 5), when gradual reduction over a few days is best achieved with oral therapy such as a beta-blocker or diuretic. In hypertensive encephalopathy (p. 214) rapid control of blood pressure is required, usually with titrated doses of intravenous labetalol, nitroprusside or hydralazine; the BP should be gradually reduced over several hours and sudden extreme falls *must* be avoided. Extreme hypotension (systolic less than 100 mmHg) should be treated, usually by eliminating the cause.

Intracranial pressure may be raised by large intracranial haemorrhages or cerebral infarcts as a result of cerebral oedema, haemorrhagic infarction, brain shift and hydrocephalus. Therefore, in a drowsy and deteriorating patient with CT evidence of brain shift or hydrocephalus it is reasonable to give mannitol (p. 264), although this is seldom helpful in the long run.

Anticoagulation with heparin, followed on with warfarin a few days later, may be helpful if a cerebral infarct appears to be progressing in a series of presumed embolic or thrombotic 'steps', particularly if it is in the brainstem. However, other general and neurological causes of deterioration must not be forgotten (p. 223).

Rehabilitation

Most of the functional improvement after stroke occurs in the first few weeks but it can continue for about 6 months, after which it is mostly due to adaptation to disability rather than any change in impairment. Improvement begins within a few days of the onset. At 6 months about 60% of the survivors are independent (Table 8.1) and many have no symptoms at all, making secondary prevention important (p. 251). Recovery is *least* likely in one-month survivors in the following circumstances:

- persisting severe motor deficit
- persisting urinary incontinence
- persisting confusion and cognitive disorder
- impairment of joint position sense
- previously disabled
- increasing age
- total anterior circulation infarction (p. 231)

The general aim is to return the patient to as near normal as possible as quickly as possible. This is facilitated by decent housing, a caring family, friends and good domiciliary services. Rehabilitation requires the combined efforts of a team:

- Physiotherapy can start at once with passive exercises leading on to active rehabilitation, control of spasticity, prevention of contractures and advice on walking aids, etc. The physiotherapist is in the best position to train all other staff (and carers) in how to lift and handle stroke patients properly.
- Occupational therapy is needed to help disabled patients adapt to their environment. At some stage a home visit may be required to assess any need for aids and adaptations.
- Speech therapy has a part to play with severe dysarthria, and severe swallowing difficulties, but less of a role in dysphasia. However, speech therapists are ideally placed to explain to dysphasic patients and their carers what the problems are likely to be and how they can be overcome. Voluntary stroke clubs also support dysphasic patients.
- Social workers may be needed to arrange housing, benefits, and to support patients and their carers.
- Stroke clubs have an important role in supporting patients, helping rehabilitate them towards normal life, and providing a forum for discussion and counselling. They also take the pressure off carers.

- Counselling so that patients' questions can be answered about the cause of their stroke, return to normal life, encouragement, etc.

Note: Patients need not necessarily 'give up' anything except perhaps cigarette smoking and overeating; normal sexual activity can continue within the limits of any physical disability. For driving, see Appendix 1.

The transfer from hospital to home can be stressful and is facilitated by:
- good liaison between hospital and domiciliary professionals
- a liaison nurse
- pre-planned provision of domiciliary services and aids
- early involvement of carers, relatives, etc. before discharge
- a trial home visit with occupational therapist, physiotherapist, social worker
- a gradual return home, first for the day, then a weekend, then permanently
- back–up from the hospital (outpatient review, day hospital care, respite care, etc.)
    During rehabilitation it is essential to:
- identify and measure patients' impairments, disabilities and handicaps
- identify patients' needs and resources (home, finance, carers, etc.)
- assess prognosis
- set realistic goals for patients, therapists and carers
- review progress regularly with relevant measurements (e.g. Barthel scale, p. 60) and reset goals as appropriate

Note: Avoid using inappropriate drugs which may make sedation, confusion, constipation and hypotension worse. Avoid the temptation to ascribe all post-stroke symptoms to the stroke itself or depression, and consider adverse effects of drugs which may have been started in the aftermath of stroke (e.g. diuretics, beta-blockers, etc.).

Note: Withdraw active rehabilitation slowly and provide some kind of long-term support if necessary. Review needs, resources and secondary prevention (p. 251) at one year post-stroke.

'Thalamic' pain is extraordinarily difficult to treat but usually resolves in a matter of months or years. Transcutaneous nerve stimulation, a vibrator, amitriptyline and carbamazepine can all be tried along with routine analgesics.

Secondary prevention of cerebral infarction

After cerebral infarction or transient ischaemic attacks the risk of a recurrent stroke is much the same, about 10% in the first year and 5% per annum thereafter. This risk is greatest in those who have vascular risk factors (p. 208), the greatest extent of arterial disease in the neck, and probably those with very frequent TIAs. Myocardial infarction is a more common cause of death than recurrent stroke and occurs at the rate of about 5% per annum. The overall death rate is between 5% and 10% per annum. For secondary prevention there is no need to wait; treatment should start almost as soon as the TIA or stroke has been diagnosed and it is almost certainly going to be required for life.

Vascular risk factors

All individuals, whether they have had a stroke or not, benefit from the sensible management of vascular risk factors. TIA and cerebral infarction survivors benefit more than patients without vascular disease because their risk of serious vascular events is higher.

• *Sustained* hypertension should be treated by slowly lowering the blood pressure over a few weeks to about 160–180 mmHg systolic, and 100 mmHg phase 5 diastolic. Weight reduction, alcohol reduction, possibly some reduction in salt intake and relaxation can all be helpful. Drug treatment may be necessary but limited by adverse effects, particularly in the elderly. Caution is required to avoid symptomatic hypotension because cerebral blood flow autoregulation may be impaired by stroke, severe stenosis or occulsion of large arteries in the neck may be already compromising cerebral blood flow, and there may be interactions with other drugs such as vasodilators for angina.

Note: A reduction in diastolic blood pressure by 5–10 mmHg reduces the relative risk of stroke by about 50% within 2–3 years.

• Smoking should be strongly discouraged.
• Excessive weight should be reduced.
• Symptomatic diabetes mellitus should be treated while asymptomatic abnormal glucose tolerance can probably be kept under review unless it is severe.
• Cholesterol level should, if possible, be reduced to below about 6.5 mmol/l by diet and, perhaps only in younger patients, by cholesterol-lowering drugs.
• Sensible exercise should be encouraged, e.g. walking, swimming.
• If the haematocrit is greater than 50, it should be remeasured without venous occlusion. If it is still raised, then any diuretics should be stopped, weight reduced, cigarettes stopped, alcohol consumption reduced and any cause for anoxia dealt with (e.g. chronic obstructive airways disease, a right-to-left intracardiac shunt, pulmonary arteriovenous malformation, etc.). If these measures fail, venesection may be required, 250 ml at a time, and with particular care if there is pulmonary disease. Polycythaemia rubra vera (p. 458) should be treated on its merits.

Antithrombotic drugs

Aspirin, 75 mg daily orally, after *ischaemic* stroke or TIA reduces the risk of serious vascular events by about 25% (stroke, myocardial infarction, vascular death). If indigestion occurs, the aspirin can be given enteric-coated; alternatively, ticlopidine (oral, 250 mg twice daily) can be used but the white blood cell count must be monitored and diarrhoea and skin rashes can be a problem.

Warfarin, preceded by heparin for a few days if quick anticoagulation is required, is indicated in the following cases:
• TIA/ischaemic stroke within a few weeks of acute myocardial infarction if the mechanism is thought to be embolic rather than haemodynamic. In 3–6 months anticoagulation can be gradually withdrawn over a few weeks and replaced by aspirin.
• TIA/ischaemic stroke in prosthetic heart valve patients.
• TIA/ischaemic stroke in cardiomyopathy patients.
• TIA/ischaemic stroke in atrial fibrillation with rheumatic valvular disease or cardiomyopathy.
• Frequent TIAs (i.e. daily) unresponsive to aspirin. If the attacks stop, then anticoagulation can be gradually substituted by aspirin in 3–6 months.

Note: Warfarin should be controlled by keeping the International Normalized Ratio at 3–4.5.

Note: If indicated at all, anticoagulation should be started as soon as possible after the onset of acute cerebral infarction.

Anticoagulation is *definitely* unwise, and aspirin *probably* unwise, in a stroke patient unless cerebral haemorrhage has been ruled out by CT scanning within 1–2 weeks of onset.

Surgery

Carotid endarterectomy

Carotid endarterectomy, to remove an atherothrombotic stenosing and/or ulcerating lesion at the origin of the internal carotid artery, reduces the risk of ipsilateral ischaemic stroke in a patient who has recovered from a *carotid* ischaemic event if the stenosis is very tight (greater than 70% of arterial diameter). In rare patients with very frequent carotid TIAs, carotid endarterectomy may stop the attacks whether or not it prevents a subsequent stroke. The main risk of surgery is a stroke (5–10% of cases) but other complications occur: neck haematoma, myocardial infarction, peripheral nerve injury at the operation site (hypoglossal, facial, superior laryngeal, vagus).

Therefore, carotid endarterectomy should be considered only if all of the following are present:

- carotid ischaemic event with recovery
- stenosis of more than 70% of the lumen diameter at the origin of the symptomatic internal carotid artery
- no other more likely source of embolism to the brain, e.g. cardiac, proximal arterial disease, intracranial arterial disease
- low institutional risk of cerebral angiography
- experienced anaesthetist
- low institutional risk of surgery (under 10% stroke and/or death)
- patient fit enough for surgery: stable neurologically, controlled blood pressure, no recent myocardial infarction, controlled angina
- patient accepts surgery

Extracranial to intracranial bypass surgery

This surgery by anastomosing a branch of the superficial temporal artery through the skull to a distal branch of the middle cerebral artery, has no definite place. It may just possibly help patients who have recurrent symptoms due to low cerebral blood flow.

It may be worth while to relieve vertebral origin stenosis in patients with very frequent vertebrobasilar TIA unresponsive to medical treatment. Frequent symptoms due to subclavian steal may be relieved by surgery or angioplasty of the subclavian artery.

Keep management of other likely vascular disorders under review:
- angina
- cardiac failure
- claudication/rest pain
- aortic aneurysm

as well as the common disorders of the elderly:
- poor vision
- poor hearing
- poor teeth
- bad feet

Useful address

Chest, Heart and Stroke Association
CHSA House
Whitecross Street
London EC1Y 8JJ
Tel: 071-490-7999

9 Raised intracranial pressure and tumours

Raised intracranial pressure

After complete contact of the skull bones at about the age of 5, the skull becomes a rigid box so that any increase in volume of one of its three contents (brain, blood, CSF) eventually leads to raised intracranial pressure. The most common cause is increased cerebral blood volume. Obstruction of CSF flow is another important mechanism. Many of the clinical features of space occupying lesions (see below) are due to brain shift rather than the raised intracranial (and CSF) pressure itself (e.g. headache).

Causes of raised intracranial pressure

- space occupying lesions:
  intracranial tumour (p. 266)
  abscess (p. 503)
  intracerebral (p. 227), subdural (p. 235) and extradural haematoma
  cerebral infarction (if large) (p. 223)
  subarachnoid haemorrhage (p. 228)
  giant aneurysm (p. 231)
- intracranial infection:
  meningitis (p. 489)
  encephalitis (p. 498)
  granuloma (e.g. tuberculosis, p. 512, fungal, p. 531)
- hydrocephalus (p. 259)
- 'benign' intracranial hypertension (p. 264)
- venous outflow obstruction or anomaly:
  dural sinus thrombosis (p. 224)
  superior vena cava obstruction
  dural arteriovenous malformation (p. 233)
- respiratory failure and hypercapnia
- hypertensive encephalopathy (p. 214)
- very raised CSF protein:
  Guillain–Barré syndrome (p. 398)
  spinal cord tumour (p. 325)
- any cause of cerebral oedema (p. 263)
- metabolic encephalopathies (p. 124)
- ischaemic/anoxic brain damage (p. 123)

Clinical features

These depend on the speed of development (e.g. intracranial haemorrhage may lead to coma within minutes) and the size and site of the causative lesion. Not all of the following features are seen in all patients:

- Headache is very common and characteristically present on waking, tending to resolve after getting out of bed. Eventually it is constant and severe, sometimes 'bursting'. Its location, if localized, usually relates to the site of any focal lesion, e.g. occipital if posterior fossa tumour. It is largely due to stretching of the dura and intracranial blood vessels (e.g. as a result of a space occupying lesion) or meningeal inflammation, rather than raised intracranial pressure itself.
- Papilloedema (p. 172) is usually bilateral but can be unilateral and even not present at all. Transient visual obscurations are common in the later stages. It is due to transmission of the raised intracranial pressure to the CSF around the optic nerve, resulting in obstruction of venous return from the eye.
- Drowsiness leading on to coma.
- Meningism (p. 492), particularly if there is a posterior fossa mass with cerebellar tonsillar herniation (p. 259) through the foramen magnum (cf. meningitis, p. 489, and subarachnoid haemorrhage, p. 228).
- Nausea and vomiting are usually late signs but, with posterior fossa tumours, vomiting can be early and projectile without warning.
- 6th nerve palsy (uni or bilateral) is a false localizing sign due to compression of the nerve at the apex of the petrous temporal bone during transtentorial herniation (p. 257).
- Increasing head circumference and separation of the sutures in children (normal head circumference, see Fig. 9.1).
- Acute intracranial hypertension can occasionally cause pulmonary oedema.
- The signs of the underlying lesion.
- *Transtentorial herniation* of the medial temporal lobe(s) is the result of a large supratentorial space occupying lesion. This herniation can be spontaneous or precipitated by lumbar puncture (p. 43). It causes:

    Deepening coma.

    Ipsilateral 3rd nerve palsy if there is unilateral herniation of the uncal part of one temporal lobe compressing the nerve.

    Further herniation causes progressive brainstem compression from above downwards, causing 'squeeze haemorrhages' within it. This leads to paralysis of up-gaze, small but reactive pupils, an abnormal respiratory pattern, and then medium-sized and fixed pupils with dysconjugate eye movements and decerebrate rigidity and finally fixed dilated pupils with no reflex eye movements or response to pain. Respiration becomes progressively affected with a Cheyne-Stokes pattern to begin with, then possibly hyperventilation, followed by irregular respirations and finally 'gasping' respiration and respiratory arrest.

    Occasionally hemiparesis occurs *ipsilateral* to the supratentorial mass due to compression of the contralateral cerebral peduncle against the tentorium (Kernohan's notch syndrome).

    Pressure from the tentorium on the ipsilateral posterior cerebral artery

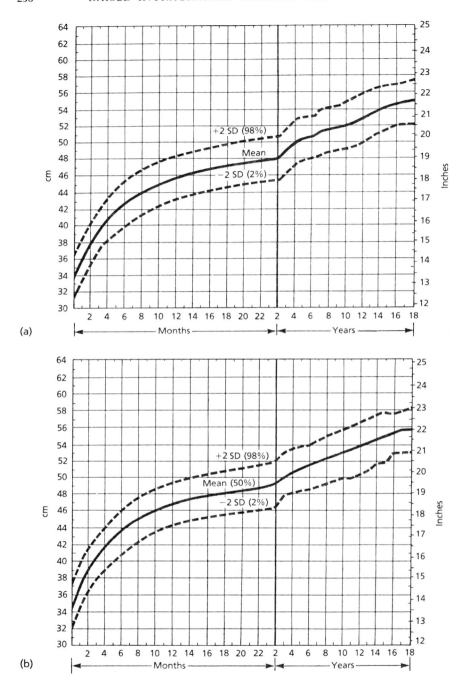

Fig. 9.1 Normal range of head circumference; (a) girls and (b) boys.

causes infarction (often haemorrhagic) in the occipital lobe. This is uncommon.

Increasing blood pressure and falling pulse rate as the brainstem becomes progressively perturbed.

• With posterior fossa space occupying lesions, and with extreme transtentorial herniation, the cerebellar tonsils and medulla are displaced through the foramen magnum (*tonsillar herniation or coning*), causing meningism and brainstem compression with deteriorating conscious level and finally respiratory arrest. Sometimes there is upward herniation of the brainstem through the tentorial hiatus as well.

The *skull X-ray appearances* include:

• erosion of the pituitary fossa (also seen in osteomalacia and hyperparathyroidism)

• 'copper beating' pattern of the vault (if onset in childhood)

• separation of the sutures (children)

• signs of the underlying cause (calcification in a tumour, shift of the pineal gland), etc.

However, in most cases the skull X-ray is normal.

Measurement of intracranial pressure

The normal intracranial pressure is less than 15 mmHg; above 20 mmHg is definitely abnormal.

The most common method of measuring intracranial pressure is by lumbar puncture (p. 41) but this is inaccurate in cases of transtentorial herniation as well as dangerous due to subsequent leakage of CSF through the dural hole, reduced CSF pressure, and hence an increase in the transtentorial pressure gradient (p. 43).

Monitoring of intracranial pressure, but not directly of cerebral oedema, is not necessarily required during treatment but can be performed by sensors in the extra or subdural space, or in the lateral ventricles. Inaccuracy is caused by leakage of CSF, blocked catheters or transducers, wrong positioning and faulty calibration. Intraventricular pressure monitoring is the most accurate but requires brain puncture which may be difficult if the ventricles are small, and can be complicated by haemorrhage and infection.

Hydrocephalus

CSF is secreted by the choroid plexuses of the lateral, 3rd and 4th ventricles at the rate of about 500 ml per day. The total CSF volume is approximately 150 ml. The CSF flows caudally through the ventricular system and exits from the 4th ventricle through the foramina of Luschka and Magendie into the subarachnoid space. It then flows down around the spinal cord and up through the tentorial hiatus and over the surface of the brain to be absorbed by the dural arachnoid granulations into the venous system. Therefore, the site of any obstruction of flow is revealed on CT scan by observing which ventricles are dilated (those 'upstream' of the block). The CT may also reveal the cause (e.g. intracranial tumour, etc.).

Hydrocephalus means dilatation of part or all of the intracranial ventricular system due to obstruction of CSF flow, impaired CSF absorption or very rarely excessive CSF secretion. The main clinical questions are:

- where is the block?
- what is it due to?
- can it be relieved?

Note: Large ventricles may be the result of loss of brain tissue ('compensatory' hydrocephalus or hydrocephalus ex-vacuo) and intracranial pressure is then normal.

Causes of hydrocephalus

- Obstruction of CSF flow distal to the outlets from the 4th ventricle and/or impaired absorption by the arachnoid granulations leading to enlargement of all the ventricles (so-called *communicating hydrocephalus*) due to:
  inflammatory exudate in the subarachnoid space (acute or chronic meningitis, p. 491)
  haemorrhage (acute or organized) after trauma (including craniotomy) or as a result of spontaneous subarachnoid haemorrhage (p. 228)
  malignant meningitis (p. 227)
  defect of absorption at arachnoid granulations (idiopathic)
- Obstruction of CSF flow within the ventricular system (*obstructive hydrocephalus*) may occur anywhere from the lateral ventricles to the outlet of the foramina of the 4th ventricle. The causes are:
  congenital
  aqueduct stenosis
  Arnold–Chiari malformation (p. 202)
  Dandy–Walker syndrome (p. 202)
  aneurysm of the vein of Galen
  haemorrhage (acute or organized) after trauma (including craniotomy) or as a result of spontaneous subarachnoid haemorrhage (p. 228)
  mass lesions; tumour (p. 266), haematoma (p. 227), colloid cyst of the 3rd ventricle (p. 275), abscess (p. 503), etc.
  inflammatory exudate in the subarachnoid space (acute or chronic meningitis, p. 491)
  malignant meningitis (p. 277)
  transtentorial herniation (p. 257)
- Excess production due to choroid plexus papilloma (p. 275) is extremely rare.

• A very high CSF protein as in the Guillain–Barré syndrome (p. 398) or spinal tumour (p. 325); the mechanism of raised intracranial pressure, papilloedema and inconstant hydrocephalus is uncertain but may be due to the excess protein 'blocking' the arachnoid granulations.

Clinical features

These depend on:
• the symptoms and signs of the underlying cause of the hydrocephalus
• the rate of development of the hydrocephalus; acute block causes raised intracranial pressure and coma
• the general clinical features of hydrocephalus, some of which are due to periventricular interstitial oedema (p. 263) and neuronal death. These include:
  drowsiness
  unsteady gait
  bilateral pyramidal signs
  mental retardation or dementia
  urinary incontinence

Note: The features of 'normal' pressure hydrocephalus are described on p. 262.

• in children hydrocephalus causes expansion of the skull (normal head circumference, see Fig. 9.1).Other causes of an enlarged head in children are:
  subdural haematoma (p. 235)
  macrocephaly
  arachnoid cyst
  intracranial tumour
  hydranencephaly
• and in adults:
  Paget's disease of bone

Hydrocephalus may arrest, the intracranial pressure normalize and, in children, mental development can be surprisingly normal. Later, this compensation may be upset by trivial head injury or physical illness, so precipitating acute symptomatic hydrocephalus.

Treatment

In symptomatic, and particularly in deteriorating, cases despite treatment of the underlying cause, the treatment is diversion of CSF flow by a ventricular drain followed, if necessary, by a ventriculo-peritoneal, lumbo-peritoneal or, rarely, ventriculo-atrial shunt with relief of the raised intraventricular pressure.

There are several important complications of shunts and these are particularly frequent in frail elderly patients:

- subdural haematoma (p. 235)
- intracranial infection (Chapter 18)
- intracerebral haemorrhage (p. 227)
- low pressure headache (p. 42)
- shunt obstruction by infection, thrombosis, ventricular wall, choroid plexus or omentum
- seizures

'Normal' pressure hydrocephalus

This rare clinical syndrome is due to progressive dilatation of the entire ventricular system (i.e. communicating hydrocephalus) without significant cortical atrophy. This is the consequence of failure of normal CSF absorption over the surface of the cerebral hemispheres due to various factors which have in common the presence of old blood or inflammatory exudate in the CSF pathways:

- head injury
- subarachnoid haemorrhage (p. 228)
- meningitis (bacterial, tuberculous, fungal but not viral, p. 491)
   However, in most cases no cause is discovered.

The *clinical features* insidiously develop some months or years after any putative precipitating cause and slowly progress:

- apathy and dementia
- difficulty in walking is particularly prominent. On the bed, power and coordination of the legs are normal and there are no abnormal neurological signs, but the gait is unsteady with frequent falls
- urinary incontinence occurs early with little awareness or concern

Diagnosis

The diagnosis depends on the appropriate clinical syndrome being associated with a CT scan showing ventricular dilatation, often with periventricular flare of low density, and with little corresponding cortical atrophy. The lumbar CSF pressure is normal but monitoring may reveal transient pressure rises; the CSF composition must be checked and should be normal unless there is an active underlying process such as chronic meningitis. In doubtful cases various tests have been proposed but none is universally accepted (e.g. monitoring the CSF pressure in the lateral ventricles or subdural space and recording its response to increasing the volume of CSF, etc.).

Treatment

Occasionally an underlying cause can be treated (e.g. chronic meningitis), but otherwise a ventriculo-peritoneal or lumbo-peritoneal shunt will relieve the hydrocephalus and the symptoms in the *correct* patient, i.e. one with the full clinical syndrome and with the typical CT appearance.

Cerebral oedema

Cerebral oedema is defined as an increase in brain volume caused by an increase in brain water content. It accompanies a wide range of pathological processes and leads to:
- increasing intracranial pressure (p. 256)
- shift and distortion of brain if the oedema is localized
- cerebral ischaemia in the region of the oedema

There are five basic types, but more than one can be present at the same time depending on the underlying pathophysiology:

Vasogenic oedema

This is caused by damage of the blood–brain barrier (i.e. 'leaky' capillaries). Usually it is localized, the oedema fluid is protein-rich and extracellular. It forms around tumours, brain abscesses, brain contusions and cerebral infarcts.

Cytotoxic oedema

This is caused by damage of cell membranes (i.e. 'leaky' cells). It is intracellular and the excess oedema fluid consists mostly of water and sodium. The main cause is focal or generalized ischaemia and hypoxia.

Hydrostatic oedema

This type is caused by increased transmural vascular pressure. The oedema fluid is mostly water and is extracellular and diffuse. It occurs when there is arterial hypertension or vasodilatation in conjunction with a reduction in extravascular pressure such as occurs during craniotomy or after the removal of a large space occupying lesion.

Interstitial oedema

This is caused by obstructive hydrocephalus. The raised intraventricular pressure causes CSF to move into the periventricular white matter.

Osmotic oedema

Osmotic oedema is usually diffuse and is caused by low plasma osmolality. It is associated with conditions causing hyponatraemia (p. 464) or hypoproteinaemia.

Treatment of cerebral oedema and raised intracranial pressure

General measures:
- remove the cause
- avoid hypercapnia, hypoxia and hyponatraemia
- avoid pyrexia
- avoid extremes of hyper and hypotension since it is likely that cerebral autoregulation (p. 208) is impaired in areas of cerebral oedema

Hyperventilation to reduce $PaCO_2$ to about 3.5 kPa, and thus reduce cerebral blood volume and rate of oedema formation, is usually appropriate only if the patient is already on a ventilator. It causes a general reduction in brain volume, although the oedematous area(s) may not shrink if their blood vessel reactivity to $PaCO_2$ is impaired.

Hypertonic solutions withdraw water from the brain to the blood, so lowering brain volume and intracranial pressure. The effect is temporary for a few hours and most obvious where the blood–brain barrier is intact and there is a rich blood supply. It may not, therefore, have a specific effect on focal areas of brain damage and oedema. However, it can help by reducing the volume of normal brain and so give an oedematous and damaged area of the brain more room, making it less likely to be compromised further by ischaemia. This treatment is, therefore, only used pending more definitive treatment of the underlying cause.

The most commonly used agent is intravenous mannitol (p. 270). The addition of intravenous frusemide may prolong and intensify its effect.

Corticosteroids reduce vasogenic oedema, particularly around tumours. They do not influence the diffuse brain swelling caused by cytotoxic and hydrostatic oedema. The usual drug is dexamethasone (p. 270).

Benign intracranial hypertension (BIH) or pseudotumour cerebri

This is an unusual and poorly understood condition which usually affects obese young women and children. The intracranial pressure is raised but the reason is unknown, the ventricles are of normal size or small, there is no obvious obstruction to CSF flow nor abnormality of its content, and no intracranial mass.

Causes

In some otherwise typical cases the underlying cause is obstruction of the sagittal or transverse sinus (p. 225). Otherwise, most patients are obese although sometimes there is an associated condition, possibly causal:

- vitamin A intoxication
- drugs:
corticosteroids or corticosteroid withdrawal
danazol
nalidixic acid
nitrofurantoin
oral contraceptive
tetracyclines
- hypoparathyroidism (p. 457)
- hypothyroidism (p. 456) and/or thyroxine treatment
- pregnancy and the puerperium
- iron deficiency anaemia (p. 460)

Clinical features

The major symptom is obscuration or blurring of vision due to papilloedema which is usually bilateral (p. 172). Since there is no brain shift, headache is usually mild or absent, there is little nausea and no vomiting, and the patient is alert and generally well. Very occasionally a 6th cranial nerve palsy may be present as a false localizing sign of raised intracranial pressure but there are *no* other focal neurological signs.

The diagnosis is confirmed after a normal enhanced CT scan (which may show somewhat small ventricles) when it is then safe to perform a lumbar puncture to show a raised CSF opening pressure (greater than 200 mmHg of CSF, although in some normals pressure may be as high as 250 mmHg, p. 41). CSF should be removed until the pressure is normal, since this alone may relieve the symptoms; its composition must be normal to support the diagnosis.

Dural sinus thrombosis may be suspected on CT scan (p. 225) and confirmed by MRI; the risk of making the diagnosis by carotid angiography with late venous views is not worth taking unless anticoagulation is being seriously considered for threatened vision (see below).

Treatment

Many patients recover spontaneously in a few weeks. Mild cases, with little headache and modest papilloedema, can be treated conservatively by removing any underlying cause if possible (e.g. weight reduction) and giving chlorthalidone, oral, 100 mg daily.

However, if the clinical picture is more severe, then corticosteroids (dexamethasone 4 mg 4 times daily) should be started at once but tailed off in 2–3 weeks if there is no effect on the papilloedema, size of the blind spots, or intracranial pressure as measured by repeat lumbar puncture. If effective, the steroids can be reduced and tailed off over several months as recovery occurs.

Repeat lumbar punctures (every 2–3 days) to remove CSF and return the closing pressure to normal are needed for a quick therapeutic effect before corticosteroids begin to work, particularly if vision is threatened. The main concern is progressive or even sudden blindness due to increasing papilloedema with enlargement of the blind spot to include central vision, retinal haemorrhage and ischaemic optic neuropathy (p. 175).

If repeated lumbar punctures and/or corticosteroids do not keep the intracranial pressure down, then more permanent measures are needed:

- lumbo-peritoneal (or cisternal-jugular) CSF drainage using a shunt (complications, p. 262)
- full anticoagulation if dural sinus occlusion demonstrated radiologically
- fenestration of the optic nerve sheath to relieve pressure on the optic nerve may preserve vision
- subtemporal decompression of the brain as a last resort

Progress is monitored by recording the symptoms, visual acuity, visual fields including the blind spots, the retinal appearances and, if necessary, by repeat lumbar punctures to measure the CSF pressure.

Intracranial tumours

Tumours inside the head arise from:

- Skull:
  osteosarcoma
  ivory osteoma
- Meninges:
  meningioma (p. 271)
  sarcoma
  melanoma
- Brain:
  astrocytoma (p. 271)
  glioblastoma multiforme (p. 271)
  oligodendroglioma (p. 272)
  ependymoma (p. 272)
  medulloblastoma (p. 273)
  choroid plexus papilloma/carcinoma (p. 275)
  lymphoma (p. 275)
  neuroblastoma
- Cranial nerve sheath:
  neurilemmoma (neurinoma, schwannoma) (p. 272)
- Pituitary:
  adenoma (p. 273)

- Pineal:
  pineocytoma/pineoblastoma (p. 274)
- Vascular structures:
  haemangioblastoma (p. 272)
  arteriovenous malformation (p. 233)
- Developmental tumours:
  craniopharyngioma (p. 274)
  epidermoid and dermoid (p. 274)
  colloid cyst of 3rd or 4th ventricles (p. 275)
  chordoma (p. 275)
  germinoma (p. 274)
  teratoma (p. 274)
  lipoma (p. 275)
- Secondary deposits from:
  carcinoma bronchus
  carcinoma breast
  carcinoma stomach
  hypernephroma
  melanoma
  choriocarcinoma
  lymphoma (p. 275)
  leukaemia (p. 459), etc.
- Direct spread from:
  carcinoma of the nasopharynx/sinuses
  glomus tumour (p. 198)

The overall incidence of primary intracranial tumours is about 15/100000 per annum. About two-thirds are 'benign', a proportion of which are only discovered at postmortem, or are very small and of only functional significance (such as pituitary adenoma). The incidence of intracranial metastases is at least 15/100000 per annum but many are never discovered in patients with widespread secondary cancer, except in the event of postmortem.

In *adults* the most common tumours are supratentorial: astrocytoma (p. 271), pituitary adenoma (p. 273), secondary carcinoma (p. 276) and meningioma (p. 271).

In *children* the most common tumours are infratentorial: astrocytoma (p. 271), medulloblastoma (p. 273) and ependymoma (p. 272).

Clinical features

Usually the clinical picture develops progressively. This progression may occur over many years with the more benign tumours or over a matter of days with highly malignant tumours. Sometimes seizures are the only symptom for many years. Occasionally the neurological deficit appears suddenly and may even be followed by recovery, so mimicking a TIA or stroke; haemorrhage into the tumour is one possible cause, particularly in malignant astrocytoma (p. 271), oligodendroglioma (p. 272), medulloblastoma (p. 273), haemangioblastoma (p. 202), hypernephroma, endometrial carcinoma, choriocarcinoma and melanoma.

The symptoms and signs are some combination of those due to:
* raised intracranial pressure (p. 256) due to obstruction of CSF flow, usually in the posterior fossa causing hydrocephalus, or brain shift as a result of the tumour itself; obstruction of the dural venous sinuses; and cerebral oedema surrounding the tumour
Note: Intracranial pressure rises exponentially so that eventually the symptoms may be abruptly precipitated by a small rise.
* pressure on nerve roots, e.g. optic chiasm from pituitary adenoma, causing bitemporal hemianopia (p. 168), 8th cranial nerve from acoustic neuroma (p. 272), 3rd cranial nerve from sphenoidal ridge meningioma (p. 271), etc.
* local pressure on the brain causing a focal neurological deficit or seizures (partial or secondarily generalized in supratentorial tumours)
* local infiltration and destruction of the brain (mostly by histologically malignant tumours) to cause a focal deficit depending on the site and size of the tumour and any surrounding oedema; also partial or generalized seizures
* secretion of hormones, e.g. from pituitary adenoma (p. 273)
* non-metastatic effects of any primary extracranial tumour (p. 475)
* secondary spread by seeding in the CSF; ependymoma (p. 272, medulloblastoma (p. 273), germinoma (p. 274), choroid plexus carcinoma (p. 275), lymphoma (p. 275)
* extracranial metastatic spread of intracranial tumours only occurs with medulloblastoma (p. 273) and lymphoma (p. 275)

Investigations

CT scan

CT scan is the most practical investigation to show tumour position, size and sometimes pathology; brain shift; cystic areas within or associated with the tumour; peritumoural oedema; and hydrocephalus. The tumour density on CT may be less than, the same as, or greater than normal brain density and often there is surrounding oedema shown as low density. Most histologically malignant and metastatic tumours enhance after intravenous contrast, as do many benign tumours. Above the tentorium almost all tumours are demonstrated, particularly if intravenous contrast is given, but below the tentorium accuracy is not so high. Here tumours may reveal themselves by obstructive hydrocephalus or displacement of the 4th ventricle. Sometimes contrast material (e.g. metrizamide or air) introduced by lumbar puncture is needed to outline structures in the posterior fossa; for example, expansion of the brainstem or an acoustic 'neuroma'. This should not be done if there is raised intracranial pressure (p. 256).

MRI

MRI is more sensitive than CT, particularly in the posterior fossa, but it is not widely available.

Skull X-ray

This may still be a useful screening test if CT is not immediately available because it may show:
- features of raised intracranial pressure (p. 259)
- displaced pineal gland if calcified
- calcification within the tumour is usually associated with more benign tumours but malignant change can still occur in such cases
- bone hyperostosis adjacent to meningioma (p. 271)
- enlargement and erosion of pituitary fossa by adenoma (p. 273), craniopharyngioma (p. 274) and very occasionally by carotid aneurysm (p. 231)
- osteolytic lesions in the skull (secondary carcinoma, myeloma, primary bone tumour, etc.)
- prominent vascular markings due to the enhanced blood supply to meningioma (p. 271)
- erosion and widening of the internal auditory meatus by an acoustic 'neuroma' (p. 272)

Chest X-ray

This is important to eliminate an obvious primary or secondary tumour.

Tumour biopsy

This is controversial. If there is a known histologically confirmed primary tumour and the CT scan shows multiple deposits characteristic of metastases, then usually no further biopsy is necessary. If not, and if there is clinical and CT scan evidence of solitary or even multiple *intracerebral* lesions which *might* be tumour, one should probably be biopsied to exclude treatable lesions such as meningioma (p. 271), lymphoma (p. 275), cerebral abscess (p. 503) or even tuberculoma (p. 513); stereotactic brain biopsy is relatively safe provided a vascular malformation (p. 233) is not a diagnostic possibility. *Extracerebral* space-occupying lesions should always be explored to exclude a meningioma (p. 271). If the patient has *only* seizures, particularly if they are mild or controlled by drugs, and a solitary *intracerebral* lesion is discovered, then biopsy is usually withheld until something more develops (sequential CT may be helpful here to monitor any change in size).

Lumbar puncture

This is contraindicated because of the risk of transtentorial herniation and/ or brainstem coning in the presence of an intracranial mass lesion (p. 43). In these circumstances the CSF pressure recorded is usually, in any case, an underestimate of the intracranial pressure because of obstruction of CSF flow at the tentorium or foramen magnum.

Treatment

Medical

For urgent control of raised intracranial pressure, transtentorial herniation and incipient brainstem coning mannitol should be given to gain time for diagnostic and therapeutic decisions. It is given as an i.v. infusion: 0.5–1.0 g/kg as a 10–20% solution over about 10–20 min. Acute cardiac failure can occur, particularly in the elderly, due to circulatory overload. Infusions cannot be repeated more than about 5 times in 48 hours because of problems with electrolyte balance.

Dexamethasone (loading dose 12 mg, then 4 mg 4 times daily, oral, or i.m.) is highly effective in reducing peritumoural vasogenic oedema and symptoms are often dramatically improved in a matter of 24–48 hours. This treatment may remain effective for several weeks.

Specific antitumour medical treatments are available only for lymphomas (p. 275) or leukaemias (p. 459), choriocarcinoma and sometimes for pituitary adenoma (bromocriptine, p. 273).

Anticonvulsants should be used in the normal way for seizures, but not as routine prophylaxis if seizures have not occurred (p. 82).

Radiotherapy

This has a definite role in eradicating lymphoma (p. 275) and leukaemic (p. 459) deposits. It can be palliative in the solid malignant tumours but this is temporary and survival is not increased more than a few months. It can be argued that this treatment is not worth while for high grade astrocytoma. However, pineal region tumours (p. 274) and brainstem astrocytomas are often radiosensitive. For hazards of radiotherapy, see p. 486.

Surgery

If an intracranial tumour can be removed without much in the way of further neurological damage this should normally be attempted, especially for benign tumours such as pituitary adenoma (p. 273), meningioma (p. 271) and acoustic 'neuroma' (p. 272). Some low grade astrocytomas can be removed, particularly the cystic variety which occurs in the cerebellum in childhood (p. 271). A solitary metastasis can often be removed successfully; the worst prognosis appears to be for secondary deposits from the gastrointestinal tract, bronchus and melanoma and the best for breast and kidney. Partial removal of a tumour may help in the control of raised intracranial pressure and local pressure on structures such as the optic chiasm. Aspiration of large cystic lesions is worth while for the temporary control of symptoms but usually cysts quickly refill. Obstructive hydrocephalus can be relieved by a ventriculoperitoneal shunt.

Features of specific tumour types

Astrocytomas

These are the most common primary brain tumour in adults and are usually supratentorial; in children, they arise mainly in the pons or cerebellar hemisphere where they tend to be cystic and histologically benign. They rarely occur in the spinal cord. They vary from histologically benign to highly malignant tumours with a correspondingly long (many years) to short (weeks) survival. Different parts of the same tumour may vary in histological malignancy, so making interpretation of biopsy material difficult. On CT they are usually of low density without enhancement if low grade, but with irregular enhancement if high grade. The tumours infiltrate into normal brain, so complete resection is rarely, if ever, possible.

Glioblastoma multiforme

In this type the cell origin is unrecognizable although many such tumours are presumably highly malignant astrocytomas and behave in the same way.

Meningiomas

These are the second most common intracranial tumour. Women are affected more than men in a ratio of 3:1. They grow from the meninges and are histologically benign in most cases. The most common sites are parasagittal from the falx cerebri, frontal from the olfactory groove or suprasellar area, temporal from the sphenoid wing, and from the skull vault. Tumours arising from the lateral ventricle, tentorium, clivus, spinal canal, orbit and the foramen magnum are much less common. Occasionally they spread over the surface of the brain (meningioma en plaque). Sometimes they are multiple when neurofibromatosis is a likely explanation (p. 277). On CT they enhance uniformly and strongly with considerable oedema of the surrounding white matter. If complete surgical removal is technically possible, recurrence is unusual.

Neurilemmomas

Neurilemmomas (neurinoma, neurofibroma, schwannoma) most commonly arise on the vestibular branch of the 8th cranial nerve (acoustic 'neuroma') in the internal auditory meatus, occasionally on the trigeminal nerve, and rarely on other cranial nerves. They are slow growing benign tumours which exert their effects by pressure on adjacent structures.

Acoustic 'neuromas' usually present in middle or old age with slowly progressive, unilateral sensorineural deafness, often with tinnitus and later with imbalance (very seldom vertigo), ipsilateral impaired corneal response and mild facial weakness. Eventually all the other features of a cerebello-pontine angle mass develop (p. 194). If diagnosed early, they can be reasonably easily removed and facial nerve function spared. Complete deafness is usually permanent but if any hearing is present before surgery it may sometimes be preserved.

Bilateral acoustic 'neuroma' and multiple neurilemmomas on cranial and spinal nerves are usually due to neurofibromatosis (p. 277).

Oligodendrogliomas

These are relatively slow growing tumours which often contain calcium. In adults they are almost all supratentorial (at least half arise in the frontal lobes). They are rare in children. Survival is variable, from weeks to years, after surgical confirmation of the histological diagnosis.

Ependymomas

These may be histologically benign or malignant and arise from the 4th ventricle in children, and in adults they are supratentorial or involve the spinal cord or cauda equina. Occasionally they seed through the CSF path-ways. They are difficult to remove completely, particularly if locally malignant, but may be radiosensitive.

Haemangioblastomas

Such tumours are benign and often cystic in older children and adults occurring mainly in the cerebellum but sometimes in the brainstem or spinal cord. They may be multiple. Sometimes they are associated with poly-cythaemia and are often part of the von Hippel–Lindau syndrome (p. 202). On CT they enhance and an associated cyst may be visible. Occasionally they present with subarachnoid or intracerebral haemorrhage rather than as a mass lesion.

Medulloblastomas

These are malignant tumours which usually arise from the cerebellar vermis in children and infiltrate the 4th ventricle, brainstem and cerebellar hemispheres. Less often they arise in the cerebellar hemisphere in adults. They metastasize via the CSF to other parts of the brain, spinal cord, cauda equina and meninges and are the only intracranial tumour to metastasize extracranially (to bone, peritoneum, lymph nodes, etc.). Clinical presentation is usually subacute with raised intracranial pressure, vomiting and ataxia due to a mass obstructing the 4th ventricle. Treatment is operative removal as far as is feasible, usually a ventriculo-peritoneal shunt to relieve hydrocephalus, and radiotherapy to the brain and spinal cord.

Pituitary adenomas

These are benign slow growing tumours which cause:
• hypersecretion of one or occasionally several hormones. Excessive prolactin production is the most common and causes infertility, secondary amenorrhoea, sometimes impotence in males and rather unusually galactorrhoea. Modest hyperprolactinaemia up to about 1500 mu/l may be merely due to distortion or damage of the hypothalamus or pituitary stalk from a functionless pituitary adenoma. Excessive growth hormone production causes gigantism in children and acromegaly (p. 458) in adults. Excessive ACTH production is rare and causes Cushing's disease, one cause of Cushing's syndrome (p. 455)
• local pressure on the optic chiasm (p. 168), optic nerves or rarely the optic tract (p. 168); cavernous sinus (p. 184); pituitary to cause hypopituitarism; and sometimes the temporal lobes to cause seizures. Headache is inconstant, nonspecific and seldom severe. Obstructive hydrocephalus and CSF rhinorrhoea are unusual
• haemorrhage into, or infarction of, a pituitary adenoma (pituitary apoplexy) is rare and causes sudden headache, often with nausea and vomiting, and sometimes leading on to drowsiness and coma; acute or subacute visual failure due to chiasmal compression; extraocular muscle palsies; and sometimes hypopituitarism with acute or delayed adrenal failure. The CSF may contain red and/or white blood cells. Clearly the differential diagnosis is subarachnoid haemorrhage (p. 228), meningitis (p. 491) and chiasmal haemorrhage (p. 168)

Note: Occasionally adenomas expand in pregnancy.

Skull X-ray may show the enlarged pituitary fossa but a contrast enhanced high resolution CT scan is more sensitive in revealing even small adenomas confined to the fossa. However, small tumours can still be invisible. Carotid angiography is often a wise prelude to surgery since an aneurysm of the carotid siphon (p. 231) may cause identical clinical, plain X-ray and CT features to those of an adenoma. Preoperative endocrine evaluation is essential since bromocriptine reverses the symptoms of prolactinomas and the tumours often shrink. Postoperative evaluation is needed to plan endocrine replacement therapy. Adenomas compressing the chiasm are usually removed surgically (often with preoperative bromocriptine to reduce their size if prolactinomas, and postoperative radiation to reduce the risk of recurrence); most operations are performed by the trans-sphenoidal route.

Craniopharyngiomas

These are rare tumours arising from embryological remnants above the pituitary fossa. They are cystic, infiltrate locally and present in children and young adults with progressive (or confusingly sometimes intermittent) optic chiasm compression (p. 168), retro-orbital optic nerve compression (p. 167), hypopituitarism, obstructive hydrocephalus (p. 260) and frontal lobe symptoms (p. 19).

Calcification is often seen on skull X-ray and CT. They are difficult to remove completely.

Pineal region tumours

Pineal region tumours (loosely refered to as pinealomas) are uncommon. They present with upper midbrain compression (Parinaud's syndrome, p. 179) and obstructive hydrocephalus (p. 259). The diagnosis is made by CT scan.

Teratomas contain various cell types and on CT are of mixed density ranging from that of fat to calcification; some are malignant. Germinomas resemble seminoma of the testis and are malignant, sometimes with CSF seeding. They are more uniform on CT. Serum human chorionic gonadotrophin and alphafoetoprotein may be raised. Pineocytoma, pineoblastoma, astrocytoma and ependymoma are rarer.

Since biopsy and/or resection are difficult, and most tumours are radiosensitive, it is usual to treat these tumours with radiotherapy without a tissue diagnosis, plus a ventriculo-peritoneal shunt if necessary. If there is no response, surgery may then be required.

Epidermoid and dermoid tumours

These are benign cystic lesions derived from embryonic inclusions of epidermis and dermis respectively. They usually arise at the base of the brain and in the cerebello-pontine angle. They look 'pearly' and contain cholesterol crystals (so called *cholesteatomas*), hair follicles and glandular tissue. They may calcify. In addition to the usual effects of intracranial tumours they may rupture to release cholesterol debris and cause chemical meningitis (p. 491) which can be recurrent. Posterior fossa tumours may communicate with the skin through a bony defect and lead to recurrent bacterial meningitis (p. 496). Despite their benign nature histologically, they are often difficult to remove completely.

Choroid plexus tumours

These are very rare, usually benign and arise in the lateral, 3rd or 4th ventricles of both children and adults. The presentation is usually with obstructive hydrocephalus, causing raised intracranial pressure. Cerebellar or brainstem signs are present if the tumour is in the 4th ventricle. Excessive CSF production is a minor cause for any hydrocephalus. The CSF protein is raised. Occasionally there is carcinomatous transformation with CSF seeding and malignant meningitis (p. 277). These tumours can be difficult to resect.

Colloid cyst

Colloid cyst of the 3rd ventricle is rare, histologically benign and usually small. It can be an entirely asymptomatic chance finding on CT or at postmortem. It may present with paroxysms of generalized headache, perhaps with loss of consciousness, due to acute hydrocephalus. The headache can be markedly affected by head position. Chronic hydrocephalus may lead to dementia and gait disturbance. On CT the cyst is usually hyperdense and may enhance with i.v. contact.

Chordomas

These are rare tumours arising from notochord remnants, usually on the clivus or in the sacrococcygeal region. In the former site they present with multiple cranial nerve palsies; the skull X-ray and CT may show bone erosion and a partly calcified mass.

Lipomas

Lipomas are rare fatty tumours which may be found in the corpus callosum or in the vertebral canal associated with spina bifida. Rarely, corticosteroid therapy and Cushing's syndrome (p. 455) can lead to spinal cord compression by masses of extradural fatty tissue.

Lymphoma

Lymphoma affects the nervous system primarily (so-called microglioma) and sometimes subsequently spreads, or as part of systemic lymphoma, either early or late in the course. It is one complication of immunosuppression as a result of AIDS, azathioprine, etc.

Lymphoma may cause:
- intracerebral deposits presenting with focal deficits, seizures, raised intracranial pressure, etc. CT shows one or more, usually enhancing, lesions indistinguishable from metastases and sometimes from meningiomas. Other visible lesions might be opportunistic infections (tuberculoma, p. 513, toxoplasmosis, p. 536, etc.)
- malignant meningitis (p. 277). The diagnosis can often be made from specific stains of the cells in the CSF
- extradural compression of spinal cord/root and sometimes the brain
- orbital deposits
- granulomatous angiitis of the nervous system (p. 451)
- opportunistic infections of the CNS (p. 490)

Late in systemic disease only palliative treatment is appropriate. Otherwise biopsy may be necessary, and perhaps surgical decompression of spinal cord or brain. The disease must be staged, local radiotherapy is often effective, and systemic chemotherapy used for widespread disease.

Malignant angioendotheliosis

This is now thought to be an intravascular lymphoma rather than endothelial cell malignancy. It affects many organs and there is widespread vascular occlusion by malignant cells which cause foci of necrosis and infarction, although it is usually confined clinically to the nervous system. It may present with subacute dementia, stroke or TIA-like episodes, focal cerebral signs and spinal cord dysfunction, leading to death in a matter of months. The ESR and CSF protein may be raised with a few excess lymphocytes in the CSF. CT is normal or non-specifically abnormal with low density area(s) which usually do not enhance. During life, biopsy is the only means of diagnosis.

Lymphomatoid granulomatosis

This may be a variant of lymphoma. There are widespread granulomatous lesions and the neurological complications include subacute encephalopathy, cranial neuropathies, seizures and stroke-like syndromes.

Cerebral metastases

In many patients the primary cancer is well known or readily diagnosed. A diagnostic problem arises when one or more intracranial low density lesions are found on CT, usually but not always showing ring enhancement with i.v. contrast, in a patient with no known primary. Clearly toxoplasmosis must be considered in patients at risk of AIDS (p. 526) and, in third world countries, tuberculomas (p. 513) and cysticercosis (p. 538). Examination of breasts, thyroid, prostate, chest X-ray, sputum cytology, mammography, faecal occult bloods, urine examination, pelvic examination, bone scan, acid phosphatase level, human chorionic gonadotrophin level, etc. may reveal the primary source of tumour. Further screening investigations outside the head are unwise (unless suggested by faecal occult blood, enlarged lymph nodes, etc.) and a diagnosis is more readily and safely achieved by intracranial biopsy, particularly stereotactically. Even if an intracranial mass is a metastasis, its removal may well be worth while if it is single, its position favourable, and the patient's general prognosis reasonable. Radiotherapy may also help.

Malignant meningitis

This is due to the seeding of tumour cells in the CSF with, or more often without, a solid intracranial or spinal primary or secondary tumour. The usual primary tumours are carcinoma of the bronchus and breast, melanoma, lymphoma and leukaemia, and these are usually already known or readily apparent at presentation with the meningitis. Carcinoma of the nasopharynx may also present with malignant meningitis by direct spread. Primary intra-cranial tumours rarely seed through the CSF (p. 268).

The clinical features include multiple cranial nerve palsies (p. 198), headache due to obstructive or communicating hydrocephalus, confusion, difficulty walking and dementia; spinal root pain and focal motor/sensory loss also occur. The diagnosis is made by CSF examination which, although almost always showing non-specific abnormalities such as raised protein and lymphocytes, and occasionally a low glucose, may reveal malignant cells on microscopy, most likely to be seen if the CSF is fresh and is collected on several occasions. The source of the malignant cells can often be deduced from special histological and immunological stains. Other causes of chronic meningitis (p. 497) must be excluded, particularly treatable conditions such as fungal infection in these frequently immunocompromised hosts.

Malignant meningitis and the primary tumour are seldom treatable and death occurs in weeks or months.

Neurofibromatosis

There are two main types, and possibly more, which are inherited as auto-somal dominant conditions.

Type I

Type I is the most common (von Recklinghausen's disease). Half the cases appear to be new mutations and clinical expression is very variable. It is carried on chromosome 17.

  Clinical features include:
- skin:
  multiple café-au-lait patches
  neurofibromas
  plexiform neurofibromas
  axillary and inguinal freckling
- iris hamartomas (Lisch nodules)
- neurilemmomas (p. 272):
  acoustic (not bilateral)
  other cranial nerves
  spinal roots
  peripheral nerves
- optic nerve astrocytoma (p. 176)
- macrocephaly
- bone:
  scoliosis
  subperiosteal neurofibromas
  hypertrophy
- mental retardation

Type II

Type II has a much higher penetrance, is carried on chromosome 22, and the hallmark is bilateral acoustic 'neuroma' (p. 272). Other features include:
- multiple CNS tumours:
  neurilemmomas on cranial and spinal nerves
  intracranial and intraspinal meningiomas (p. 271)
  astrocytoma of the optic nerve (p. 176), brainstem, spinal cord, etc.
- cataracts
- skin changes are less common than in Type I

Useful address

LINK, The Neurofibromatosis Association
Surrey House, Office No. B09
34 Eden Street
Kingston-Upon-Thames
Surrey KT1 1ER
Tel: 081-547-1636

10   Disorders of movement and posture

Movement disorders are conditions where there is slowness of voluntary movement (bradykinesia), involuntary movements (dyskinesias) and sometimes both. Muscle power, postural sensation and cerebellar function are often normal.

All involuntary movements are worse under stress and, apart from palatal myoclonus (p. 308), attenuate markedly during sleep. Patients may have more than one type of involuntary movement and, without easily defined criteria, there is often disagreement over how to classify a particular movement. However, it is more important to describe the movements, look for the cause and find a treatment than to debate definitions. If there is a pathological substrate to be found, it usually lies in the basal ganglia and extrapyramidal motor system. The conditions can be approached by considering specific diseases (e.g. Parkinson's disease) or symptoms (e.g. tremor).

Parkinsonism

Parkinson's disease is but one, albeit the most common, cause of the parkinsonian syndrome (i.e. parkinsonism) which is characterized by some combination of tremor, rigidity, bradykinesia and postural instability.
- Parkinson's disease (p. 280)
- drugs and toxins (p. 288)
- post-encephalitic parkinsonism (p. 290)
- akinetic-rigid syndromes with parkinsonian features (p. 290)
- akinetic-rigid syndromes in childhood (p. 292)
- intracranial tumour (p. 282)
- head injury
- cerebral anoxia (p. 292)
- cerebrovascular disease (p. 292)
- Fahr's syndrome (p. 293)
- hypoparathyroidism (p. 457)

Parkinson's disease (paralysis agitans)

This is a fairly common sporadic disorder of unknown cause affecting males and females equally. It is almost the only disease which is less common in smokers. The incidence is about 20 per 100 000 population per annum, the prevalence 150 per 100 000 population and both increase with age.

It is characterized pathologically by loss of pigmented neurones in the substantia nigra and locus coeruleus, degeneration of the dopaminergic nigrostriatal pathway, and Lewy bodies (eosinophilic cytoplasmic inclusions) in the brainstem and other parts of the brain.

Clinical features

Patients usually present at the age of 50–70 years. Typically progression is slow over several years and, unless there is an intercurrent cause of death, patients eventually become bedbound and die of pneumonia, urinary tract infection or septicaemia.

Sometimes the very earliest features include fatigue, restlessness and unilateral or bilateral sensory symptoms such as coldness, burning, numbness and tingling. Presentation with writer's cramp (p. 305) or foot dystonia is well known, but rare. These early symptoms persist or become submerged in the three cardinal motor features of the disease (tremor, rigidity and bradykinesia) which start in one limb, may remain largely unilateral for a few years or spread to the other side at an early stage. Even in the late stages there is asymmetry of motor involvement in most cases.

Tremor has a frequency of 4–6 Hz, is typically present at rest, and attenuates or disappears with movement of the affected part; the tremor may persist during a sustained posture. It is worse in public, under stress and when other body parts are moved voluntarily. Usually it starts distally in one limb (arm more often than leg) and spreads to the other ipsilateral limb and to the other side. Tremor may also affect the lips, tongue, jaw, vocal cords but not the head. It is often a social embarrassment but seldom causes severe handicap.

Rigidity of the 'cogwheel' or 'lead pipe' type affects the limbs, neck and trunk. Like tremor, it can begin very asymmetrically and be brought out by voluntary movement of the contralateral limb.

Bradykinesia is poverty and slowness of voluntary movement in the absence of muscle weakness. It affects the facial, pharyngeal, limb and trunk muscles. As a consequence the face is expressionless and mask-like. Blinking is infrequent. Speech is soft, monotonous and sometimes festinating and almost incomprehensible. Swallowing may become difficult; rather rarely there is upper respiratory obstruction. Fine manipulative finger movements are slow and laboured, writing becomes shaky and small. The posture is flexed and there is difficulty initiating walking, turning, getting out of a chair and turning over in bed. The gait is slow and festinating with a marked tendency to fall unexpectedly due to impaired postural reflexes, and to be rooted to the spot; the steps are small and arm swing is reduced. The poor gait and immobility lead to dependent ankle oedema.

Other features may include:
- joint and muscle pain due to immobility and rigidity (frozen shoulder is a common presentation)
- excessive sebum production causing a greasy and shiny face
- dribbling due to defective swallowing of saliva
- jerky eye movements, poor convergence and impaired up-gaze
- blepharospasm (p. 304)

• eyelid apraxia; difficulty initiating eyelid opening without active contraction of the orbicularis oculi or weakness of eyelid elevation
• dementia: probably somewhat more frequent than expected in similar aged patients, particularly in the *later* stages of the disease. It must be distinguished from adverse effects of drug treatment (see below), depression and physical slowness (p. 154)
• constipation
• postural hypotension in some patients
• depression, although more patients look depressed than actually are

A positive glabellar tap is both insensitive and nonspecific, being found in some normal elderly individuals and others with generalized brain disorders. Taps on the root of the nose between the eyebrows at about two per second cause reflex blinks; the sign is positive if blinking fails to habituate after about five taps.

There is no weakness until late in the disease when the rigidity and bradykinesia make any movement extremely difficult. There are no corticospinal, cerebellar or sensory signs. Vision, hearing and taste are normal but smell may be impaired.

Investigations and diagnosis

The diagnosis is based on the clinical picture which, except perhaps in very early cases, is characteristic. Sometimes only two of the three cardinal features are present, tremor quite often being conspicuously absent. If there is only one cardinal feature, then Parkinson's disease may not be the diagnosis. Also non-parkinsonian features (e.g. failure of horizontal gaze, pyramidal signs, cerebellar features, etc.) usually rule out the diagnosis; however, such features may appear later, so the diagnosis of Parkinson's disease should be kept under review, *particularly* if there is a poor therapeutic response to L-dopa.

The differential diagnosis of tremor is discussed on p. 293.

Extrapyramidal rigidity must be differentiated from spasticity (p. 7). The akinetic/rigid form of Huntington's disease (p. 298) and other akinetic/rigid syndromes with parkinsonian features (p. 290).

General slowing up with some fragmentary parkinsonian features can be found in depression, normal pressure hydrocephalus (p. 262), dementing conditions (p. 150) and widespread cerebrovascular disease.

Other causes of parkinsonism (p. 280) should be apparent from any history of exposure to drugs and toxins (p. 288) or past history of encephalitis lethargica (p. 290). An intracranial tumour (usually convexity meningioma, p. 271) can occasionally cause contralateral hemi-parkinsonian features but there is some additional non-parkinsonian feature as well (e.g. pyramidal signs, raised intracranial pressure or seizures); in cases of doubt or no response to treatment, a CT scan is needed. Occasionally an infarct, haemorrhage, arteriovenous malformation (p. 233) or trauma to the basal ganglia causes contralateral hemi-parkinsonism or other extrapyramidal features (e.g. chorea, p. 301, dystonia, p. 306, tremor, p. 293).

Juvenile parkinsonism (progressive pallidal atrophy) presents in adolescence as a parkinsonian syndrome with pyramidal signs and sometimes dystonia.

Treatment

Drug treatment does not slow the progression of the disease and is not required until the symptoms are definitely interfering with normal activities. Any drug should be introduced in a low dose and slowly increased over a few weeks until either an adequate therapeutic response is achieved or adverse effects appear. Sudden drug withdrawal is unwise, even if it was ineffective, because this may cause severe akinetic rigidity, sometimes akin to the neuroleptic malignant syndrome (p. 289); therefore, the dose should be reduced slowly over weeks.

Patients should be started first on long-term L-dopa to restore dopamine to the depleted striatum. The less effective anticholinergic drugs should be avoided in the elderly, but in younger patients are still useful if tremor and rigidity are the predominant problems, and occasionally in other patients who do not respond to L-dopa. Anticholinergics and L-dopa can be given together.

No drug is curative and any beneficial effect is lost within hours of its being withdrawn. As the disease progresses, drug treatment eventually becomes ineffective.

L-Dopa

Dopamine does not cross the blood–brain barrier. However, dihydroxy-phenylalanine (L-dopa), its precursor, enters the brain where it is decarboxy-lated to dopamine. L-dopa is also decarboxylated in the gut and elsewhere, leading to peripheral dopaminergic adverse effects such as nausea, vomiting, postural hypotension, cardiac arrhythmias and glaucoma; these can be partly avoided, and the dose of L-dopa reduced considerably, by concurrent admin-istration of an extracerebral dopa-decarboxylase inhibitor which does not penetrate the brain (carbidopa in Sinemet and benserazide in Madopar). L-dopa *alone* is no longer used.

L-dopa is best but not necessarily taken after food to minimize nausea and vomiting, although after large meals there can be unpredictable reduc-tion or delay in absorption. It should *never* be given with non-selective and type A monoamineoxidase inhibitors, and avoided in combination with methyl dopa.

About 80% of patients with Parkinson's disease improve, some remark-ably, whereas L-dopa is unlikely to help in other akinetic-rigid syndromes

p. 290). Bradykinesia, rigidity and tremor are all improved but postural instability is seldom helped.

Sinemet. Starting dose is Sinemet-110 (containing 100 mg L-dopa), half a tablet twice daily after food (usually breakfast and tea), or use Sinemet LS containing 50 mg L-dopa. Increase slowly over a matter of weeks until symptoms are controlled, usually with a twice to 4 times daily regimen. Maximum tolerated dose is usually no more than Sinemet-275 (containing 250 mg of L-dopa), 2 tablets 4 times daily; occasional patients appear to respond to higher doses. Patients must have their dose carefully tailored to suit them, their activities and any effect of meals.

Madopar. Similar prescribing principles apply although Madopar is available as dispersible tablets as well as capsules, which is useful if swallowing is a problem, and controlled release (CR) capsules containing 100 mg L-dopa to smooth out fluctuations. There is no difference in the therapeutic or adverse effects.

    Madopar-62.5 contains 50 mg L-dopa
    Madopar-125 contains 100 mg L-dopa
    Madopar-250 contains 200 mg L-dopa

The central adverse effects of L-dopa are dose dependent and reversible, although this may take several weeks:

• Involuntary movements occur in any body part. Restlessness, chorea and athetosis are common dose-related adverse effects which can occur as the drug begins to relieve the parkinsonism, at the time of peak drug effectiveness, and sometimes as the effect wears off. Dystonia is rather less common at the same times. Often the patients are not worried by or even aware of the movements if they are mild.

• Pain; the dystonic movements can be painful and misinterpreted as cramp. Sometimes paroxysmal pain in one or more body part occurs *without* dystonia (or rigidity) as the drug effect wears off, or unpredictably.

• Dystonic foot postures have a particular tendency to occur on waking and are usually related to too little L-dopa even though they disappear if the drug is stopped for a few days.

• Psychiatric disorders: confusion, agitation and mania, nightmares, hallucinations, paranoia and psychosis.

    These central adverse effects usually do not become a problem for perhaps 2 or 3 years when the dose has to be increased to maintain a therapeutic effect.

    The duration of the therapeutic effect of a single dose appears to decrease from about half to 6 hours after a dose to half to perhaps 4 hours (the 'wearing off' effect or 'end of dose deterioration') and there can be marked fluctuation from a rigid parkinsonian state ('off') to a mobile ('on') but often dyskinetic state; if this happens very quickly over seconds or minutes, it is called the 'on–off' effect. Sometimes such fluctuations can be avoided by giving smaller but more frequent doses of L-dopa, selegiline (see below), bromocriptine (see below) or possibly Madopar CR (see above), but eventually each individual dose has to be lowered so much to avoid the adverse effects that it becomes impossible to control the parkinsonian symptoms. Occasionally *raising* the dose can push the patient quickly through a period of dyskinesia to a period, sometimes lasting some hours, of reasonably normal mobility. Another tactic is to try an extremely low protein breakfast and lunch (less than 7 g) and give almost all the daily protein requirement in the evening which may help a few patients who can tolerate the diet. Eventually some patients have such severe fluctuations in performance and/or central adverse effects that they may prefer to stop L-dopa completely and live in a severe rigid but at least stable parkinsonian state.

Rarely L-dopa causes a rash and altered taste sensation and, extremely rarely, an autoimmune haemolytic anaemia (Coombe's positive). It does not influence the development of malignant melanoma.

Selegiline

This is a centrally acting monoamineoxidase B inhibitor which reduces the breakdown of dopamine within the brain. In a proportion of patients with L-dopa-induced fluctuations it can smooth out the response. The dose of L-dopa may have to be reduced a little to avoid dose-related adverse effects. Dietary restriction of tyramine is not necessary.

It should be given as a single morning dose of 10 mg, or 5 mg on rising and 5 mg in the middle of the day.

Note: This drug can also delay the need for starting L-dopa in untreated patients by about a year or so; whether this delays the problems eventually associated with L-dopa therapy and later disability is unknown.

Bromocriptine

This is a dopaminergic agonist with a longer duration of action than L-dopa (6–12 hours) but it is considerably less effective. It has similar adverse effects, particularly psychiatric disturbance and postural hypotension, although dyskinesias and fluctuations are less common. In addition, it may cause:
• erythromelalgia-like symptoms with tender, warm and uncomfortable erythema of the lower legs and feet
• Raynaud's phenomenon
• livedo reticularis
• blurred vision
• nasal congestion
• hair loss?
• pleural infiltrates and effusion?

It is not a first line drug but can be tried, usually unsuccessfully, when: L-dopa is ineffective, causes intolerable adverse effects, or the response fluctuates unacceptably, particularly if the duration of benefit is very short.

Usually it is introduced slowly in patients already taking L-dopa which itself may have to be reduced to avoid adverse effects, or sometimes withdrawn; test dose of 2.5 mg in case of marked postural hypotension. Then, 2.5 mg twice daily, increasing by 5 mg/week or so to the minimum effective dose. The maximum tolerated dose can be as high as 20 mg 4 times daily.

Note: A bedtime dose of bromocriptine may prevent the early morning 'off-dose' dystonia (typically in the foot) in patients taking L-dopa. Alternatively, an extra dose of L-dopa can be taken in the middle of the night. Lithium is also said to help in the usual doses (p. 142) but sometimes the pain is so severe that L-dopa has to be abandoned.

Lysuride

This is another dopaminergic agonist which has only just been introduced into clinical practice. It has similar actions and adverse effects to bromocriptine. It should be started in low dose (200 μg at bedtime) and increased slowly and as necessary, up to a maximum of 5 mg daily in 3 divided doses, preferably taken after food.

Apomorphine

This is another dopaminergic agonist but is short acting and has to be given by subcutaneous injection, or via an infusion pump; the nausea and vomiting can be avoided by giving oral domperidone (20 mg 3 times daily starting 24 hours earlier) for a few weeks when usually it can be withdrawn.

Dose: from 1–20 mg daily depending on response.

The main uses are to relieve 'off periods' in patients having to take frequent doses of L-dopa and for positive 'off period' phenomena such as dystonia and pain.

Anticholinergic drugs

Several are available and all are similar. They tend to cause peripheral atropine-like adverse effects (dry mouth, urinary hesitancy and retention, dizziness, constipation, tachycardia, dilated pupils and blurring of near vision, glaucoma) and central adverse effects (confusion, forgetfulness, drowsiness, hallucinations) particularly in the elderly. Drying up saliva can, however, be an advantage if dribbling is a major problem.

Benzhexol: oral, 1 mg twice daily, increasing to 5 mg 3 times daily if necessary.

Orphenadrine: oral, 50 mg twice daily, increasing to 100 mg 4 times daily if necessary.

Amantadine

Amantadine, an antiviral drug, has a rather poorly sustained therapeutic effect. It can cause confusion, psychosis, ankle oedema and livedo reticularis.

Dose: oral, 100 mg twice daily, increasing if necessary to 200 mg twice daily.

Surgery

This has a minor role, mainly in patients with intractable and disabling upper limb tremor for whom a stereotactic contralateral thalamotomy can be helpful. Rigidity is also improved but not bradykinesia. Bilateral thalamotomy is dangerous, tending to cause dysarthria and pseudobulbar palsy.

General care

- Keep patient under regular review.
- Be patient; parkinsonian patients can be irritatingly slow, self-conscious and look miserable (which is often misleading), so raising negative feelings in the doctor.
- If drug regimens are at all complicated, write them down for the patient.
- Explain the difference between the symptoms of the disease and the adverse effects of treatment, so that drug timing and dosage can be adjusted by the patient within limits set by the doctor.
- Nausea and vomiting occasionally occur as a result of L-dopa and bromocriptine. Therefore, give these drugs after meals if possible and, if necessary, use metoclopramide as an antiemetic (10 mg twice daily, oral) or domperidone (10–20 mg twice daily, oral). Usually tolerance develops and the antiemetic can be stopped (prolonged treatment can itself cause parkinsonism, p. 288).
- Warn patients about postural hypotension (disease or drug-induced).
- Avoid neuroleptics and other drugs likely to cause parkinsonism (p. 288).
- Intercurrent infections and surgery can cause a surprisingly large deterioration. Antiparkinsonian drugs should *not* be interrupted under these circumstances.
- Regular exercise and occasional courses of physiotherapy can be helpful.
- Difficulty starting walking can be helped by providing a visual stimulus for the patient to step over (e.g. one's own foot, or an inverted walking stick with a handle).
- Falls are usually unexpected and seldom respond to treatment.
- Aids to reduce handicap, advice from occupational therapists, etc.
- Oral hygiene; salivation may be excessive because of the disease or deficient because of anticholinergic drugs. Parotid irradiation is in rare cases required for uncontrollable salivation.
- Speech therapy in selected patients with speech or swallowing problems.

- If there is severe dysphagia, there are now available liquid or dispersible formulations of some of the antiparkinsonian drugs.
- Constipation is common and should be dealt with in the normal way; if possible, constipating drugs (e.g. anticholinergics) should be stopped.
- Holiday admissions to hospital can be useful to give the carer a rest, the patient some physiotherapy, and to allow reassessment of medication and aids.

Measuring the effect of the disease and its treatment

On treatment with L-dopa there is so much daily and even hourly variation in an individual's disability and handicap that it can be difficult to measure the response to treatment satisfactorily. Patients, if educated to do so, may keep useful daily diaries of 'on' and 'off' periods which can then be related to drug dosage, meals, time of day, etc. However, any indication of overall worsening or improvement over weeks or months is rather subjective and relies very much on the views of the patients and their carers. Depending on an individual's particular disability one or more of the following can be measured:

- time to walk 10 m, turn and return
- time to place pegs in a standard board
- writing name and address, drawing a spiral

A rather rough overall staging of the disease (Hoehn and Yahr) is:

Stage I: unilateral involvement only, usually with minimal or no functional impairment

Stage II: bilateral or midline involvement without impairment of balance

Stage III: first sign of impaired righting reflexes. Some restriction in activities, disability mild to moderate but still leading independent life

Stage IV: severe disability but still able to walk and stand unassisted

Stage V: confined to bed or wheelchair unless aided

Useful address

Parkinson's Disease Society
36 Portland Place
London W1N 3DG
Tel: 071-255-2432

Parkinsonism caused by drugs and toxins

Long-term use of certain drugs (many of which block dopamine receptors) can cause a typical parkinsonian syndrome, sometimes with additional features of tardive dyskinesia (p. 309) and akathisia (p. 306). The drugs may also unmask or exacerbate Parkinson's disease itself. The patients are mostly middle-aged or elderly:

- phenothiazines
- butyrophenones (haloperidol, droperidol, etc.)
- flupenthixol
- metoclopramide
- reserpine
- tetrabenazine
- pimozide
- methyl dopa
- flunarizine
- cinnarizine
- domperidone
- phenylamine

Usually the parkinsonism remits within 12 months of stopping the drug (if that is feasible). L-dopa and the anticholinergics are seldom helpful but are still worth trying, particularly the latter.

Neuroleptic malignant syndrome

Neuroleptic malignant syndrome is an idiosyncratic and particularly acute and severe form of drug-induced parkinsonism. The offending drug may have been taken for only some hours, or for years. Muscle rigidity and akinesia develop over a few days and may become so severe that respiration, eating and swallowing are compromised. The rigidity can cause muscle necrosis, raised plasma creatine kinase levels and myoglobinuria. The patients also develop:

- high fever, tachypnoea
- neutrophil leucocytosis, raised liver enzymes
- peripheral circulatory failure, metabolic acidosis
- hyponatraemia and acute renal failure
- autonomic instability; labile blood pressure, profound vasoconstriction, tachycardia, sweating
- drowsiness leading to coma

Differential diagnoses include other causes of high fever, catatonia (p. 313), malignant hyperpyrexia (p. 430), heat stroke (p. 485) and meningism due to meningitis (p. 491).

The causative drug must be stopped; high temperature controlled and assisted ventilation may be required. Intravenous diazepam, benztropine (i.m. or i.v. 1–2 mg as necessary), or particularly dantrolene (i.v. 1–2 mg per kg 6-hourly and then oral 25 mg 4 times daily) may reduce the rigidity. Bromocriptine (2.5–10 mg 3 times daily, oral) is also helpful and can be combined with i.v. dantrolene as the first choice treatment.

Rechallenging the patient with the same drug is unwise but, if therapeutically necessary, a low potency neuroleptic can be used in a low dose (e.g. thioridazine).

Exposure to the following toxins may cause parkinsonism:
- carbon monoxide (p. 549)
- MPTP (methylphenyl tetrahydropyridine), a compound which has been used by i.v. drug abusers, produces a subacute, severe and pure parkinsonian syndrome which is persistent although it does respond to L-dopa
- manganese (p. 548)
- carbon disulphide (p. 546)

Post-encephalitic parkinsonism

Encephalitis lethargica was epidemic in the first part of the twentieth century and sporadic cases still occur. The acute illness, lasting days or months, is characterized by:
- fever, lethargy and malaise
- headache
- drowsiness, stupor and coma
- ophthalmoplegia
- hyperactivity and involuntary movements
- reversal of sleep rhythm

During the acute illness, or up to several years later, a parkinsonian syndrome sometimes develops, progresses and then becomes static. However, unlike Parkinson's disease, there are additional features such as oculogyric crises (sustained ocular deviation, usually upwards, for minutes or hours), tics, chorea, blepharospasm, myoclonus, personality change, compulsive and psychotic behaviour, and corticospinal tract signs.

Akinetic-rigid syndromes with parkinsonian features

Steele–Richardson–Olszewski syndrome

This syndrome (progressive supranuclear palsy) is a rare degenerative disorder (prevalence 1.4 per 100 000) primarily of the brainstem, basal ganglia and cerebellum. It starts in late middle age and progresses to death in about 5 years. The characteristic feature is gradual paralysis of voluntary (and eventually reflex) eye movement, first in the vertical and then in the horizontal plane, but this may not be obvious at presentation. Patients often complain of difficulty walking downstairs because they cannot look down, reading, and moving their eyes, less often of diplopia. Other features include:
- increasing parkinsonism with an emphasis on unsteadiness of gait and sudden falls, axial and neck rigidity often with neck hyperextension. Tremor is mild or absent
- pseudobulbar palsy, dysarthria, dysphagia and mild bilateral corticospinal tract signs in the limbs
- mild dementia

- lid retraction, infrequent blinking, blepharospasm, apraxia of eye lid opening
- absent or poor ocular convergence

Antiparkinsonian drugs are seldom effective.

Shy–Drager syndrome

This syndrome (multisystem atrophy) is a multisystem degenerative disorder affecting mainly the brainstem, basal ganglia and central autonomic neurones. It starts in middle age and is fatal in a few years. The patients present with a combination of the following, of which postural hypotension is the most characteristic:
- autonomic failure:
  postural hypotension
  impotence
  urinary hesitancy, retention or incontinence
  constipation
  dry eyes and mouth
  impaired sweating
  pupillary abnormalities; poor reaction to light and accommodation, Horner's syndrome
- increasing parkinsonism but with little or no tremor
- pseudobulbar palsy with mild corticospinal tract signs in the limbs
- mild cerebellar features
- laryngeal obstruction due to vocal cord palsy leading to loud snoring and sleep apnoea (p. 115)
- iris atrophy
- poor ocular convergence
  There is little or no dementia.
  Antiparkinsonian treatment is seldom effective, but symptomatic treatment can help the postural hypotension (p. 404), sleep apnoea (p. 117) and urinary problems.

Striatonigral degeneration

This is clinically identical to Parkinson's disease except that it does not usually respond to L-dopa. The corpus striatum degenerates as well as the substantia nigra.

Olivo-ponto-cerebellar atrophy

This is a gradually progressive degenerative disorder with parkinsonian features along with cerebellar signs, dementia and some corticospinal tract features. It can be familial. Diagnosis can be made only at postmortem. Antiparkinsonian drugs are seldom effective.

Akinetic-rigid syndromes in childhood

- Wilson's disease (p. 310)
- juvenile Huntington's disease (p. 298)
- cerebral palsy
- Hallervorden–Spatz disease (p. 292)
- Pelizaeus–Merzbacher disease (p. 292)
- Lesch–Nyhan syndrome (p. 482)
- progressive pallidal atrophy or 'juvenile parkinsonism' (p. 305)
- drugs (p. 288)

Hallervorden–Spatz disease

This is a very rare, sometimes familial, condition of progressive rigidity, bradykinesia, dystonia, dysarthria and dementia in childhood, or occasionally in adult life. Chorea, seizures, cerebellar ataxia, muscle atrophy and retinitis pigmentosa have also been reported. Iron-containing pigment is deposited in the globus pallidus and substantia nigra and can be identified by MRI.

Pelizaeus–Merzbacher disease

This is a rare familial leucodystrophy. In childhood there is progressive dementia, parkinsonism, dystonia, spasticity, optic atrophy, ataxia and nystagmus.

Cerebral anoxia

From whatever cause, cerebral anoxia occasionally causes disproportionate basal ganglia damage which tends to become clinically obvious days or weeks after regaining consciousness. There is severe bradykinesia, rigidity, dystonia, choreoathetosis, some degree of cognitive damage and bilateral corticospinal tract involvement.

Cerebrovascular disease

Patients who have had several ischaemic or haemorrhagic strokes can develop parkinsonian features but almost always in addition to obvious effects of the strokes on the pyramidal system, language, visuospatial function, etc. An isolated basal ganglia infarct or haemorrhage may very rarely cause the abrupt onset of parkinsonian features contralateral to the lesion with a tendency for spontaneous improvement.

Fahr's syndrome

This is rare. Pathologically it consists of bilateral calcification of the basal ganglia, cerebellar dentate nuclei and sometimes the subcortical white matter. It is a progressive neurological disorder with various combinations of rigidity, dystonia, chorea, dementia, seizures, dysarthria and cerebellar ataxia. Occasionally it is familial; a cause is rarely found but it is worth considering other reasons for basal ganglia calcification:

- hypoparathyroidism (p. 457)
- pseudo hypoparathyroidism (p. 457)
- pseudo pseudo hypoparathyroidism (p. 457)
- mitochondrial cytopathy (p. 430)
- cerebral anoxia
- Cockayne syndrome (p. 482)

Calcification of the basal ganglia (particularly in the globus pallidus) is seen on CT in about 1% of normal asymptomatic individuals; apart from a plasma calcium, it is not worth investigating if it is an incidental finding.

Tremor

Tremor is involuntary, oscillating and rhythmic movement of one or more parts of the body. It may occur when the body part is relaxed and at rest (e.g. parkinsonism, p. 280), during voluntary movement of the part (e.g. intention tremor as a result of cerebellar disease, p. 14) or during a sustained posture (e.g. benign essential tremor, p. 294). Thus, there are 'rest' or 'static', 'intention' or 'action' and 'postural' tremors but quite often more than one type is present in a single individual. The causes are:

- physiological (p. 294)
- excessive sympathetic stimulation (p. 294)
- benign essential tremor (p. 294)
- senile tremor (p. 295)
- task-specific action tremors (p. 295)
- parkinsonism (p. 280)
- asterixis (p. 296)
- cerebellar/brainstem disease (p. 199)
- Wilson's disease (p. 310)
- peripheral neuropathy (p. 393)
- hysteria
- drugs:
  sympathetic stimulation (p. 294)
  causing parkinsonism (p. 288)
  causing cerebellar syndrome (p. 200)
  alcohol (p. 542)
  amiodarone

cimetidine
cyclosporin
ergot alkaloids
fluoxetine
lithium
mexiletine
phenytoin (p. 88)
sodium valproate (p. 91)
tocainide
tricyclic antidepressants
vidarabine
- toxins:
  mercury (p. 547)

Physiological tremor

Physiological tremor is universal and is the small amplitude and rapid (about 8–12 Hz) tremor best seen in the outstretched hands. It persists but attenuates through voluntary movement and is usually absent at rest.

Excessive sympathetic stimulation

This exaggerates physiological tremor and can be troublesome. Usually the deep tendon reflexes are symmetrically exaggerated, often with a brisk jaw jerk as well. Causes include:
- anxiety, stress, fatigue
- hyperthyroidism, including factitious thyroxine administration (p. 456)
- hypoglycaemia (p. 108)
- phaeochromocytoma (p. 109)
- withdrawal of sedatives, alcohol, opiates
- drugs:
  sympathetic stimulants (e.g. isoprenaline, salbutamol, oxymetazoline, ephedrine, phenylpropanolamine)
  amphetamines
  caffeine
  diethylpropion
  fenfluramine
  mazindol
  methylphenidate

Benign essential tremor

This is a coarse tremor (about 5–8 Hz) during a sustained posture, persisting or worsening during action. Usually it is absent at rest and worse under observation or stress, and sometimes prevented or relieved by alcohol. It tends to affect the hands, arms and head (titubation) and the onset may be unilateral. Bringing a glass of fluid to the lips is particularly troublesome. There are *no* other neurological symptoms. The prevalence is about 300 per 100 000. It is often familial (autosomal dominant) and appears in middle age. There is an occasional association with blepharospasm (p. 304) and other dystonias. Progression is slow or sometimes negligible but the tremor persists for life. It rarely causes a serious physical or social problem but some difficulty with writing and drinking liquids is quite common and leads to embarrassment.

Management:
- Reassurance that the tremor is not due to Parkinson's disease may be all that is required.
- Alcohol (in moderation) may control the tremor at times of embarrassment.
- Beta-blockers. Non-selective beta-blockade helps a few patients. A single dose can be used when required, or medication can be regular. Dosage must be individualized.

   propranolol: 40–120 mg as a single oral dose when needed, or 20 mg 3 times daily, slowly increasing to full beta-blockade if necessary; or long–acting propranolol in a similar but once daily dosage.

   nadolol: oral 80 mg, increasing to 240 mg daily. Useful because it can be given as a single daily dose.

   metoprolol. This beta-one blocker may help those who respond to propranolol but cannot tolerate it because of bronchospasm. However, in tremor-suppressing doses, it may block beta-2 receptors and cause wheezing. Dose: oral, 150 mg as a single dose, or 50 mg twice daily, increasing to 100 mg 3 times daily if necessary.

- Primidone. Test dose of 62.5 mg oral and then up to 250 mg 3 times daily if necessary (adverse effects, p. 93).
- Phenobarbitone, dosage as for epilepsy (p. 92).
- A combination of primidone and beta-blockers may be better than either alone.
- Contralateral stereotactic thalamotomy is rarely needed to control incapacitating tremor of the dominant hand; it is a final resort.

   Most patients do not seem to get enough functional help from drug treatment to make continuation worth while and very few ever require surgery.

Senile tremor

This is probably a variant of benign essential tremor. 'Tremulousness' in the elderly is common.

Task-specific action tremors

Like occupational cramps (p. 305), these occur only when a specific task is attempted (e.g. writing). There are no other neurological signs. They are very rare, the cause is unknown, and the treatments for benign essential tremor sometimes help.

Asterixis

Asterixis (or negative myoclonus) is an irregular flapping tremor of the outstretched hands with the wrists extended. It is seen in some metabolic encephalopathies:
- hepatic encephalopathy (p. 467)
- uraemic encephalopathy (p. 465)
- respiratory failure

Chorea

Chorea is one category of involuntary movement. The patient is restless and fidgety. There are fleeting and irregular fragments of coordinated movements which are purposeless. These tend to be rather abrupt and unpredictable and the patient may try to disguise them by turning the involuntary movements into something which looks purposeful. Chorea may affect any or many parts of the body and is often brought out by asking the patient to maintain a posture, e.g. tongue out, hold arms out. Severe chorea can interfere with normal function, leading to dysarthria, dysphagia, unsteady gait, falls and clumsy hands. Chorea can be confused with myoclonus and cerebellar ataxia.

Causes of chorea
- Huntington's disease (p. 298)
- chorea acanthocytosis (p. 299)
- Sydenham's (rheumatic) chorea (p. 300)
- pregnancy, the oral contraceptive pill (p. 300)
- systemic lupus erythematosus (p. 444)
- Wilson's disease (p. 310)
- hyperthyroidism (p. 456)
- hypocalcaemia (p. 457)
- polycythaemia rubra vera (p. 459)
- kernicterus (p. 300)
- cerebral palsy
- Fahr's syndrome (p. 293)
- cerebral anoxia (p. 292)
- carbon monoxide poisoning (p. 549)
- encephalitis lethargica (p. 290)
- ataxia telangiectasia (p. 202)

- dominant and idiopathic cerebellar ataxia (p. 201)
- xeroderma pigmentosum (p. 203)
- tardive dyskinesia (p. 309)
- focal paroxysmal kinesigenic choreoathetosis (p. 300)
- familial paroxysmal choreoathetosis (p. 300)
- stroke (p. 300)
- Hallervorden–Spatz disease (p. 292)
- Lesch–Nyhan syndrome (p. 482)
- drugs:
  amiodarone
  amphetamines
  antihistamines
  bromocriptine (p. 285)
  butyrophenones
  carbamazepine (p. 90)
  flunarizine
  flupenthixol
  L-dopa (p. 283)
  metoclopramide
  nomifensine
  phenobarbitone (p. 92)
  phenothiazines
  phenytoin (p. 88)

Treatment

The underlying cause should be removed if possible. Sometimes chorea can be controlled by drugs, but often only at the price of adverse effects: depression, drowsiness and parkinsonism.

- tetrabenazine, oral, 12.5 mg twice daily, increasing gradually if necessary and, if tolerated, to 50 mg 3 times daily
- haloperidol, oral, 5 mg 3 times daily, increasing gradually if necessary to 10 mg 3 times daily, or more if tolerated
- thiopropazate, oral, 5 mg 3 times daily, increasing if necessary to 30 mg 3 times daily
- pimozide, oral, 2 mg daily, increasing as necessary to 20 mg daily

Approach to the diagnosis of the cause of chorea

- past history; cerebral palsy, kernicterus, stroke
- family history; chorea, dementia, suicide
- pregnant? oral contraceptives?
- drugs and duration of exposure
- full blood count (polycythaemia rubra vera?) and film (acanthocytes?)

- ESR, antinuclear factor, lupus anticoagulant (?systemic lupus ery-thematosus)
- thyroid function
- copper studies (see Wilson's disease, p. 310)
- ASO titre (rheumatic chorea?)
- serum calcium (hypocalcaemia?)
- CT scan (basal ganglia infarct, haemorrhage, tumour, calcification, ect.)

Huntington's disease

This is an autosomal dominant disorder affecting males and females equally. The prevalence is about 6/100 000 population. There is degeneration and atrophy of the basal ganglia, particularly the caudate nucleus and putamen, and cerebral cortex.

The patients usually present in middle life with the gradual onset of chorea, often preceded or accompanied by behavioural, affective or psychotic disorders. As the disease progresses it becomes clear that the patient is de-menting and, within a few years, the patient is hopelessly demented, incontinent, mute, cachectic and has generalized chorea. CT scanning rarely shows obvious caudate nucleus atrophy except in advanced cases. The duration of the disease from onset to death is about 15 years. Suicide is common. A certain *clinical* diagnosis can only be made if there is an appropriate family history, but sometimes this is deliberately obscured. New mutations are excessively rare. It must be distinguished from autosomal dominant cerebellar ataxia of late onset (p. 201) and chorea-acanthocytosis (p. 299).

Onset during childhood is rare (3%). The clinical picture is of progressive akinesia, rigidity, dystonia, dementia and sometimes seizures. There is no chorea. The inheritance is usually from the father.

There is no cure but sometimes the chorea can be controlled (p. 297).

Prevention depends on well-organized and sympathetic genetic counselling. Until recently there was no reliable and available presymptomatic or prenatal diagnostic test and individuals at risk were advised not to have children. The risk of developing the disease in the child of an affected parent declines with age (Fig. 10.1) but not until after the all important child-bearing years. However, there is now a DNA probe to detect the approximate location of the Huntington's gene on the short arm of chromosome 4 in white blood cells. This allows the detection of presymptomatic individuals (provided DNA is available from at least one grandparent which is not often possible at present because their generation is dead) and, of wider applicability, prenatal prediction since grandparents of the fetus are much more likely to be living. For a fetus it should be possible to ascribe a risk from 0 to 50%, but not more, and this does not influence the risk situation for the parent.

The crucial point is that patients with, or at high risk of, Huntington's disease should be referred to a clinical genetics service and have blood taken

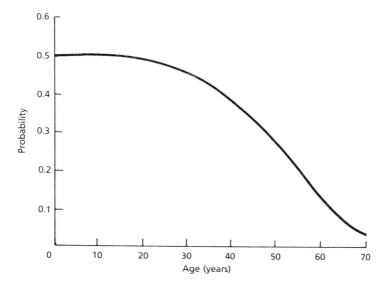

Fig. 10.1 Probability that the offspring of a parent with Huntington's disease will develop the disorder at a given age.

and stored for DNA analysis which will then allow more accurate genetic counselling for later generations.

Useful address

Association to Combat Huntington's Chorea
108 Battersey High St.
London
SW11 3HP
Tel: 071-223-7000

Rare causes of chorea

Chorea-acanthocytosis

This is very rare but important because, although it has some features of Huntington's disease, it has a more benign course, dementia does not occur, and inheritance is probably recessive. Onset is in early middle age with orofacial dyskinesia and then chorea, dystonia and tics of the limbs. Tendon reflexes are depressed and there is a subclinical motor neuropathy. More than 10% of the red blood cells are acanthocytes. The serum lipids are normal. Seizures occasionally occur. CK levels may be raised.

Sydenham's (rheumatic) chorea

This is an extremely rare complication of beta haemolytic streptococcal infection. The association with rheumatic fever is somewhat uncertain and can be occult. Even the antistreptolysin O titre is not necessarily raised. It occurs subacutely in children and adolescents, females more often than males. It usually resolves in a matter of months but may recur spontaneously, during pregnancy or while taking oral contraceptives.

Pregnancy and oral contraceptives

Chorea is a rare complication of pregnancy and when it occurs may be due to underlying systemic lupus erythematosus (p. 444) or recurrent rheumatic chorea (see above). It can be extremely severe but stops within weeks of delivery, and may recur in subsequent pregnancies. Also, chorea may complicate the use of oral contraceptives; this is very rare and fortunately is reversible.

Kernicterus

Neonatal hyperbilirubinaemia damages the basal ganglia and during childhood progressive chorea and athetosis develop. In addition, there may be mental handicap, seizures and corticospinal tract signs.

Focal paroxysmal kinesigenic choreoathetosis

Brief paroxysms of tonic, dystonic or choreoathetoid movements are precipitated by sudden movement or startle. The attacks last no more than a minute or two and may be unilateral or bilateral. They are controlled with phenytoin (p. 88).

Familial paroxysmal choreoathetosis

This is usually a dominant condition in which attacks of choreoathetosis and dystonic posturing, lasting several minutes, are provoked by alcohol, stress, emotion and caffeine. Clonazepam (p. 93) may be helpful.

Stroke

Rarely cerebral infarction or haemorrhage in the basal ganglia (often but not always in the subthalamic nucleus) causes acute contralateral chorea. This can be exceptionally wild and the proximal flinging movements of the arm or leg are then called hemiballismus. This normally resolves in a matter of weeks or months. Untreated, it can lead to injury and exhaustion.

Choreoathetosis, and dystonia, are more likely to complicate stroke in children than adults. Hemichorea is also occasionally caused by trauma or tumour of the contralateral basal ganglia.

Athetosis

Athetoid movements are involuntary writhing and snake-like movements of any part of the body. Usually they are worse during voluntary movement of the affected part which becomes clumsy. Often there is chorea as well and the causes of both movement disorders are more or less identical. *Pseudo-athetosis* is the writhing movement of the outstretched fingers, when the eyes are shut, due to impaired joint position sense (p. 15).

Dystonia

Dystonia is sustained muscle contraction causing an abnormal posture or movement which can be painful. Usually it is intermittent, at least to begin with, and it may be associated with chorea and other abnormal movements.
  Dystonic movements and postures may:
- be confined to one body part (e.g. arm): *focal dystonia*
- spread to at least two parts of the body: *segmental dystonia*
- spread to all four limbs and axial muscles: *generalized dystonia*
- be confined to the neck or back: *axial dystonia*
- be confined to more than one body part on the same side: *hemidystonia*

Causes

- acute drug-induced dystonia (p. 302)
- chronic drug induced dystonia: L-dopa (p. 283), bromocriptine (p. 285), phenytoin (p. 88), phenobarbitone (p. 92), carbamazepine (p. 90), tetrabenazine (p. 297)
- tardive dystonia (p. 309)
- primary dystonias:
  torsion dystonia (dystonia musculorum deformans, p. 303)
  cranial dystonia (Meige's syndrome, p. 303)
  spasmodic dysphonia (p. 303)
  spasmodic torticollis (p. 304)
  blepharospasm (p. 304)
- symptomatic secondary dystonias:
  metabolic
    Wilson's disease (p. 310)
    hypoparathyroidism (p. 457)
    homocystinaemia (p. 481)

Lesch–Nyhan syndrome (p. 482)
metachromatic leucodystrophy (p. 478)
hexosaminidase deficiency (p. 479)
akinetic rigid syndromes
   juvenile Huntington's disease (p. 298)
   chorea-acanthocytosis (p. 299)
   Parkinson's disease (p. 280)
   juvenile parkinsonism (p. 305)
   Hallervorden–Spatz disease (p. 292)
   Pelizaeus–Merzbacher disease (p. 292)
   Fahr's syndrome (p. 293)
focal basal ganglia lesions (stroke, etc., p. 305)
multiple sclerosis (p. 346)
cerebral palsy
cerebral anoxia (p. 292)
carbon monoxide poisoning (p. 549)
head injury
post-encephalitic parkinsonism (p. 290)
ataxia telangiectasia (p. 202)
focal paroxysmal kinesigenic choreoathetosis (p. 300)
familial paroxysmal choreoathetosis (p. 300)
dystonia with marked diurnal variation (p. 305)
occupational cramps (p. 305)

Acute drug-induced dystonia

Acute drug-induced dystonia, a rare adverse effect, is more common in children and adolescents than adults. It tends to occur after one or a few normal doses of the offending drug (most often given as an antiemetic):
- phenothiazines (e.g. chlorpromazine, prochlorperazine)
- butyrophenones (e.g. haloperidol, droperidol)
- metoclopramide
- antihistamines
- tetrabenazine
- domperidone
- chloroquine, amodiaquine

The dystonia is usually of the head and neck muscles with neck retraction, spasmodic torticollis, tongue protrusion, trismus, opisthotonos, choking and oculogyric crisis. It can be painful and frightening and often there is tachycardia and fever. It usually resolves in an hour or two. The main differential diagnosis is tetanus.

Treatment: i.v. diazepam 10 mg or i.v. benztropine 1–2 mg (proportionately less in children)

Torsion dystonia (dystonia musculorum deformans)

This type is rare, can be familial, and usually starts in childhood or adolescence. The cause is unknown. It is progressive but may eventually become static. Remission is most unusual. The dystonic writhing postures and movements affect the trunk, arms, legs and neck and there is a marked tortional component. It may be impossible for the patient to sit down. Grotesque and unlikely postures are taken up. Walking backwards or running may be easier than walking forwards. Blepharospasm (p. 304), spasmodic torticollis (p. 304) and writer's cramp (p. 305) may be additional features.

Treatment: occasionally large doses of a number of different drugs can help, at least temporarily, but to achieve this without intolerable adverse effects may be impossible, particularly in adults. The dose must be built up very slowly over many weeks:

- benzhexol, oral, up to 120 mg daily in 3 divided doses (or other anticholinergics) is the most effective and the dose should be increased by about 2 mg every 1 or 2 weeks, starting with 2 mg twice daily. Children are more likely than adults to be tolerant of adverse effects (p. 286)
- lithium, oral, up to 1500 mg daily in divided doses (p. 142)
- drugs as for chorea (p. 297)
- baclofen (p. 352), oral, up to 120 mg a day in 3 divided doses
- L-dopa (p. 283) or bromocriptine (p. 285)
- diazepam, oral, up to 100 mg daily in 3–4 divided doses
- carbamazepine (p. 90)

Stereotactic thalamotomy can help contralateral hemidystonia. Psychological treatments are usually unsuccessful (e.g. hypnotherapy, psychotherapy, behaviour therapy).

Cranial dystonia

Cranial dystonia (Meige's syndrome) is rare. It starts in middle age and tends to progress. There are dystonic and choreiform movements of the facial (blepharospasm, blinking, pouting), jaw, tongue, palate, larynx, neck and respiratory muscles. Functional blindness, dysarthria, dysphonia and dysphagia can be severe. It may be associated with torsion dystonia (above) and essential tremor (p. 294).

Spasmodic dysphonia

This may be isolated or part of a more widespread dystonic syndrome. There is laryngeal dystonia and spasm during speaking so the voice becomes hoarse, strained and eventually temporarily lost. Sometimes this is hysterical.

Spasmodic torticollis

This type is characterized by intermittent tilting or turning of the head to one side, sometimes neck extension (retrocollis), due to abnormal contractions of neck muscles. The movements are involuntary, forced and can be painful. Patients often develop tricks to straighten their head, e.g. touching the chin. Eventually the attacks become prolonged and even sustained throughout waking hours and the involved neck muscles hypertrophy. It tends to start in middle age, progress and sometimes improve or even remit. Usually no cause is found; a psychological one is suspected but seldom proven. Sometimes it is associated with:

- torsion dystonia (p. 303)
- writer's cramp (p. 305)
- essential tremor (p. 294)
- post-encephalitic parkinsonism (p. 290)
- acute drug-induced dystonia (p. 302)

There are no abnormal neurological or other signs apart from the movement disorder.

Treatment is unsatisfactory but can be explored along the lines of that for torsion dystonia (p. 303). Injection of botulinum toxin (see below) into the most overactive muscles (about 25 ng) may help some patients but has to be repeated every few months; transient dysphagia and voice change may occur. Surgical division of the upper cervical nerve roots bilaterally may help but can cause instability of the neck followed by arthritis and pain.

Blepharospasm

This denotes involuntary, repeated and sustained contractions of the eyelids bilaterally. It may be an intermittent problem or progressive and sometimes causes functional blindness. It occurs in isolation and/or occasionally in association with:

- cranial dystonia (p. 303)
- torsion dystonia (p. 303)
- Parkinson's disease (p. 281) but, more often, other akinetic rigid syndromes (p. 290)
- post-encephalitic parkinsonism (p. 290)
- Wilson's disease (p. 310)
- rostral brainstem lesions (multiple sclerosis, stroke, etc.)
- acute drug-induced dystonia (p. 302)
- essential tremor (p. 294)
- kernicterus (p. 300)

Medical treatment is the same as for torsion dystonia and is usually ineffective. Injection of botulinum toxin into the eyelid muscles has a reasonable effect after a week or so but has to be repeated every few months which may be unpleasant. It can cause ptosis and diplopia, usually transiently. The dose is about 1.5 ng (Porton Down type A botulinum toxin) in 2 ml saline around each eye. Section or avulsion of the peripheral branches of the facial nerve destined for the orbicularis oculi muscles can help in severe cases, but at the risk of facial weakness, and relief is not necessarily permanent.

Dystonia with marked diurnal variation

This is usually a dominantly inherited disorder in which children develop generalized dystonia, usually starting in the legs, in the afternoon and evening. It responds to low doses of L-dopa.

Hereditary juvenile dystonia-parkinsonism

This is usually autosomal dominant. It starts in childhood with difficulty walking and dystonia in the lower limbs, and progresses with more widespread dystonia and parkinsonism. A small dose of L-dopa is very effective.

Focal brain lesions

Focal brain lesions, i.e. tumour, arteriovenous malformation, head injury, stroke (usually only if in childhood) in the basal ganglia and thalamus region, occasionally cause dystonia in the contralateral arm and/or leg (hemidystonia) or spasmodic torticollis. There may be associated pyramidal signs. After acute brain injury the dystonia may not appear for some months.

Occupational cramps

Repetitive movements of the hands (and sometimes of the lips of instrument players) of people who use them a great deal at work (clerks, typists hairdressers, etc.) may lead to, or perhaps reveal, a general deterioration and loss of skill in a single specific movement, usually writing (so-called writer's cramp) or sometimes typing, harp playing, using scissors, morse code operating, violin playing, etc.

Onset is in adult life and the course is intermittent or progressive. If the specific activity involved is abandoned, the symptoms either resolve or at least become insignificant. In some people there may be progression to various dystonic syndromes, including torsion dystonia (p. 303), and also to Parkinson's disease (p. 280).

Typically writer's cramp causes the hand and forearm muscles to tighten and ache when writing. Grip becomes involuntarily tighter, abnormal and inappropriate. The hand is clumsy when writing and the pen may be jerked across the page. However, in most patients other activities are performed normally and there are no other neurological signs. Differentiation from

Parkinson's disease (p. 280), benign essential tremor (p. 294), task-specific action tremor (p. 295) and spasticity is usually straightforward.

The cause is unknown. It may be one of the dystonias and physically determined in some way or it may be psychological. Neither drug treatment as for torsion dystonia (p. 303) nor various psychological treatments are very successful. Even changing hands may merely transfer the problem to the previously unaffected side.

Useful address

Dystonia Society
Omnibus Workspace
39–41 North Road
Islington
London N7 9DP
Tel: 071-700-4594

Akathisia

Akathisia is a subjective feeling of restlessness or a 'need to move' which may be generalized or confined to one body part. It occurs at any time of day and may be relieved by lying down (cf. restless leg syndrome below). The restlessness may remain a subjective feeling or be associated with actual movements of the affected part, usually of a fidgety kind, although sometimes the movements may be stereotyped or semipurposeful. Often no cause is found but it can be an early symptom of parkinsonism (p. 280) or a result of drugs which cause tardive dyskinesia (p. 309). Indeed, drug-induced akathisia and tardive dyskinesia can be difficult to distinguish.

Restless legs (or Ekbom's) syndrome

This is a form of akathisia in which one or more often both legs feel uncomfortable (described rather variably as pain, pins and needles or burning usually in the muscles below the knees). There is an irresistible desire to move them. It is most noticeable when relaxing in the evening or in bed while trying to sleep. It is relieved by moving the legs, getting up and walking about. The patients may also have nocturnal myoclonus (p. 120). It tends to wax and wane in severity and nuisance to the patient, sometimes over many years. Usually no cause is found, but occasionally the patient is uraemic (p. 465), pregnant, iron deficient (p. 460) or has a peripheral neuropathy (p. 392), Parkinson's disease (p. 280) or multiple sclerosis (p. 344). It may also be a non-specific effect of fever, too much caffeine and possibly calcium blockers.

The treatment is of the underlying cause (if any) and the following possible drugs:

- clonazepam up to 2 mg, oral, if necessary, at bedtime, but only if really required, not for long periods
- carbamazepine, up to 300 or 400 mg, oral, if necessary, at bedtime
- L-dopa (p. 283), 50–100 mg, oral, at bedtime

Myoclonus

Myoclonic movements are involuntary, very brief, sudden, shock-like contractions of muscles, or groups of muscles which usually produce movement about the associated joints. They do not have the random flow of chorea nor the stereotyped features of tics. They can occur at rest or be precipitated by movement (action myoclonus). They may be isolated, repetitive and irregular, or rhythmic (e.g. palatal myoclonus). They are caused by an abnormal electrical discharge in the brain or spinal cord.

Myoclonus occurs in a huge variety of neurological and general medical disorders:

Progressive myoclonic encephalopathies

These are characterized by myoclonus with or without seizures as part of a progressive brain disorder.

- infections:
  subacute sclerosing panencephalitis (p. 525)
  Creutzfeldt–Jakob disease (p. 531)
  post-encephalitic parkinsonism (p. 290)
- inborn errors of metabolism:
  Gaucher's disease (p. 478)
  hexosaminidase deficiency (p. 479)
- Progressive myoclonic epilepsies (p. 75)
- Alzheimer's disease (p. 160)
- metabolic disorders:
  renal failure (p. 465)
  dialysis dementia (p. 467)
  hepatic encephalopathy (p. 467)
  respiratory failure
  hyponatraemia (p. 464)
  hypocalcaemia (p. 457)
- toxins:
  bismuth (p. 548)
  methyl bromide (p. 550)

Static myoclonic encephalopathies

These are characterized by myoclonus after an acute cerebral insult.

- post-anoxic action myoclonus (p. 309)
- post head injury

Myoclonic epilepsies

These are characterized by seizures accompanied by myoclonus
- infantile spasms (p. 74)
- Lenox–Gastaut syndrome (p. 75)
- juvenile myoclonic epilepsy (p. 75)

Benign hypnagogic myoclonus

On falling asleep almost everyone at some time experiences an occasional jerk of the whole body accompanied by arousal or startle reaction.

Essential familial myoclonus

This is autosomal dominant, appears before the age of 30, is not usually disabling or associated with other problems apart from essential tremor (p. 294) in some cases.

Focal myoclonus

This is myoclonus restricted to one group of muscles or body part.
- palatal myoclonus (below)
- segmental myoclonus (below)
- hemifacial spasm (p. 191)
- nocturnal myoclonus (p. 120)
- cortical myoclonus (p. 70)

Palatal myoclonus. This is a rhythmic (1–3 times per second) contraction of the soft palate throughout the day and night. Myoclonus is, therefore, a misnomer and palatal nystagmus more accurate. It causes difficulty with speaking and swallowing and also an irritating rhythmic clicking in the ear. Some patients have associated movements of the ocular muscles and diaphragm. It can be caused by an infarct or other lesion in the brainstem but usually there is no explanation.

Segmental myoclonus. Segmental myoclonus is restricted to one part of the body innervated by the brainstem or spinal cord. The causes include tumour, arteriovenous malformation (p. 233), trauma and transverse myelitis (p. 332). It must be distinguished from cortical myoclonus (p. 70), simple partial motor origin seizures (p. 70) and epilepsia partialis continua (p. 70) which are due to cortical epileptic discharges which may be evident on the EEG.

Post-anoxic action myoclonus. This can appear after recovery from severe anoxia. The myoclonus is precipitated by a voluntary movement and sometimes by noise. There may be no other evidence of brain damage.

Treatment

No specific treatment is required if the underlying cause can be treated (e.g. renal failure) or the myoclonus is no more than a trivial nuisance. Some patients require anticonvulsants to control other more disabling types of seizure and the myoclonus often responds as well. Specific treatments for myoclonus itself are not always successful but include:
- clonazepam, oral (for dosage, see Table 2.1 and p. 93).
- sodium valproate, oral (for dosage, see Table 2.1, and p. 91)

Drug-induced movement disorders

Certain drugs produce idiosyncratic and dose-related movement disorders, the most common being phenothiazines. The same drug may cause a number of different and overlapping disorders. They are described under the preceding sections, i.e. drugs causing:
- parkinsonism (p. 288)
- neuroleptic malignant syndrome (p. 289)
- tremor (p. 293)
- chorea (p. 297)
- dystonia (p. 301)
- akathisia (p. 306)
- tardive dyskinesia and dystonia (below)

Tardive dyskinesia and dystonia

Involuntary, choreoathetoid movements around the mouth and of the face (grimacing, chewing, tongue protrusion, lip smacking, etc.), and sometimes involving the neck and limbs, may occur when certain drugs have been taken for months or years (perhaps as a consequence of dopamine receptor supersensitivity) or after withdrawal of long-term medication:
- phenothiazines
- butyrophenones
- antihistamines
- flunarizine
- flupenthixol
- metoclopramide

   Less commonly the movements are dystonic (tardive dystonia) and affect any body part or are generalized. Some patients have both tardive dyskinesia and dystonia.

The condition is more common in the elderly and perhaps in brain-damaged patients. The problem is persistent and may worsen with continued drug exposure. Most patients do not, at least at first, notice the abnormal movements but sometimes they are distressing, embarrassing and interfere with speaking and eating.

Note: Consider other causes of involuntary movements before necessarily incriminating drugs. Also, tardive dyskinesia-like movements occasionally appear in the normal elderly.

Treatment

If possible the offending drug should slowly be withdrawn, but the movements may worsen transiently and take months or years to disappear, if ever. If they are distressing, or show no sign of disappearing, or the causative drug has to be continued, it is very uncertain how patients should be treated. As a last resort, increasing the dose of the offending drug may help for a while. Occasionally tetrabenazine (up to 25 mg 3 times daily), the cholinergic drug deanol (up to 300 mg 4 times daily), or *anti*cholinergic drugs (see torsion dystonia, p. 303) are helpful. Other possibilities include sulpiride, pimozide and vitamin E.

Prevention depends on avoiding inappropriate prescribing of the potentially causative drugs.

Wilson's disease (hepatolenticular degeneration)

Although very rare, it is important to recognize Wilson's disease because it is treatable and, if left untreated, fatal. It is an autosomal recessive condition with abnormal copper deposition in the brain (particularly the basal ganglia), liver, cornea and other organs. The 'hepatic' onset tends to occur in children, causing cirrhosis, and the 'neurological' onset is usually in adolescence and almost never over the age of 40.

The neurological symptoms are insidious and progressive. Often a psychiatric diagnosis is made initially because the first symptoms may merely be some clumsiness of the arms and legs, personality change, and a mild fall-off in mental performance. Eventually the full blown disease develops with increasing and progressive:

• tremor (postural and intention), titubation of the head
• rigidity and bradykinesia
• dystonia and chorea
• incoordination, limb ataxia
• dysarthria, dysphagia, drooling
• dementia
• seizures rarely

Aminoaciduria, abnormal liver function and thrombocytopenia are common at the time of neurological presentation.

The diagnosis of neurological disease will not be missed if Kayser–Fleischer rings are diligently sought, if necessary by slitlamp examination of the cornea. The brown ring of copper deposition is at the edge of the cornea, in the upper and lower parts first, and is most easily seen at the bedside by using an auroscope without the earpiece. Biochemically, the diagnosis is confirmed by a low plasma caeruloplasmin (the copper binding plasma protein), less than 20 mg per 100 ml. Serum copper tends to be low and urine copper excretion high. Liver copper concentration is high but seldom needs to be measured. CT may show low density in the basal ganglia, cortical atrophy and hydrocephalus.

Treatment

- Usually a low copper diet is unnecessary.
- Penicillamine, oral, 1.0–2.0 g daily in 2–4 divided doses before food, plus pyridoxine 25 mg daily to counter the anti-pyridoxine effect of penicillamine; adverse effects include rash, nausea, taste loss, anorexia, fever, proteinuria, nephrotic syndrome, lymphadenopathy, thrombocytopenia, agranulocytosis, myasthenia, lupus erythematosus, polymyositis. Tolerance to adverse effects can be achieved by starting with a low dose (250 mg twice daily) and increasing it slowly over a few weeks.
- Trientine, for those intolerant of penicillamine; oral, 1.2–2.4 g daily in 2–4 divided doses before food. Adverse effects: nausea.
- Oral zinc sulphate (200 mg 3 times daily), particularly if toxicity on penicillamine or trientine, has been suggested since it blocks copper absorption from the gut. It can cause indigestion.

Monitor clinical response, full blood count, proteinuria and urine copper excretion.

Note: Early after starting treatment the condition may worsen and any improvement can take weeks or months. If caught early, the prognosis is excellent but treatment *must* be lifelong. 10% of patients do not respond to treatment. The family should receive genetic advice and presymptomatic siblings should be identified and treated.

Tics

Tics are abrupt, repetitive, rather stereotyped, coordinated but inappropriate and involuntary jerk-like movements. They are relatively easy to imitate and can be voluntarily suppressed for a time, usually at the expense of mounting inner tension. Muscles around the eye, face, neck and shoulders are the most commonly affected and the tics are worse at times of stress or anxiety, and when being observed.

Males are three times more often affected than females. The onset is in childhood or adolescence. A single tic occurs in about 10% of children but usually disappears in adolescence. It is unusual to find a cause, even an overtly psychological explanation. Occasionally tics are part of an organic disease (post-encephalitic parkinsonism, p. 290, Sydenham's chorea, p. 300).

Treatment is reassurance, explanation and occasionally psycho- or behaviour therapy.

Gilles de la Tourette syndrome

This is a rare and sometimes familial disorder. Multiple tics develop in childhood or adolescence and are accompanied by explosive stereotyped verbal utterances (usually swear words, coprolalia) and sounds (grunts, throat clearing, sniffs, barks, etc.), repetition of the last word or sentence of others' (echolalia) or their own speech (palilalia), obsessional/compulsive behaviour and sometimes obscene (copropraxia) and other gestures. Males are more frequently affected than females. It tends to persist in adult life but the severity often declines. It is probably not an organic disease, but psychological treatments are seldom helpful.

Some patients respond to haloperidol: starting dose, oral, 0.5 mg 3 times daily, increasing to as much as 10 mg 3 times daily if necessary. Pimozide is an alternative; starting with 1 mg daily, oral, slowly increasing to 10 mg daily if necessary. Clonidine may help a few: increasing up to 6 µg per kg daily, oral, in 3 divided doses, but sedation can occur. Withdrawal must be slow, to avoid rebound hypertension.

Hiccups

Hiccups are due to intermittent uncontrollable and sudden contractions of the diaphragm and other respiratory muscles. They are usually short-lived and self-limiting but are sometimes intractable, particularly in males. They may be spontaneous and idiopathic, due to excessive alcohol or food consumption, high doses of corticosteroids, renal failure, general anaesthesia, brainstem lesions, stimulation of the relevant reflex arc (afferent vagal and efferent phrenic nerves among others) or to some pathological condition 'irritating' the diaphragm. There are numerous suggested cures:

Folk cures

- drinking from the wrong side of a cup
- swallowing granulated sugar

- breath holding
- irritation of the pharnyx and gag reflex
- sudden fright
- induced sneezing (e.g. by pepper)

Drugs

- chlorpromazine, 50 mg i.v., and then oral maintenance if necessary, 75 mg, 3 times daily or possibly more
- haloperidol, 5 mg, 3 times daily, oral, increasing as necessary to 60 mg daily
- metoclopramide, 10 mg, 3 times daily, oral
- sodium valproate (p. 91)
- nifedipine, 10–20 mg, 3 times daily, oral
- other suggested drugs include amantadine, apomorphine, amitriptyline, baclofen, phenytoin

Catatonia

Catatonia is a syndrome characterized by posturing and waxy flexibility of one or more body parts (which tend to stay where they are put) often associated with psychosocial withdrawal, excitement, bizarre repetitious movements, fever, circulatory failure and sometimes leading to stupor and death. Although it occurs mainly in schizophrenia and affective disorders, various organic causes should also be considered:
- encephalitis (p. 498)
- non-convulsive status epilepticus (p. 97)
- multiple sclerosis (p. 342)
- neuroleptic malignant syndrome (p. 289)
- typhoid fever (p. 509)
- systemic lupus erythematosus (p. 444)

In many cases no cause at all is found. Symptomatic treatment is electroconvulsive therapy.

11 Disorders of the spinal roots and cord

The spinal cord extends from its junction with the brainstem at the foramen magnum to its termination as the conus medullaris opposite the first lumbar vertebra (Fig. 11.1). In neonates and infants the cord extends further down the lumbosacral vertebral canal. A pair of nerve roots emerge at each segmental level of the spinal cord: an anterior root carrying efferent motor fibres from the anterior horn cells of that spinal segment and a posterior root carrying afferent sensory fibres to the dorsolateral part of the cord. Each pair of roots unites near its corresponding intervertebral foramen through which the

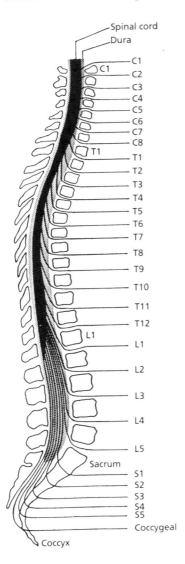

Fig. 11.1 Diagram to show the relationship between the vertebrae, spinal cord and spinal roots. The cord and proximal roots are surrounded by cerebrospinal fluid (shown shaded) contained in the dural sac.

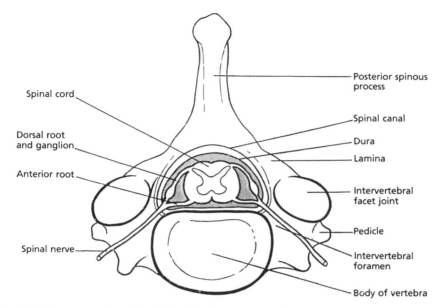

Spinal cord

Dorsal root
and ganglion

Anterior root

Spinal nerve

Posterior spinous
process

Spinal canal

Dura

Lamina

Intervertebral
facet joint

Pedicle

Intervertebral
foramen

Body of vertebra

Fig. 11.2 Diagram to show the relationship between vertebra, spinal cord, nerve roots and spinal nerves. Shading represents CSF in the subarachnoid space.

roots pass out of the spinal canal as a mixed motor and sensory spinal nerve (Fig. 11.2).

Since there are eight cervical nerve root pairs, but only seven cervical vertebrae, the first cervical spinal nerve emerges above the first cervical vertebra and the eighth below the seventh cervical vertebra. Thereafter the spinal roots leave the spinal cord with increasing downward angulation and, below the first lumbar vertebra, the lumbar and sacral roots of the cauda equina fill the spinal canal but are still covered by the blind termination of the dural sac as far down as the sacrum (Fig. 11.1). In the thoracic region the spinal cord and vertebral levels are not the same: the T10 vertebra corresponds to the T12 cord and the L1 vertebra to the sacral cord segments (Fig. 11.1).

Disorders of nerve roots (radiculopathies)

Lesions tend to affect both the sensory and motor nerve roots together at any one particular segmental level. Causes include:
- trauma
- compression (see spinal cord compression, p. 320)
- neuralgic amyotrophy (p. 368)
- infections:

herpes zoster (p. 523)

Guillain–Barré syndrome (p. 398)

• peripheral neuropathies (p. 389) also involving nerve roots (i.e. poly-radiculopathies)

A *motor (anterior) root lesion* causes lower motor neurone weakness and wasting, perhaps with fasciculation, of the group of muscles (myotome) it supplies. If the efferent arc of a tendon reflex is subserved by that root, then it is likely to be depressed or lost (p. 12). From the practical clinical point of view one needs to know which movements are subserved by which motor roots and their associated myotomes (see below) and the root and peripheral nerve supply of individual muscles (Table 1.2). Thus, weakness of a particular movement, or muscle(s), which is of a lower motor neurone type (p. 8) allows one to deduce which motor root (or peripheral nerve) is involved. For example, weakness of shoulder abduction along with weakness and wasting of the deltoid, supraspinatus, infraspinatus and biceps muscles is most likely due to a C5 root lesion (Table 1.2 and below).

Relationship between specific motor roots and the movements for which they are responsible. This is approximate since there is overlap between the muscles innervated from individual roots. Also, note that T2 to L1 motor root lesions are not usually detectable because of the difficulty in examining individual intercostal and abdominal wall muscles and overlap of the muscle territories of supply between individual roots.

C5	shoulder abduction and some elbow flexion
C6	elbow flexion in semiprone position (i.e. brachioradialis)
C7	extension of elbow, wrist and fingers
C8	flexion of wrist and fingers, grip
L2	small muscles of the hand
L3	hip flexion
T3	hip adduction and knee extension
T4	ankle dorsiflexion and inversion
L4/L5	hip extension
L5/S1	great toe dorsiflexion and knee flexion
S1	ankle plantar flexion and eversion

A *sensory (posterior) root lesion* causes diminished or absent cutaneous sensation, affecting light touch over a more extensive area than pain, in the corresponding skin dermatome (Fig. 11.3). The pattern is somewhat variable between individuals and, because of overlap between adjacent dermatomes, sensory loss from damage to a single nerve root may be slight or even absent.

Thus, knowledge of the dermatomes and the pattern of sensory loss from individual sensory nerve lesions (Chapter 14) allows one to localize a lesion in the peripheral sensory pathway. On the trunk the dermatomes are

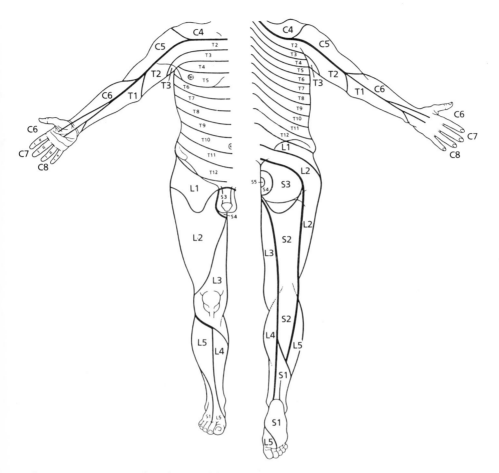

Fig. 11.3 Approximate distribution of dermatomes on the upper and lower limb. (Reproduced with permission from *Aids to the Examination of the Peripheral Nervous System*, Ballière Tindall.)

arranged in bands between T3 and T12, with T6 at about the xiphisternum and T10 at the umbilicus. There is no C1 sensory root representation on the skin so that numbness on the back of the head and upper neck is due to a C2 root lesion (Fig. 7.3). The dermatomes do not cross the midline.

Sensory root lesions also can cause pain which tends to be felt rather diffusely in the corresponding myotome (e.g. 'sciatica' in low lumbar root lesions). Impaired joint position sense is unpredictable, e.g. a C8 root lesion can cause impairment in the little finger, but not always. A tendon reflex subserved by a particular sensory root will be depressed or absent (p. 12).

S2–S4 root lesions may impair bladder and rectal function (p. 31) and cause impotence in the male (p. 33). A T1 root lesion may cause an ipsilateral Horner's syndrome (p. 178).

Spinal cord and root compression

This can be an emergency; surgical decompression is sometimes curative and it is, therefore, important to recognize it quickly. The possible causes are:

Diseases of vertebrae and discs

- fracture or dislocation
- prolapsed intervertebral disc (p. 326)
- spondylosis (p. 327)
- primary, and more often secondary, tumours (p. 321)
- infection (osteomyelitis, TB and Pott's disease of the spine, p. 513, etc.)
- osteoporotic vertebral collapse
- Paget's disease of bone (p. 483)
- atlanto-axial dislocation (trauma, rheumatoid disease, p. 448)
- Down's syndrome
- psoriatic arthropathy
- ankylosing spondylitis (p. 450)
- sickle cell disease/trait (p. 460)
- fluorosis
- congenital anomalies (Arnold–Chiari malformation, p. 202; basilar impression, p. 202; spinal dysraphism, p. 329; achondroplasia, p. 484; multiple hereditary exostoses; Klippel–Feil syndrome, p. 202)
- spinal hyperostosis due to taking retinoids
- kyphoscoliosis

Extradural conditions

- epidural abscess (p. 505)
- secondary tumours (p. 321)
- epidural haemorrhage:
  trauma
  haemostatic failure (p. 462)
  anticoagulants
  haemangioma of vertebral body
  epidural spinal arteriovenous malformation (p. 335)
  epidural anaesthesia (p. 44)
  lumbar puncture in anticoagulated patients (p. 44)
  idiopathic (the majority)
- extramedullary haematopoiesis (p. 461)
- epidural fat (Cushing's syndrome, p. 455)

Meningeal conditions

- primary or secondary tumour (below)
- arachnoiditis (p. 335)
- arachnoid cysts
- infections:
  tuberculosis (p. 512)
  syphilis (p. 515)
  fungal granuloma (p. 532)
  cysticercosis (p. 538)
  schistosomiasis (p. 539)
- sarcoid granuloma (p. 472)

Disorders of the nerve roots or cord

- primary or secondary tumour (below)
- arteriovenous malformation (p. 335)
- trauma

Classification of tumours in this region

- Extradural (usually metastatic):
  secondary tumours from
      bronchus (usually single spinal lesion)
      breast (often multiple extradural deposits)
      prostate
      kidney
      gastrointestinal tract, etc.
  neuroblastoma
  lymphoma (p. 275) and leukaemia (p. 459)
  myeloma/plasmacytoma (p. 460)
  primary bone tumours
  sarcoma
  haemangioma of bone
- Intradural but extramedullary:
  neurofibroma
  meningioma (commonly thoracic, p. 271)
  sarcoma (female more often than male)
  chordoma (commonly sacral region, p. 275)
  dermoid (usually sacral region, p. 274)
  lipoma (p. 275)
  secondary tumour (rare)
  malignant meningitis (p. 277)
- Intramedullary (uncommon):
  ependymoma (cauda equina or cord, p. 272)
  astrocytoma (mostly cervical, p. 271)

haemangioblastoma (p. 272)
oligodendroglioma (p. 272)
secondary tumour (very rare)

Spinal tumours are most often metastases rather than primary benign or malignant tumours. Metastases usually spread from the vertebral body into the anterior and anterolateral parts of the dural space. They tend to occur in the thoracic region and are distinctly unusual in the cervical spine except when due to local spread from the nasopharynx, etc.

Clinical features

The spinal cord and roots are vulnerable to compression since they are contained within the rigid vertebral canal (Fig. 11.2). The canal width varies so that individuals with constitutionally narrow canals are most likely to be affected by cord compression. From Fig. 11.2 it can be seen that the spinal cord is particularly vulnerable to posterior intervertebral disc protrusion, and the spinal nerves to posterolateral disc protrusion and bony overgrowth around the intervertebral facet joints.

The clinical features depend on the location and speed of progression of the compressive lesion. Acute onset suggests trauma, prolapsed intervertebral disc (p. 326), vertebral body collapse, epidural haemorrhage (p. 320), etc.; subacute onset, tuberculosis (p. 512), epidural abscess (p. 505), etc; and, slow insidious progression, neurofibroma, meningioma (p. 271), spondylosis (p. 323), etc.

Compression of the cord causes an upper motor neurone deficit below the level of the lesion which is almost never unilateral, although it may be very asymmetrical in its clinical manifestations. Thus, a high cervical cord lesion will cause symptoms and/or signs in the arms as well as in the legs but a thoracic cord lesion will affect only the legs.

Sensory loss to some or all modalities occurs below the level of the lesion but may be slight or even absent at times depending on whether and which ascending spinal cord pathways are involved; sensory symptoms and signs tend to start in the feet and spread up to just below the anatomical level of the lesion. Cervical cord compression may cause Lhermitte's symptom (p. 18), ipsilateral Horner's syndrome, but rather unusually (p. 178), and sometimes particularly prominent loss of joint position sense in the fingers even when other sensory signs and corticospinal features are slight or absent. Occasionally, early cord lesions cause cerebellar-looking ataxia even when joint position sense is normal.

In acute cord lesions there is 'spinal shock' and the affected limbs are weak and flaccid, deep tendon reflexes are lost below the lesion, but the plantar responses are extensor and usually there is a sensory level and sphincter involvement.

Acute cord compression causes a painless atonic distended bladder with overflow incontinence (p. 31), whereas an incomplete or slowly progressive lesion tends to cause a small spastic bladder with urgency of micturition (p. 31). Bladder involvement occurs only with bilateral cord lesions; there is often associated impotence in males (p. 33) and sometimes rectal sphincter disturbance with constipation, but rarely faecal incontinence (p. 33).

Acute and major high cervical cord lesions above the segmental supply of the diaphragm (C3, C4, C5) may paralyse ventilation.

Spinal root and nerve compression causes segmental motor, sensory and sphincter symptoms and signs (p. 318) which are extremely useful for localizing the site of the lesion. Below the L1 vertebra only spinal roots can be involved, whereas above this level compressive lesions may affect either the cord, or the roots, or both. For example, a compressive lesion at the 5th cervical vertebra may cause a combination of segmental motor and sensory signs implicating the C5 nerve root (perhaps only an absent biceps and supinator reflex on the side of the lesion), along with corticospinal tract signs in the legs with or without a sensory level below C5. A lesion at the T12 vertebra may cause a combination of lumbosacral root signs and, by compressing the sacral segments of the cord (conus medullaris), extensor plantar responses (see also p. 35).

The non-neurological features may point to the cause of the lesion:
• spinal pain and/or tenderness (epidural abscess, p. 505, acute prolapsed disc, p. 326, epidural haemorrhage, p. 320, metastasis, vertebral collapse, etc.)

Note: spinal pain at night is highly suggestive of a tumour

• impairment of straight leg raising (lumbosacral root irritation)
• spinal angulation due to vertebral body collapse (TB, p. 513, tumour, etc.)
• skin lesions, e.g. café-au-lait spots in neurofibromatosis (p. 277)
• sacral dimple (spinal dysraphism, p. 329)
• malaise, fever, loss of weight (metastasis, infection)
• spinal bruit (arteriovenous malformation, p. 335)
• known primary cancer present, or removed in the past, makes metastatic cord compression likely

Diagnosis

It is important to think of cord or root compression in any patient becoming weak in the legs and/or arms, particularly if there is loss of sensation in the limbs and sphincter disturbance. In acute cases *urgent* investigation is required followed by treatment if possible since the prognosis for recovery is poor once there is complete paralysis of the legs (and arms) or urinary retention.

The diagnosis depends on the history, bothering to do a simple neurological examination which is so easily omitted if the patient is in bed postoperatively or with cancer, and a general medical examination. In urgent cases one does not wait for the results of the simple investigations before proceeding directly to myelography, CT or MRI.

Investigations should normally include:

- full blood count and ESR
- syphilis serology
- chest X-ray for:
  primary or secondary tumour
  tuberculosis
  paravertebral shadow (Pott's disease, neurofibroma)
- spinal X-ray at the appropriate level suggested by the neurological lesion
for:
  erosion of vertebral bodies or pedicles by tumour
  paraspinal mass (TB)
  vertebral body collapse (osteoporosis, infection, tumour)
  intervertebral disc space narrowing (spondylosis) or destruction (infection)
  osteophytes, subluxation, spondylolisthesis, width of spinal canal
  scalloping of posterior margin of vertebral body (long-standing tumour)
  instability of neck (flexion and extension views required)
  intervertebral exit foramina (oblique views required in neck) diminished in
    spondylosis, enlarged by neurofibroma

Myelography

This is usually required unless there is an *obvious* non-compressive cause for the cord/root syndrome (p. 330). It is *always* required in an acute cord syndrome apart perhaps from trauma. Since cord compression may require surgery, the patient should normally be transferred to a neurological centre before myelography.

Myelography can reveal distortion and/or obstruction of the CSF space around the cord and roots. The clinical site of the lesion will direct the radiologist's attention to a particular location, but, unless a lesion is found to explain the clinical picture, it is usually necessary to pass the contrast medium up to and through the foramen magnum to avoid missing a meningioma or Arnold–Chiari malformation in this region. A common mistake is to image only from the L1 vertebra downwards in a patient with a lumbosacral root lesion, but the lumbar roots arise as high up as the 10th thoracic vertebra.

If the lumbar puncture to introduce contrast medium fails (for example the needle passes straight into a tumour), then the contrast must be injected into the subarachnoid space by the lateral cervical approach (or cisterna magna).

Note: Widening of the spinal cord in the antero-posterior view may be due to anterior or posterior cord compression, but if it is also present in the lateral view then the possibilities are a cord tumour (p. 321), transverse myelitis (p. 332) or a syrinx (p. 334).

CT scanning

CT scanning of the vertebral canal is increasingly used either by itself to demonstrate disc lesions and spondylosis; with contrast enhancement to visualize tumours; immediately after myelography to clarify details of cord compression, particularly in the occipito-cervical region, lateral disc protrusions, extraspinal extent of tumours; delayed after myelography to demonstrate uptake of contrast into a syrinx; and sometimes after puncture of a spinal cord cavity to show greater anatomical detail (endomyelography).

MRI

MRI is rapidly becoming the preferred method of investigating spinal cord syndromes. Not only does it display the bones and soft structures impinging on the spinal cord and roots better than myelography and CT, but it also shows cord cavitation (e.g. syringomyelia), inflammation (transverse myelitis, multiple sclerosis) and intramedullary tumours.

Lumbar puncture

This alone is not only unhelpful but can be counter-productive since it makes subsequent myelography more difficult if it causes CSF pooling in the sub- and extradural spaces, and it may precipitate acute deterioration if there is spinal cord compression.

CSF

CSF obtained at myelography must *always* be examined for protein, glucose and cells and then stored, particularly in case the myelogram does not indicate a surgical approach (e.g. a normal myelogram, equivocal changes of spondylosis, etc.). The CSF may reveal the underlying cause of the spinal cord or root problem:
- malignant cells in malignant meningitis (p. 277)
- oligoclonal bands in multiple sclerosis, etc. (p. 348)
- positive culture in chronic infection (TB, fungus, etc.)

If there is a spinal block, the CSF protein will be very high (perhaps over 5 g/l) and occasionally this may cause raised intracranial pressure (p. 261).

The management of spinal tumours

In patients with known primary malignant disease, clearcut clinical features of progressive spinal cord and/or root compression *and* plain X-ray changes of a secondary deposit in the appropriate place for the neurological lesion, there is probably no need for myelography, particularly if there are multiple secondaries and the overall prognosis is poor. In this situation the chance of neurological improvement and enhanced quality of life from neurosurgical decompression is negligible, no better than after treatment with radiotherapy, which is often useful to control local pain.

If there is no known primary malignancy, then a myelogram or MRI must be performed and, if a compressive mass lesion is found (and definitely does not look like spondylosis, thoracic disc, etc.), then a tissue diagnosis may be possible by CT-guided percutaneous biopsy. Otherwise, surgery is required to obtain biopsy material and perhaps to decompress the cord and/or roots; such decompression is, however, probably no more effective than radiotherapy, chemotherapy or hormonal therapy (depending on tumour type) and should be avoided except perhaps in acute cases of malignant tumour compression. Of course, if the tumour is benign, it should be removed if technically possible. If unremitting pain is due to spinal instability, particularly in the neck, then operative fixation of the vertebral column may be helpful.

If a secondary deposit is found without a known primary, then further investigation assists in the general management of the patient and helps to indicate specific treatment possibilities:

- mammography
- pelvic examination
- serum acid phosphatase
- bone scan (skeletal survey is more sensitive in myeloma)
- faecal occult bloods and, if positive, barium studies
- urine occult blood and, if positive, renal imaging
- liver ultrasound
- plasma protein electrophoresis

Degenerative disorders of vertebrae and discs

The acute 'slipped disc'

Acute extrusion of the nucleus pulposus of the intervertebral disc may be spontaneous, or precipitated by lifting, sudden back movement and straining. The prolapse is usually posterolateral rather than central. The lumbar discs are most often affected (L4–S1), cervical discs occasionally (C4–T1), and thoracic discs rarely. The patients are usually young adults or middle-aged.

The clinical consequences are some combination of the following:

- Acute pain, local tenderness and paraspinal muscle spasm at the level of the prolapse. The pain is worse on moving or coughing and relieved by certain postures and rest. Spinal pain which is *worse* at rest is more likely to be due to a tumour or abscess.
- Acute nerve root compression, which is usually unilateral, affecting one or perhaps two roots. On the other hand, a central prolapse of a lumbar disc may compress most of the cauda equina, causing multiple lumbosacral

root lesions and sphincter disturbance. Root pain and sensory disturbance is exacerbated by movement, coughing and straining; root 'irritation' can be tested in the legs by straight leg raising (lower lumbar and sacral root compression) and the femoral stretch test (upper lumbar roots although they are rarely affected by a disc prolapse).

Note: In the Guillain–Barré syndrome nerve stretch tests may cause pain (p. 399).

In the cervical region a prolapsed disc affects the root at its own level, but in the lumbar region the roots are angulated and bear an inconstant relationship with the prolapsed disc whose site can be more accurately determined from imaging (generally myelography or CT) than the clinical features which are best used to direct the radiologist to approximately the correct place. On balance, a prolapsed disc damages the root passing to the foramen below, i.e. an L4/L5 disc usually affects the L5 root.

• Acute spinal cord compression (thoracic and cervical discs only), see p. 322.

Treatment

Treatment is almost always conservative at first since the symptoms usually settle in a few days or weeks with appropriate analgesia, avoiding unwise activities (bending and lifting for lumbar discs) and bed rest on a firm mattress or board. Further immobilization may help; a cervical collar must be rigid enough to prevent neck movement, particularly if flexion and extension are painful. At night a softer collar may be more tolerable. A lumbar corset must be firm enough to limit painful back movements. Traction and manipulation can be effective in the right hands.

Surgical decompression is occasionally indicated:
• acute cord compression
• acute bladder disturbance as a result of a central prolapse of a lumbar disc
• continuing root pain from a prolapsed lumbosacral or cervical disc which has not responded to about six weeks' conservative treatment
• progressive loss of motor function; trivial root signs such as an absent tendon reflex are not an indication for surgery

Spondylosis

This has several features: bony overgrowth around the intervertebral facet joints, osteophyte formation and bony bars at the intervertebral spaces, thickening of the intervertebral ligaments and slipping of one vertebral body on the next (spondylolisthesis) with narrowing of the disc spaces. These bony changes are almost universal on mid to low cervical spine and lower lumbosacral X-rays in elderly people and cannot be regarded as the definite cause of neurological symptoms and signs unless myelography, CT or MRI shows cord and/or root compression in a place appropriate to the neurological lesion. Thoracic spondylosis occurs but is seldom symptomatic. The cause of spondylosis is a combination of vertebral instability, perhaps due to a prolapsed disc in the past, repetitive spinal trauma and 'ageing'.

The clinical consequences usually appear from late middle age and are some combination of:

• Pain and stiffness locally, which is often intermittent, lasting days or weeks with months or years of freedom. This is usually exacerbated by movement, posture, coughing, straining, etc. However, pain can be completely absent even with severe disease and neurological complications.

• Acute disc protrusion is unusual, although it may have occurred in the past.

• Subacute or chronic cervical cord compression (and perhaps ischaemia) at one or more levels, and aggravated by a congenitally narrow cervical canal. The onset may be rather acute after an apparently trivial neck injury (e.g. whiplash or even after just a trip) and progression is probably accelerated by frequent extension and flexion of the neck. Bladder symptoms are rather unusual. Cervical spondylotic myelopathy may remit and there can be long periods of neurological stability, or even freedom from symptoms, or there may be progressive disability.

• Subacute and chronic nerve root compression and perhaps ischaemia which may remit, stabilize or progress. Sensory symptoms are usually exacerbated by movement. The common roots affected are C5, C6 and C7 in the neck and L5 and S1 in the back.

• Claudication of the cauda equina which is probably the result of lumbosacral spondylosis along with a congenitally narrow canal and possibly ischaemia due to atheroma of the lower aorta. There is often a recent or past history of lumbar pain, back injury or 'sciatica'. The patient complains of pain, numbness and maybe weakness of the buttocks and legs (usually bilaterally), which appears on standing up or when walking for a while, and is relieved by bending forwards, lying down or sitting down rather than by merely standing still and erect. Ischaemic *muscle* claudication comes on only after walking and is relieved by standing still, not necessarily by bending forward. Lumbosacral root signs are often absent or can only be found after exercise (absent tendon reflex, weakness, etc.), and straight leg raising can be surprisingly normal. On myelography there is total or subtotal obstruction of CSF flow at one or more lumbar levels.

• Possibly syncope (p. 105) or brainstem TIA (p. 219) due to vertebral artery compression.

Treatment

Treatment is usually conservative in the first instance with appropriate analgesia, rest and immobilization if possible (p. 327) along with avoidance of heavy lifting, bending, etc. in the case of lumbar spondylosis. Surgery may be indicated:

• Progressive cervical myelopathy with disability is sometimes helped by cervical decompression and/or fusion of the involved vertebrae.

- Persistent nerve root pain, or progressive loss of motor root function, may be helped by laminectomy and decompression.
- Claudication of the cauda equina is often relieved by a wide lumbar laminectomy but the symptoms tend to recur.

Pain in the low back is very common and its important causes include:

Acute low back pain:
- prolapsed intervertebral disc (p. 326)
- spontaneous vertebral collapse (osteoporosis, corticosteroids, tumour, etc.)
- epidural haemorrhage (p. 320)
- 'lumbosacral strain', the majority

Subacute low back pain:
- osteomyelitis
- epidural abscess (p. 505)
- spinal tumours (p. 321)
- spinal arteriovenous malformation (p. 337)
- lumbar spondylosis (p. 327)
- pelvic tumours
- diskitis
- osteoporosis

Chronic low back pain:
- lumbar spondylosis (p. 327)
- spinal tumours (p. 321)
- pelvic tumours
- arachnoiditis (p. 336)
- osteoporosis
- ankylosing spondylitis (p. 450)
- polymyalgia rheumatica (p. 450)

Note: Pain in the low back may be referred from the abdomen, kidneys and pelvis.

Spinal dysraphism

During fetal development there may be some degree of failure of the folding and fusion of the neural plate with its normal covering of meninges, bone and skin. This may be associated with hydrocephalus as a result of aqueduct stenosis or abnormalities in the posterior fossa. In the spine, dysraphism is most common in the lumbosacral area and presents as the following:

Spina bifida occulta

This is usually asymptomatic and is found in about 5% of the normal population. It may be revealed when an incidental X-ray shows failure of fusion of one or more vertebral arches, or suspected if there is a tuft of hair, skin dimple or vascular anomaly over the low back in the midline. Occasionally a sinus communicates from the skin to the lumbar CSF sac through which meningeal infection occurs, one cause of recurrent bacterial meningitis (p. 496). Rarely mild dysraphism can be associated with lipomas or dermoids in the cauda equina region and these may not become symptomatic until later life. Abnormal tethering of the spinal cord may become symptomatic in children or sometimes adolescents.

Meningocoele

Meningocoele is a cystic CSF-filled protrusion of the dural sac through the defective vertebral arch, but there are seldom any neurological consequences.

Myelomeningocoele

This is when the dural sac contains spinal cord or roots and then there are usually motor, sensory and bladder disturbances.

Rachischisis

Rachischisis is when the dural sac is open and the neural tissue exposed on the back. There are always severe neurological deficits.

Non-compressive spinal cord disorders

Progressive spinal cord disorders may obviously be non-compressive (e.g. motor neurone disease, Chapter 13, hereditary spastic paraplegia, p. 337) or come to be considered only after imaging has ruled out what at first sight appeared to be spinal cord compression. There are many disorders which are primarily of the spinal cord, or in which the spinal cord is affected as part of a more widespread disease:

Injury:
- penetrating and non-penetrating trauma
- radiation (p. 334)
- decompression sickness (p. 485)
- epidural analgesia (p. 44)
Infections:
- transverse myelitis (p. 332)
- post-infectious encephalomyelitis (p. 502)
- tuberculosis (p. 513)

- syphilis (p. 515)
- polio (p. 522)
- herpes zoster (p. 523)
- AIDS (p. 526)
- HTLV-1 (p. 529)
- rabies (p. 529)
- gnathostomiasis (p. 537)
- schistosomiasis (p. 539)
- intra-abdominal or renal suppuration

Vascular:
- infarction (p. 333)
- arteriovenous malformation (p. 335)

Familial:
- Friedreich's ataxia (p. 336)
- hereditary spastic paraplegia (p. 337)

Metabolic:
- B_{12} deficiency (p. 470)
- folate deficiency? (p. 470)
- nicotinic acid deficiency (p. 471)
- vitamin E deficiency (p. 471)
- adrenoleucodystrophy (p. 456)
- hyperthyroidism (p. 456)

Toxic:
- lathyrism (p. 336)
- cassava poisoning (p. 553)
- nitrous oxide (p. 550)
- i.v. drug abuse (p. 551)
- subacute myelo-optico-neuropathy (p. 550)

Inflammatory:
- collagen vascular disorders (p. 444)
- sarcoidosis (p. 472)
- arachnoiditis

Others:
- multiple sclerosis (Chapter 12)
- Devic's disease (p. 346)
- motor neurone disease (Chapter 13)
- tropical 'myeloneuropathies' (p. 337)
- syringomyelia (p. 334)
- paraneoplastic syndrome (p. 476)

Note: Bilateral pyramidal signs in the legs can be due to a lesion affecting the parasagittal leg areas of both the left and right motor cortex, usually a parasagittal meningioma. However memorable, this situation hardly ever happens in practice.

Therefore, investigation of a patient with progressive spastic paraplegia and a normal myelogram should include:

- Past history: check on radiation exposure, toxins, diet, intra-abdominal sepsis and renal infection.
- Pes cavus indicates long-standing problem (e.g. Friedreich's ataxia, hereditary spastic paraplegia).
- Family history: examine parents and siblings for evidence of hereditary spastic paraplegia and, if X-linked inheritance, consider adrenoleucodystrophy.
- Look for infection: check CSF analysis including oligoclonal bands (p. 348), blood for syphilis serology, HIV, HTLV-1, schistosomiasis, angiotensin converting enzyme.
- CT for parasagittal meningioma must have cuts to the vertex.
- MRI: changes characteristic of MS in brain and/or spinal cord (p. 350, syringomyelia (p. 334), cord tumour, arteriovenous malformation.
- Visual evoked potential: delay supports diagnosis of MS (p. 349).
- Plasma B_{12} and folate: subacute combined degeneration of the cord (p. 470).
- Antinuclear factor and check for any features of sarcoidosis (p. 472).
- Consider non-metastatic effect of carcinoma (p. 476).
- Consider motor neurone disease (Chapter 13) and re-examine for lower motor neurone lesion signs and EMG to look for denervation in more than one limb.

However, even after extensive investigations, the underlying cause can remain in doubt. Some cases will be multiple sclerosis or hereditary spastic paraplegia but should not be labelled as such without good evidence.

Transverse myelitis

The clinical picture is of an acute or subacute spinal cord syndrome (usually thoracic) with a normal myelogram (or perhaps a swollen cord on imaging) and an 'inflammatory' CSF with an excess cell count (lymphocytes usually) and sometimes oligoclonal bands. Recovery may take weeks or months, or sometimes does not occur. This syndrome may be the presentation of, or occur during the course of, well-defined disorders such as:

- multiple sclerosis (p. 342)
- systemic lupus erythematosus (p. 444)
- sarcoidosis (p. 472)

or be due to diagnosable infections such as:

- brucellosis (p. 510)
- spinal tuberculosis (p. 513)
- syphilis (p. 515)
- borrelia (p. 517)
- mycoplasma pneumoniae (p. 521)
- post-infectious encephalomyelitis (p. 502)

- enteroviral infection (p. 522)
- herpes simplex type 2 (p. 523)
- herpes zoster (p. 523)
- Epstein–Barr virus (p. 524)
- rubella (p. 526)

In most cases no definite cause is found although eventually one may become obvious (e.g. multiple sclerosis).

Spinal cord infarction

Infarction of the spinal cord due to arterial occlusion, or less often venous occlusion, is rare. The main blood supply comes from the anterior spinal artery which is fed by branches of the vertebral, costocervical and radicular arteries arising from the aorta. The anterior part of the thoracic cord appears to be the most vulnerable to ischaemia, possibly because the collateral blood supply is at its most precarious at this point. The causes are:

- spinal trauma (not necessarily very severe)
- acute spinal cord compression (p. 320)
- embolism from atherothrombosis of the aorta or origins of the intercostal and lumbar arteries
- ruptured aortic aneurysm or aortic dissection
- surgical or radiological instrumentation of the aorta
- prolonged and/or severe hypotension
- inflammatory arterial disease (e.g. polyarteritis nodosa, p. 447, syphilis, p. 515, sarcoidosis, p. 472, tuberculosis, p. 513)
- haematological disease (p. 210), particularly sickle cell anaemia (p. 460)
- decompression sickness (p. 485)
- intraspinal infection
- fibrocartilaginous embolism from spontaneous or traumatic intervertebral disc rupture
- spinal arteriovenous malformation (p. 335)
- intra-abdominal or renal chronic sepsis (p. 336)
- 'hypercoagulability' (thrombocythaemia, metastatic cancer, etc. p. 462)

Onset is sudden, sometimes with back pain, and may progress over a few days. The clinical picture is of an acute cord syndrome, often with relative preservation of posterior column function (position sense). Initially the paralysis is flaccid and may remain so because of ischaemic damage to the anterior horn cells throughout a long section of cord. Usually there is little if any recovery and there is seldom specific treatment. Unless the cause is obvious (e.g. aortic surgery), a myelogram must be done to rule out acute cord compression (e.g. prolapsed thoracic disc). The CSF should be normal or there is a modest leucocytosis (<100 mononuclear cells per cm^3) and mildly raised protein content (<1 g/l).

Radiation myelopathy

The spinal cord may be exposed to excessive doses of radiation (usually more than 40 Gray or 4000 rads) during treatment of tumours in the neck, mediastinum and spinal canal. One to four years later a progressive myelopathy develops which may then become static. A transient myelopathy can occur within weeks of irradiation, causing paraesthesia in the limbs and Lhermitte's symptom.

Syringomyelia

In this rare condition (prevalence 7 per 100 000) a fluid-filled cavity (or syrinx) develops in the centre of the spinal cord, usually in the cervical region and sometimes extending down into the thoracic cord or up into the brainstem (syringobulbia). The clinical onset is in young middle age and is usually rather insidious with slow progression, sometimes rather sudden exacerbations, often with long periods of clinical stability.

The clinical picture is of a central cord lesion and may, therefore, be mimicked by a cord tumour which itself may be cystic. There is dissociated and suspended sensory loss over several cervical dermatomes extending on to the chest, often asymmetrically (Fig. 1.10); areflexia corresponding with the segmental level of the lesion; segmental muscle weakness and wasting corresponding with the level of the lesion; and eventually corticospinal tract and sensory signs below the level of the syrinx as it expands into the cord white matter. However, the signs do not bear a very close relation with the size and length of the syrinx. In syringobulbia there is clinical evidence of low brainstem involvement with loss of pain sensation over the trigeminal distribution, dysphagia, dysarthria, tongue wasting, limb and truncal ataxia and nystagmus. Often there is an associated Arnold–Chiari malformation (p. 202), causing upper cervical cord compression with pain in the occiput and neck, low brainstem signs and characteristically vertical nystagmus on down-gaze.

Sometimes a syrinx develops months or years after a severe spinal cord injury and causes increasing pain with ascending cord signs above the known site of injury.

Diagnosis

Diagnosis is best made by MRI which clearly shows the cavity and any associated abnormality at the foramen magnum. It will also show a central cord tumour. If normal, then Tangier disease should be considered (p. 398) since it can cause a very similar clinical syndrome.

Haematomyelia is a blood-filled spinal cord cavity with similar signs to syringomyelia and the causes include:

- spinal trauma
- haemostatic failure (p. 462)
- spinal arteriovenous malformation (below)
- spinal tumour (p. 321)
- acute intracranial hypertension

Treatment

Treatment of syringomyelia is controversial. If there is an Arnold–Chiari malformation, then foramen magnum decompression can relieve pain and perhaps stabilize a progressive neurological deficit. Otherwise, draining the syrinx with a syringo-peritoneal or syringo-subarachnoid shunt is said to help.

Useful address

Ann's Neurological Trust Society (ANTS)
Jocelyn Lodge
Keythorpe
Tugby
Leicester
Tel: 053-756-244

Spinal arachnoiditis

A progressive overgrowth of fibrous tissue in the subarachnoid space can occur as a consequence of:
- myelography using oil-based or ionic water-soluble contrast media (p. 46)
- subarachnoid haemorrhage (p. 228)
- trauma, including spinal surgery
- infection (TB, syphilis, bacterial meningitis, cysticerosis, etc., Chapter 18)
- ankylosing spondylitis (p. 450)

Often, it is merely an asymptomatic finding on myelography which makes the interpretation of the myelogram extremely difficult. However, it can lead to progressive vascular occlusion and ischaemia of the spinal cord and roots; cord and/or root compression with a lot of pain; and obstruction of CSF flow at the foramen magnum, possibly causing syringomyelia.

The CSF protein is usually raised and the diagnosis made by non-ionic water-soluble myelography to show obliteration of the nerve root sheaths, smooth outline of the theca and eventually attenuation and obliteration of the thecal sac. There is no effective treatment.

Spinal arteriovenous malformation

Spinal arteriovenous malformations (spinal AVMs) may present at any age;

they are more often extra- than intramedullary; and males are more often affected than females (2:1). The clinical features include:

● Gradually progressive or occasionally an acute spinal cord syndrome. Pain in the back is common, sometimes the neurological deficit is worsened by exercise and the clinical picture may be of a rather long cord lesion. This myelopathy is due to compression of the cord, venous infarction, perhaps vascular 'steal' from the cord to the AVM, or even low pressure haemorrhage.

● Spinal subarachnoid haemorrhage is unusual. Other causes include:
    haemostatic failure (p. 462)
    coarctation of the aorta
    inflammatory arterial disease (e.g. systemic vasculitis, p. 447)
    mycotic spinal artery aneurysm
    vascular spinal tumours (e.g. ependymoma)
There is sudden pain which is felt more in the back than in the head, but with cervical AVMs there can be confusion with intracranial subarachnoid haemorrhage. Meningism develops. Root pain is a clue. A localized haematoma may cause acute cord compression.

● Spinal vascular bruit (less than 10% of cases).
    The diagnosis is usually suspected on myelography, which shows dilated and tortuous vessels on the surface of the cord, or by MRI, and is then confirmed by spinal angiography.
    If the AVM has bled, or if there is progressive neurological deterioration, then it may be worth while to embolize the AVM or to remove it surgically if technically possible.

Intra-abdominal suppuration

Occasionally chronic suppuration in the abdomen or kidneys can cause infarction of the spinal cord, probably as a result of spreading septic thrombophlebitis.

Lathyrism

An acute or subacute spastic paraplegia is seen in epidemics in India, usually at times of famine. There is little sensory involvement. It is due to the ingestion of neurotoxins from the pulse crop, lathyrus sativus.

Friedreich's ataxia

This is a rare (prevalence 2 per 100 000) progressive autosomal recessive condition starting in childhood or adolescence which leads to inability to walk by about the age of 30 and death some years later. There is degeneration of the posterior and lateral columns of the spinal cord and dorsal roots; the brainstem and cerebellum are only slightly affected.
    The first symptoms are unsteadiness and clumsiness. At this stage one

usually finds ataxia of all four limbs, absent tendon reflexes in the legs and often mild dysarthria. Within a few years there is progression to truncal ataxia, impaired joint position and vibration sense in the feet, pyramidal weakness in the legs more than the arms, bilateral extensor plantar responses and eventually distal muscle wasting and weakness. There is no spasticity, seldom cutaneous sensory loss or nystagmus. Pes cavus, scoliosis and cardiomyopathy are common. Optic atrophy, sensorineural deafness and diabetes can occur. There is a variant in which the tendon reflexes are retained or brisk and the prognosis is rather better. Motor nerve conduction velocity is normal or slightly reduced (cf. hereditary motor and sensory neuropathy type I, p. 396) and sensory action potentials are very reduced or absent. Vitamin E deficiency (p. 471) and abetalipoproteinaemia (p. 479) must be excluded.

Useful address

Friedreich's Ataxia Group
Copse Edge
Thursley Road
Elstead
Godalming
Surrey GU8 6DJ
Tel: 0252-702864

Hereditary spastic paraplegia

This is a dominant or recessive condition which can start at any age and is extremely variable in severity. Walking slowly deteriorates mainly because of spasticity in the legs; there is little if any weakness. There are brisk tendon reflexes in the legs, often with clonus, and bilateral extensor plantar responses. Urinary urgency and pes cavus are fairly common and sometimes there is diminution of vibration and joint position sense in the feet along with absent ankle jerks. The arms are seldom affected, but sometimes there is an associated distal amyotrophy and sensory neuropathy.

Mild cases are asymptomatic but have brisk reflexes and extensor plantars. It is, therefore, important to examine the parents and siblings of patients with slowly progressive spastic paraplegia before assuming that the diagnosis is multiple sclerosis, although with recessive inheritance isolated cases are bound to occur and can be impossible to diagnose. If inheritance is X-linked, then the diagnosis is probably adrenoleucodystrophy (p. 456).

Tropical 'myeloneuropathies'

It is deceptively easy, and quite inappropriate, to label any patient with either a neuropathy or myelopathy in a developing country as a case of tropical 'myeloneuropathy'. So often the patients have not been properly investigated or turn out to have a reasonably certain cause for their neurological disorder (e.g. spinal tumour). It is, therefore, important to consider the normal 'Western' causes of neuropathies (p. 389) and myelopathies (this chapter) as well as in particular the following:

- infections:
  tuberculosis (p. 512)
  syphilis (p. 515)
  AIDS (p. 526)
  HTLV-1 (p. 529)
  schistosomiasis (p. 539)
- tropical malabsorption
- nutritional deficiency (beri beri, p. 468, pellagra, p. 471, etc.)
- toxins:
  lathyrism (p. 336)
  cassava poisoning (p. 553)

General management of paraplegia and tetraplegia

Acute phase

- Passive leg (and arm) physiotherapy to prevent contractures which leads on to active rehabilitation as weakness improves.
- Skin care with two-hourly turning, protection of pressure areas and avoidance of urine and faecal soiling, all of which reduce the risk of pressure sores.
- Bladder care. In acute cord lesions continuous catheterization is usually needed to empty the painless, atonic bladder with overflow. Intermittent catheterization every 4–6 hours can be substituted and eventually reflex bladder emptying may occur spontaneously and is encouraged by abdominal compression.
- Low dose subcutaneous heparin (5000 units twice daily) for some weeks as prophylaxis against peripheral venous thromboembolism but contraindicated if there is any possibility of spinal cord haemorrhage.
- Attention to social and psychological consequences of acute paralysis.

Chronic phase

- Physiotheraphy to establish the best possible walking pattern, provision of walking aids and wheelchair as necessary. Teaching patient and carers how to stand, transfer, etc.
- Management of flexor and extensor spasms (p. 352) which may be exacerbated by urine infection, pressure sores, etc.

- If reflex bladder emptying cannot be achieved, then intermittent self-catheterization is less likely to cause urine infection, urinary calculi and renal failure than permanent catheterization. In some patients a small spastic bladder develops and condom drainage may be practical in males (see also p. 353). Urinary infections should be treated if symptomatic.
- Attention to constipation which may exacerbate bladder problems; high roughage diet, laxatives, etc.
- Avoidance of prolonged sitting or lying and development of pressure sores.
- Appropriate wheelchair, cushions, mattress, etc.
- Attention to home circumstances, adaptations, rehousing, etc.
- Career or job advice and planning.
- Car adaptation.
- Advice on benefits, finance, etc.
- Advice on sexual activity (SPOD, p. 62).
- General psychological support and counselling.
- Holidays for patient and carer, respite admissions, etc.

Useful addresses

Spinal Injuries Association
Yeoman House
76 St James's Lane
London N10 3DF
Tel: 081-444-2121

Association for Spina Bifida & Hydrocephalus
ASBAH House
42 Park Road
Peterborough
Cambs PE1 2UQ
Tel: 0733-555-988

12   Multiple sclerosis (or disseminated sclerosis)

Multiple sclerosis (MS) is the most common cause of severe physical disability in young British adults. It is most prevalent in temperate regions, although rare in Japanese and Maoris, and almost unknown in the tropics. The prevalence in the UK is about 100 patients/100 000 population, with an incidence of about 5/100 000 per annum.

The cause is unknown, but the disease is probably initiated during childhood (by an infection or some other environmental factor) in genetically susceptible individuals, and has an immunological basis. In most northern and central European populations MS has a tendency to be associated with the histocompatibility antigens DR2 and DW2. Females are more often affected than males (in a ratio of about 1.5:1). Occasional familial cases occur; the probability of developing MS if a family member is affected is approximately:

monozygotic twin	0.4
dizygotic twin	0.05
sibling	0.05
children	0.01

There is no excess risk in those married to MS patients.

MS is a relapsing and remitting disease of the *central* nervous system. The early lesion consists of an area of oedema centred on a small vein, a few mm in diameter, with inflammation and an infiltrate of plasma cells, lymphocytes and macrophages. Myelin is destroyed, so nerve conduction is slowed or blocked, but axons are relatively preserved. The early inflammatory lesion is replaced later by a gliotic scar or plaque. Lesions occur in the white matter of the brain, spinal cord and optic nerves, but only some, depending on their position, cause neurological symptoms and signs. MS is not definitely associated with any other disease, autoimmune or otherwise.

Clinical features

The onset of symptoms is mostly between the ages of 20 and 40, with a peak at about 30. The clinical picture is one of episodes of neurological dysfunction, as a consequence of focal lesions in the central nervous system, which are disseminated in space and time. To make the diagnosis of MS, there must be good evidence for at least two separate lesions at different times and no likely alternative explanation; vague symptoms, particularly in the past, such as 'visual blurring', 'numbness', etc. are not good enough without well documented physical signs. It is, therefore, usually impossible to make the diagnosis after a single neurological episode, particularly if only one discrete part of the nervous system is affected. About 15% of patients present and continue with a progressive, usually spinal cord, syndrome when the diagnosis can only be made with absolute certainty at postmortem.

Almost any part of the *central* nervous system white matter can be affected.

Optic nerve

Optic (or retrobulbar) neuritis (p. 173) is a common first event and is unusual once the progressive stage of the disease has been reached. There is subacute monocular blurring of vision reaching its worst in a week or so, which is usually accompanied by, or perhaps preceded by for a few days, pain in the eye, worse on eye movement. This may progress to complete blindness. The pain subsides in about a week and almost always the vision slowly recovers in a few more weeks. Chronic progression with no improvement is very unusual and other causes should be sought (p. 170). Recurrence in the same or the other eye is not unusual; vision is less likely to recover than after a single attack.

Macular vision is most affected, causing a central scotoma and poor visual acuity, loss of colour vision and an afferent pupillary defect. If the inflammatory demyelinating lesion is close to the optic disc, papilloedema appears (p. 172) but usually the fundus is normal.

After symptomatic recovery there may be optic atrophy (with pallor particularly of the temporal side of the optic disc) and sometimes a paracentral scotoma, subtle disturbances of colour vision, distortion of depth perception (Pulfrich's phenomenon), and a relative afferent pupillary defect.

Sometimes in the acute stage, but more often during recovery, the patient may notice brief but bright flashes of light (phosphenes) precipitated by eye movement (or even unexpected sounds), particularly in the dark or with closed eyes.

Optic neuritis may be recurrent or sequentially bilateral. It is very rarely simultaneous in both eyes and in such cases MS seldom develops. MS is less likely to follow optic neuritis in childhood than in adults, and also less likely if there are no oligoclonal bands (p. 348) in the CSF than when there are, and if the MRI is normal.

Sensory features

Numbness, tingling, burning, 'tight bands', watery feelings and even itching, which tends to be more paroxysmal than persistent, may start in one limb and spread to involve the contralateral limb, the other limbs, or the face. There may be loss of vaginal, rectal, and perineal sensation as well.

Sensory symptoms spread and intensify over days or weeks and may come and go over various parts of the body for many years. It may be difficult to find objective cutaneous sensory loss and, even in advanced cases, a clearcut spinal sensory level is unusual.

Isolated joint position sense loss, particularly in one hand, is well recognized and causes considerable clumsiness which may be misinterpreted as weakness or hysteria.

Burning pain in the limbs or trunk due to spinothalamic tract involvement occurs, but is unusual. Root pain is rare.

Lhermitte's symptom (p. 18) is a common feature at any stage of MS but can occur as a result of other disorders affecting the cervical spinal cord.

Motor features

The legs are more affected than the arms by intermittent or progressive weakness with upper motor neurone signs, the latter often being found without any symptoms in the early stages of the disease. Usually both legs are affected, but often asymmetrically. Sometimes only one leg, rarely one arm, and very rarely both limbs on one side are affected. There are scarcely ever any lower motor neurone or extrapyramidal features. The onset is seldom sudden but usually progresses over days, weeks or sometimes months. Eventually spastic paraparesis may develop and then paraplegia. Flexor or extensor spasma may be frequent and/or prolonged enough to be a nuisance, particularly if they are painful or occur at night. Such spasms are exacerbated by bedsores and urinary tract infection. A complaint of restless legs (p. 306) is common.

Sometimes MS presents with a slowly progressive spastic paraparesis with no other clinical features. This is rare under the age of 30. Clinically, it is impossible to differentiate from spinal cord compression, and myelography or MRI are required to exclude this. Helpful, but not absolute, differentiating features are:
- a clearcut sensory level is unusual in MS but common in cord compression
- abdominal reflexes tend to be lost early in MS but late in spinal cord compression
- segmental root pain is rare in MS but quite common in cord compression
- segmental motor or sensory features are very rare in MS
- the visual evoked potential may be delayed in MS (p. 349)
- multiple brain white matter lesions on MRI suggest MS (p. 350)

Sphincters (see also p. 30)

If the pyramidal tracts are affected, a common problem is frequency, urgency of micturition and, eventually, urge incontinence. If these urinary symptoms occur, but with no past or present evidence of corticospinal tract disorder, they are probably not due to MS (p. 33). In MS the bladder is usually small and 'spastic' and its emptying, even when containing only a small volume of urine, is uninhibited. Urine infection is a frequent complication and makes incontinence worse, as does any constipation. Urine retention is less common. Constipation is common in advanced MS but faecal incontinence rare. In males, impotence is common but very rarely occurs without other evidence of MS. It seldom seems to recover.

Brainstem and cerebellum

Rotational vertigo is often an early but usually temporary feature. It is accompanied by nausea, vomiting, imbalance and sometimes diplopia. Horizontal, vertical, rotatory or ataxic nystagmus is found and often a unilateral or bilateral internuclear ophthalmoplegia (p. 180). These signs may also be found without any obvious corresponding symptomatic disturbance.

Cerebellar ataxia, particularly of the arms, and dysarthria are common in the later stages and nystagmus becomes a constant feature. Incapacitating postural and action tremor of the arms and titubation of the head occur in severe cases.

Diplopia is common early or late, and is due to a 6th nerve palsy and/or some form of internuclear gaze disturbance. Isolated 3rd and 4th cranial nerve palsies do not occur. Some patients complain of oscillopsia (p. 193).

Less usual features are lower motor neurone facial weakness, facial numbness, myokymia (p. 192) and very rarely deafness.

'Cerebral' features

Dementia is not uncommon in advanced cases and occasionally appears early. Seizures are rare, aphasia and homonymous hemianopia even rarer.

Miscellaneous typical features

Tiredness

This is a common but real complaint, particularly during relapse.

Heat

An increase in body temperature in hot weather, during exercise (Uhthoff's phenomenon), in a hot bath, or even after a hot drink can, in some patients, make any symptoms considerably worse, and occasionally temporarily produce symptoms not previously experienced (e.g. monocular blindness after a vigorous game of squash without any past history of optic neuritis).

Paroxysmal symptoms

These are stereotyped, can be a presenting, but are more often a later, feature, and may occur many times a day. They usually last less than a minute and are experienced over a period of weeks or months. They may be triggered by hyperventilation, movement, anxiety or touch. They are not epileptic and probably arise in the brainstem. Various types of disturbance have been described:

- Trigeminal neuralgia (p. 145) which can be bilateral.
- Unilateral and uncomfortable, if not painful, dystonic spasms of the limbs or face. Sometimes there are contralateral sensory symptoms in addition.
- Ataxia and dysarthria, often with paraesthesia or weakness of the face or limbs, and sometimes diplopia. These attacks are much briefer and more frequent than brainstem TIA (p. 220), tend to occur at a younger age, and respond to carbamazepine.

Narcolepsy (p. 114) is sometimes described in MS which may indeed be one rare cause of the narcolepsy syndrome.

Complications of MS

- urine infection
- pressure sores
- septicaemia
- contractures
- pneumonia
- depression
- suicide
- divorce
- hysterical elaboration on top of the undoubted organic disease of the nervous system

Devic's disease (neuromyelitis optica)

This is a combination of bilateral optic neuritis and a more or less simultaneous transverse myelitis (p. 332), usually in the thoracic spinal cord, causing spastic paraparesis. It is rare, occasionally due to MS, but more often it is a monophasic event without further neurological problems. The cause is unknown and recovery is unpredictable.

Prognosis

The spectrum of severity ranges from a few patients who die in the first neurological episode (usually massive demyelination of the brainstem) to occasionally finding MS at postmortem in elderly patients who have never had neurological symptoms (0.02% of unselected postmortems). Many patients have a normal life expectancy and little, if any, physical disability. Less than 10% are seriously disabled within 5 years of onset and on *average* life expectancy is reduced by about 10 years. About 50% eventually become disabled to some extent.

Normally the early stages are characterized by relapses and remissions. A relapse may last days or weeks and, at first, recovery is complete. Quite often by the time there is an established deficit, it is difficult to distinguish a relapse due to a new episode of demyelination from the effects of fatigue, intercurrent infection, depression and heat. The relapse rate is variable and tends to decline with time; initially it is about two per annum. Sometimes the relapse rate is very much less and patients remain well for years.

Once the disease has been present for a few years it is common for some residual disability to remain after a relapse. Eventually identifiable relapses stop and the patient enters a state of chronic and progressive neurological disability. Finally, in some cases there is total dependence, with spastic paraplegia, incontinence of urine, ataxic upper limbs, dysarthria, nystagmus and dementia; this leads to pressure sores, septicaemia, pneumonia and death.

In about 15% of patients the course is progressive from onset, usually with a spastic paraparesis.

In an individual the prognosis is unpredictable in the early stages, but in general the older the age of onset the worse the eventual disability. Patients with progressive paraparesis from the onset, or who have cerebellar ataxia or weakness in the first attack, tend to do badly. Patients with only sensory symptoms in the early attacks tend to do well, as do those with a first remission of 5 years or so. Patients with frequent relapses and incomplete remission in the first year or two tend to have a poor prognosis. If 10 years after the first attack the patient is still walking, the outlook is reasonably good.

Patients who have CSF oligoclonal bands and/or disseminated lesions on MRI at the time of their first attack are possibly likely to do worse than those who do not, partly perhaps because those without these findings do not actually have MS.

Diagnosis

There is no specific diagnostic test. Diagnosis depends on the clinical features and the exclusion of other disorders, particularly those which are treatable. Late in the course of the disease the diagnosis is usually easy, but it is still worth keeping under occasional review. The real diagnostic problem is in patients with their first neurological episode when, depending on which part of the nervous system is involved, other diagnoses could be:

- optic nerve:
  compression of optic nerve (p. 167) or chiasm (p. 168)
  ischaemic optic neuropathy (p. 175)
  optic nerve astrocytoma (p. 176)
  Leber's hereditary optic atrophy (p. 174)
  retinal disorders (e.g. central serous retinopathy)
  toxic optic neuropathy (p. 171)
  syphilis (p. 515)
  post viral infection (p. 502)

sarcoidosis (p. 472)
- brainstem:
vascular malformation (p. 233)
astrocytoma (p. 271)
Arnold–Chiari malformation (p. 202)
stroke (p. 239)
'viral' labyrinthitis (p. 107)
myasthenia gravis (Chapter 15)
- spinal cord:
compression/tumour (p. 320)
motor neurone disease (Chapter 13)
arteriovenous malformation (p. 335)
- multiple lesions:
systemic lupus erythematosus and other collagen vascular disorders (p. 444)
stroke (p. 237)
sarcoidosis (p. 472)
acute post-infectious encephalomyelitis (p. 502)
subacute myelo-optic neuropathy (SMON) (p. 550)
syphilis (p. 515)
migrant sensory neuritis of Wartenberg (p. 402)
subacute combined degeneration of the spinal cord (p. 470)
- hereditary conditions:
hereditary spastic paraplegia (p. 337)
idiopathic sporadic late onset cerebellar ataxia (p. 201)
Friedreich's ataxia (p. 336)
- hysteria (p. 38)

Investigations

Investigations should always include:
- full blood count and ESR
- syphilis serology
- relevant plain X-rays

The CSF

The CSF is helpful as an aid to diagnosis of both early relapsing/remitting cases and chronic progressive cases. Often there is a modest increase in the lymphocyte count (usually less than 30 and not more than 100 cells/cm^3), and about a third have a slight increase in total protein content, but almost never more than 1.0 g/1. More often the IgG component of the CSF protein is raised: more than 15% of total protein, or an IgG/albumin ratio of more than 0.27. An abnormal level of IgG in the blood makes the CSF level difficult to interpret. It is, therefore, better to calculate the IgG index, which in normals is less than 0.67 (CSF IgG/serum IgG ÷ CSF albumin/serum albumin). Perhaps more sensitive still is an oligoclonal pattern in the CSF: two or more bands representing gamma globulins (IgG) on polyacrylamide gel electrophoresis which separates the proteins on the basis of their charge and size. Provided no similar bands are present in the serum they represent locally synthesized immunoglobulin in the nervous system.

None of these changes are found in all cases; they are not closely related to clinical disease activity, nor are they specific to MS. An increase in lymphocytes or protein is common in numerous neurological conditions (e.g. meningitis, p. 491) and an increase in CSF IgG, and oligoclonal bands, has also been reported in:

- neurosyphilis (p. 515)
- meningitis (p. 491) and encephalitis (p. 498)
- acute post-infectious encephalomyelitis (p. 502)
- subacute sclerosing panencephalitis (p. 525)
- Guillain–Barré syndrome (p. 398)
- cerebral systemic lupus erythematosus (p. 444)
- myasthenia gravis (Chapter 15)
- sarcoidosis (p. 472)
- cerebral infarction (p. 244)
- intracranial tumours (p. 266)
- increased level of IgG in the blood
- contamination of the CSF by red blood cells

Therefore, the CSF changes should only be used to support the diagnosis of MS in clinically appropriate circumstances. Nonetheless, in disabled patients who appear to have clinically definite MS a completely normal CSF would raise questions about the diagnosis.

Evoked potentials (p. 55)

The averaged electrical response, detected over the head by scalp electrodes, to sensory stimuli (visual, auditory or somatosensory) is the evoked potential. A change in its shape, or more often delay in its latency, may confirm a symptomatic but clinically equivocal lesion, or reveal an asymptomatic or forgotten one. In MS this may, therefore, confirm a 'second' but subclinical lesion, and so support the diagnosis, but this use has been overtaken by MRI (see below). In practice the visual evoked potential (VEP) is the most useful; a delay of the major positive peak (P100 response) often (but not always) persists indefinitely after unequivocal optic neuritis. Also it is delayed in patients in whom optic nerve involvement has been unnoticed, long forgotten, or subclinical and who have no physical signs of optic nerve damage.

A delayed VEP is helpful in the correct clinical context but is *not* specific for MS. Other causes for delay must be considered:

- technical artifact (e.g. patient closes eyes or goes to sleep)
- impaired visual acuity (e.g. cataract, refractive error, toxic amblyopia)

- optic nerve (p. 167) or chiasm compression (p. 168)
- ischaemic optic neuropathy (p. 175)
- occasionally lesions of the optic radiation or visual cortex

Unfortunately a delayed VEP cannot be absolutely relied upon when searching for a 'second lesion' in patients with progressive spastic paraparesis. Normally a myelogram or MRI has to be carried out to exclude a compressive spinal cord lesion, and the diagnosis of MS is then one of exclusion (neurosyphilis and B_{12} deficiency being other considerations). The reasons are that MS and cervical spondylotic myelopathy (p. 327) may coexist and other disorders causing spastic paraplegia can be associated with a delayed VEP, e.g. hereditary spastic paraplegia (p. 337), Arnold–Chiari malformation (p. 202), vitamin B_{12} deficiency (p. 470), sarcoidosis (p. 472) and syphilis (p. 515).

Normal values for evoked responses must be established by each laboratory, standardized by age and sex, and checked periodically.

Note: If a sensory pathway is obviously affected clinically, then it is diagnostically pointless to measure the evoked response in that pathway since any delay does not provide further evidence for a 'second lesion'.

CT scan

Plaques of demyelination, if they are large enough, appear as areas of low density which, if acute, may enhance with intravenous contrast. High dose intravenous contrast infusion with delayed CT often reveals even more enhancing lesions. These lesions are usually seen in the white matter of the cerebral hemispheres, particularly in the periventricular regions but, if multiple, may be confused with metastases (p. 268) or even multiple infarcts (p. 242). However, MS lesions do not normally cause any mass effect. Later, the CT scan may become normal, although some low density areas persist, but no longer enhance. In advanced cases ventricular dilatation and cortical atrophy are present. It should be noted, however, that in early and possible cases of MS the CT scan is usually completely normal.

Magnetic resonance imaging

This is much more sensitive than CT in detecting MS lesions. Typically there is an irregular pattern of confluent periventricular abnormality associated with discrete lesions elsewhere in the cerebral white matter. Although multiple lesions in the white matter of the cerebral hemispheres, brainstem and cerebellum are not specific to MS, their presence does support the diagnosis in the correct clinical context. Multiple lesions can be found in patients who appear to have had only one clinical episode, even optic neuritis, and may appear and disappear with no clinical correlates. MS plaques cannot, however, be reliably distinguished from multiple infarcts (p. 242), nor the changes of acute post-infectious encephalomyelitis (p. 502). It is too early to say whether disseminated cerebral lesions on MRI can be relied upon to make myelography or MRI of the spinal cord unnecessary to exclude cord compression in patients presenting with progressive spastic paraparesis.

Imaging to exclude other diagnoses

Naturally the appropriate imaging technique may be needed to *exclude* non-MS conditions when there is diagnostic uncertainty, e.g. myelography or spinal MRI for progressive spastic paraparesis (p. 332); CT of the orbits to exclude optic nerve compression (p. 174); MRI of the brainstem and upper cervical cord to exclude Arnold–Chiari malformation (p. 202), vascular malformation (p. 233), etc.

In many patients there is, eventually, not much doubt about the diagnosis of MS on clinical grounds alone. In most, or even all, it is, however, sensible to examine the CSF and to have an MRI scan (failing that, a high dose contrast infusion CT) since both are safe, neither requires hospital admission, and if *both* are normal the diagnosis of MS should be questioned, except in patients with early clinical disease.

Treatment

There is no cure, but symptomatic treatment and prevention of complications are important, as is long-term support for chronically disabled patients and their families. Courses of physiotherapy for patients with difficulty in walking are often helpful. The time to tell the patient the diagnosis is when the physician is reasonably certain about it, and not before.

Treatment of relapse

Corticosteroids

These are used for an acute and severe relapse to hasten remission and relieve any severe pain of optic neuritis. Subsequent disability is not affected. Occasional courses in chronic progressive disease may help in a few patients, particularly those with spasticity. Long-term treatment is both ineffective and disastrous because of adverse effects.
- i.m. ACTH gel: 80 units daily, tailing off over about 3 weeks
- oral prednisolone: 80 mg daily, tailing off over about 3 weeks is probably just as effective
- very high doses of i.v. methylprednisolone (500–1000 mg infusion in 100 ml normal saline over 1 hour, daily for 5 days) may be more effective and convenient. Immediate adverse effects include facial flushing, ankle swelling, metallic taste and hiccups

Symptomatic treatments

Spasticity and flexor or extensor spasms

These usually only affect the legs and, if painful or a nuisance, can be helped by general measures such as physiotherapy, relief of constipation, urine retention and pressure sores. Useful drugs are:

baclofen: 5 mg 3 times daily, oral, increasing if necessary to a maximum of 100 mg daily. Continuous spinal intrathecal infusion of baclofen (up to 650 μg daily) may be useful for far advanced cases not helped by, or intolerant of, oral drugs

diazepam: 2 mg 3 times daily, oral, increasing if necessary to a maximum of 40 mg daily

dantrolene: 25 mg daily, oral, increasing if necessary to a maximum of 100 mg 4 times daily

If nocturnal spasms are the problem, these drugs should be used only at bedtime since they can all cause drowsiness and weakness. During the day they may be impossible to use in patients who rely on spasticity to stand up. Other adverse effects include:

baclofen: dizziness, nausea, vomiting, confusion, seizures, psychosis

dantrolene: dizziness, depression, diarrhoea, malaise, hepatotoxicity

The dose of these drugs should be slowly increased over some weeks until either the desired therapeutic effect is attained, or adverse effects limit their use. If in maximal dosage no effect occurs, the drug should be slowly withdrawn rather than stopped suddenly for fear of producing withdrawal seizures and hallucinations.

Nerve blocks (phenol, alcohol or local anaesthetic injected into the motor nerve or muscle) may help for days or months but can only be used if weakness is already so great that any further weakness will make no functional difference. Intrathecal phenol or alcohol to destroy the cauda equina can be used if there is already no bladder control.

Surgery. Neurectomy and lengthening or division of muscle tendons may be required for severe contractures.

Dorsal column stimulation of the spinal cord with epidural electrodes may help in the occasional case but is seldom practical.

The bladder

Urine infections exacerbate urgency and incontinence and should be treated with the appropriate antibiotics. Urinary urgency can sometimes be helped by anticholinergic drugs to inhibit detrusor contractions (p. 30):

propantheline: oral, 15 mg 3 times daily up to 30 mg 3 times daily
terodiline: oral, 12.5 mg twice daily up to 25 mg twice daily

These drugs have anticholinergic adverse effects such as dry mouth, dry eyes, blurred vision, glaucoma, constipation and urinary retention. If there is no symptomatic improvement with increasing doses after a month or so, the first drug should be abandoned and the other tried.

Incontinence pads, intermittent self- or permanent catheterization, an ileal conduit, or urinary appliance may eventually become unavoidable.

In the last resort, dorsal column stimulation of the spinal cord may help a small number of patients.

The bowels

Constipation responds to a high fibre diet, bulk laxatives or glycerol suppositories. In advanced cases enemas or manual evacuation may be required.

Tremor

Ataxia with postural and intention tremor of the upper limbs and head can be very disabling. A few patients seem to respond to potentially toxic doses of isoniazid (p. 514): starting at 300 mg, oral, and building up to 1200 mg daily in 3 or 4 divided doses along with pyridoxine, 100 mg daily. Adverse effects include drowsiness, dysphagia and increased bronchial secretions; liver function must be monitored. Beta-blockers may also be useful (see benign essential tremor, p. 295). Weights on the wrists can help and occasionally stereotactic surgery to the contralateral thalamus is useful. Electrical stimulation of the thalamic-midbrain junction may also be effective.

Pain

The treatment of painful spasticity is discussed above; trigeminal neuralgia responds to carbamazepine (p. 90), but 'thalamic' or central pain (p. 26) is very resistant to treatment. Often strong analgesia is required; carbamazepine or tricyclic antidepressants are worth trying and sometimes spinal cord stimulation helps. Musculoskeletal pain as a result of the physical disability can be a problem and is treated with non-steroidal anti-inflammatory drugs.

Paroxysmal symptoms

Paroxysmal symptoms (including Lhermitte's symptom) usually respond dramatically to oral carbamazepine which should be used in the lowest possible dose for satisfactory control, i.e. starting at 100 mg twice daily up to a maximum of 2 g daily. Phenytoin is less effective.

Excessive tiredness

This may be helped by amantadine (dose and adverse effects, see p. 287).

General advice

Sympathetic counselling, explanation and advice are appropriate for all patients. Depression is common and can sometimes be alleviated with anti-depressants. Small doses of amitriptyline (25–75 mg daily) may help reduce the frequency of excessive laughing and crying (emotional lability) which is seen in some very disabled patients. There is possibly some increased risk of relapse in the puerperium (not related to breast feeding), but this does not seem to have any long-term adverse effect on the course of the disease. Disabled patients should be advised to think about who will look after any planned children.

Possible precipitants of relapse

These include infection, trauma, spinal anaesthesia and emotional stress. Vaccination is not contraindicated, particularly if the risk of infection without immunization is high, *unless* it has apparently caused relapse previously. Necessary surgery, lumbar puncture, myelography and oral contraceptives are not contraindicated.

The familial risks are very small (see p. 342) but often need to be discussed. There is certainly no evidence that the disease is contagious.

Reduction of relapse rate and long-term disability

This ultimate goal is elusive. There is no certain effective long-term treatment but many treatments have been suggested. Two are of current interest:
- azathioprine: oral, 2.5 mg/kg daily. The effect is unproven but there may be a small advantage for some patients. Adverse effects include marrow suppression, infection, lymphoma, abdominal pain, nausea, vomiting, diarrhoea and hepatitis
- cyclophosphamide is more toxic but possibly more effective

A low saturated fat diet with polyunsaturated fatty acid supplementation is probably harmless and, in theory, may help. Although of unproven benefit, many patients like to take sunflower seed oil or evening primrose seed oil, both of which contain linoleic and linolenic acids.

Measuring the effect of treatment may be carried out in the usual way for any disabling disease (p. 59) and/or by the widely used Kurtzke disability status scale. This is rather heavily weighted towards physical mobility. However, serious disability and still normal physical mobility are very unusual in MS, so the scale is reasonably valid:

0   Normal neurological examination
1   No disability, but mininal signs such as extensor plantar response or impaired vibration sense
2   Minimal disability, e.g. slight weakness or mild gait, sensory, visuomotor disturbance
3   Moderate disability although able to walk, e.g. monoparesis, moderate ataxia or combinations of lesser dysfunctions
4   Relatively severe disability although able to walk, to be self-sufficient, and up and about for some 12 hours a day
5   Disability severe enough to preclude ability to work a full day without special provisions. Maximal motor function: walking unaided no more than about quarter of a mile
6   Assistance (sticks or crutches) required for walking
7   Restricted to wheelchair but able to wheel self, and enter and leave wheelchair alone
8   Restricted to bed but with effective use of arms
9   Totally helpless and bedridden
10   Death due to multiple sclerosis

Useful addresses

The Multiple Sclerosis Society
25 Effie Road
London SW6 1EE
Tel: 071-736-6267/8

Action for Research in Multiple Sclerosis (ARMS)
4A Chapel Hill
Stansted
Essex CM24 8AG
Tel: 0279-815553

13 Motor neurone disease (MND)

Motor neurone disease (MND; sometimes referred to as amyotrophic lateral sclerosis) is a sporadic, progressive and fatal group of conditions in which upper and/or lower motor neurones degenerate and disappear. The brunt may fall on the anterior horn cells of the spinal cord (causing *progressive spinal muscular atrophy*), the cranial nerve motor nuclei in the brainstem (causing *progressive bulbar palsy*), the corticospinal tracts, causing pyramidal features in the arms and legs (*primary lateral sclerosis*), or the corticobulbar tracts (causing *progressive pseudobulbar palsy*). Most commonly there is a mixture of all four components, if not at onset then later in the course of the disease. The cause is unknown.

The incidence is similar in all parts of the world, 1.5/100 000 population per annum, apart from in Guam and the Kii peninsula of Japan where it is much higher. The prevalence is about 6 patients per 100 000 population. Males are affected more often than females (about 1.5:1) and usually the onset is in late middle age and old age. The disease is fatal within about 4 years of onset although some patients survive much longer.

Inherited forms of the disease

Familial MND

About 5% of adults with MND have an affected first degree relative, but whether this is a reflection of shared genes or shared environmental exposure is uncertain. In familial cases the sex ratio is 1:1.

Werdnig–Hoffman disease

Werdnig–Hoffman disease (acute infantile spinal muscular atrophy) is an autosomal recessive condition with onset *in utero* or in neonates. There is generalized muscular hypotonia, wasting and weakness followed by death under the age of one. This is one form, therefore, of spinal muscular atrophy since degeneration of the anterior horn cells in the spinal cord leads to atrophy of the muscles supplied by the corresponding motor nerves.

Kugelberg–Welander syndrome

Kugelberg–Welander syndrome (chronic childhood proximal spinal mus-cular atrophy) presents in children with slowly progressive muscular atrophy, which is usually symmetrical and proximal, due to loss of anterior horn cells in the spinal cord and brainstem. Life expectancy is sometimes normal but progressive disability and death are more common. Usually it is autosomal recessive but occasionally dominant.

Disorders related to motor neurone disease

In some individuals there appears to be a combination of MND with dementia, usually of the Alzheimer type but sometimes with spongiform changes in the brain (p. 531) and, in Guam, with Parkinson's disease.

There is an unusual condition of progressive lower motor neurone wasting and weakness of one limb (monomelic amyotrophy) which apparently remains focal for years and perhaps always. It seems to be more common in Asia than in the West, in males than in females, and it usually starts under the age of 40.

In very rare cases patients who have had polio may, after having a stable neurological deficit for many years, become progressively weaker, but the cause is uncertain, as is any relationship with MND (p. 522).

Hexosaminidase deficiency (p. 479) may present in children and young adults with what looks very like MND, but usually there is some additional feature such as cerebellar ataxia, peripheral neuropathy or mental impairment.

Clinical features

The onset is insidious and progressive and may start in the legs or arms, usually asymmetrically and distally or, less often, with slurring of speech and dysphagia. Cramp is a common symptom in the early stages but the main problems are increasing fatigue, weakness and clumsiness (sometimes stiffness), usually with both upper and lower motor neurone signs on examination. Fasciculation is often prominent in the affected muscles, even at an early stage before any weakness and before being noticed by the patient.

Respiratory failure due to weakness of the respiratory muscles is an unusual presentation but is common in the later stages; there is orthopnoea and breathlessness, difficulty breathing, nocturnal hypoventilation and restlessness, morning headache, irritability and day-time somnolence (cf. other causes of neuromuscular respiratory failure, p. 417).

Pain is a common symptom, particularly at night, and may be due to muscular cramp; joint and muscle stiffness as a result of immobility; skin pressure due to immobility; headache as a result of respiratory failure; spasticity with painful extensor and flexor spasms; depression; and sometimes the limbs are painful for no identifiable reason.

Pseudobulbar and/or bulbar palsy are common with weakness of the muscles supplied by the lower cranial motor nerves. Emotional lability may occur. Eventually all voluntary muscle groups are affected with the exception of the extraocular muscles and the external sphincter of the bladder.

Apart from constipation late in the disease the sphincters are not involved, potency is normal in the male, there are no sensory signs although various mild sensory symptoms and pathological changes in the sensory tracts are quite common, and the special senses and intellect are always normal.

Diagnostic points to look for are:
- fasciculation and wasting of the tongue
- brisk jaw jerk
- weak neck flexion
- brisk tendon reflexes despite wasting and fasciculation in the same muscle
- normal sensation

Note: At onset the weakness can be very asymmetrical even to the extent of affecting only one limb.

Survival tends, on average, to be shorter in older patients and in those with onset in the bulbar muscles. Patients usually die of pneumonia secondary to neuromuscular respiratory failure, weak cough, aspiration, along with malnutrition and cachexia. Death during a choking attack is exceptional. Progressive spinal muscular atrophy alone without bulbar or upper motor neurone involvement, which is a rare form of MND, tends to have a much better prognosis.

Investigations

The clinical picture is usually characteristic but investigations should always include:
- full blood count and ESR
- liver function
- plasma proteins and electrophoresis (cf. predominantly motor neuropathy of plasma cell dyscrasia, p. 460, and a few MND patients have abnormal paraproteins)
- syphilis serology; syphilitic amyotrophy (p. 515) can occasionally masquerade as MND
- thyroid function; thyrotoxic myopathy, neuropathy and myelopathy (p. 455) are said to mimic MND but this must be extraordinarily rare as a serious differential diagnosis
- chest X-ray
- leucocyte hexosaminidase in young patients

Electromyography

This shows widespread denervation (p. 58) but normal or only slightly slowed motor and sensory nerve conduction velocities unless there is a complicating pressure palsy; two or more limbs should be involved by the denervating process, at least eventually (note the differential diagnosis of motor root lesions with focal myotomal weakness and wasting, p. 318). In advanced cases there may be some slowing of motor nerve conduction velocity due to fall-out of large fibres. Occasionally there is a decremental response to repetitive motor stimulation (cf. myasthenia gravis, p. 412).

CSF

A modest rise in the protein content (up to about 1 g/l) is the only abnormality but often the CSF is normal. There is no increase in the cell content.

Myelogram

Sometimes there is confusion between MND and cervical spondylotic myelopathy and radiculopathy (p. 327) and with other causes of progressive spastic paraparesis without sensory signs (p. 330). A similar problem can arise in lumbar spondylotic radiculopathy (p. 327). If there is any possibility of progressive spinal cord and root compression, a myelogram (or MRI) must be done to rule it out.

Muscle biopsy

This is necessary in patients who have only progressive lower motor neurone weakness, particularly if the course is prolonged, to exclude chronic polymyositis (p. 435), acid maltase deficiency (p. 427), limb girdle dystrophy (p. 423), etc. In progressive muscular atrophy there should only be features of denervation on the muscle biopsy. The same appearances can be found in chronic motor neuropathies but in these cases the motor conduction velocities are almost always decreased.

For an absolutely secure diagnosis there must be clearcut evidence of progression and widespread denervation in more than one limb or the bulbar muscles (preferably clinically and supported by EMG rather than relying on either alone) along with pyramidal signs in the bulbar muscles and/or in all four limbs. There should be no sensory signs and no intellectual deterioration. This situation almost certainly will not occur until some way into the natural history of many patients and until then other diagnostic possibilities, particularly if treatable, should be borne in mind. This definition excludes pure progressive spinal muscular atrophy which can only be accepted as MND if other causes of the same clinical syndrome are excluded by muscle biopsy (see above and also p. 422) and there is no evidence of a motor neuropathy or radiculopathy; chronic spastic paraparesis of no known cause (p. 332); and chronic progressive pseudobulbar palsy of no known cause (p. 203).

Note: Occasional patients have slightly raised serum anti-acetylcholine receptor antibodies and in some the plasma CK levels are slightly elevated.

Management

There is no cure but much can be done to help patients and their carers. It is worth reassuring them that intellect and personality remain normal, as does sphincter control.

- Cramp can be treated with quinine (p. 419).
- Saliva, which may be difficult to swallow, can be dried up with anticholinergic drugs or, if absolutely necessary, by parotid radiation.

  atropine, oral 0.6 mg up to 4 times daily

  propantheline, oral 15 mg 3 times daily up to 30 mg 4 times daily

  hyoscine, transdermal patch behind ear; slow release over 72 hours

Finding the best head posture for most effective swallowing is important.

- Choking attacks should be treated by tilting the patient forwards, clearing the mouth, and training the carer to use a portable sucker if appropriate. Reassure that death from choking is exceptional.
- Poor sleep may be due to pain, saliva pooling in the throat, hypoventilation, depression, anxiety or excessive sleeping during the day. Appropriate measures can usually be taken and night sedation prescribed if necessary. An electric fan often seems to help and many patients find sitting up to be the best position for sleeping.
- Splints for the support of weak joints and a collar to support a weak neck along with correct support in a wheelchair with a head rest and adjustable back rest may be helpful.
- Physical and drug treatment of spasticity if this is painful or a nuisance (p. 352).
- Aids and adaptations in the home with advice and help from occupational and physiotherapists. In the later stages frequent turning, correct mattress and beds, etc. are important.
- Speech therapy to help with communication and swallowing problems, including the use of communication aids and palatal supports.
- Attention to the diet so that food is of the best consistency to be swallowed and is nutritious; weight loss is inevitable and can be alarming for the patient. Fluids are often most easily swallowed as jellies.
- Pharyngeal spasticity may be helped by holding an ice cube in the mouth, or an ice pack on the throat, before a meal.
- Nasogastric tube feeding or gastrostomy may be needed in some patients. Severe dysphagia in a patient who is otherwise reasonably well can occasionally be helped by a cricopharyngeal myotomy to relieve pharyngeal spasticity provided lower motor bulbar function is adequate. However, the operative mortality is high.

- Management of constipation is important; glycerin suppositories and enemas are usually preferable to laxatives.
- Non-steroidal anti-inflammatory analgesics and eventually morphine (5–10 mg oral as necessary) for limb aches and pains. Opiates are also very useful for night sedation.
- Assisted ventilation should usually be avoided apart from at night in the occasional patient with neuromuscular respiratory failure who is otherwise reasonably well, or whose symptoms of nocturnal apnoea (confusion, headache, etc.) are otherwise uncontrollable. Rather than ventilation a rocking bed can sometimes be effective in this situation.
- Terminal nursing care in hospital or hospice is often necessary unless the family can cope.
- Ensure benefits are taken up: mobility, attendance and invalid care allowances.
- Bedsores are very rarely a problem, presumably because of normal skin sensation.

Useful address

Motor Neurone Disease Association
PO Box 246
Northampton MN1 2PR
Tel: 0604-22269/250505

14 Disorders of peripheral nerves

Nerve plexuses

The brachial (Fig. 14.1) and lumbosacral nerve plexuses are formed by the union of spinal nerves and they give rise to peripheral nerves. They are complicated structures but are seldom damaged except by trauma.

Non-traumatic lesions

Tumours

Malignant axillary lymph nodes and tumours at the apex of the lung may invade the lower trunk of the brachial plexus to cause C8 and T1 root lesions and, if the cervical sympathetic ganglia are involved, an ipsilateral Horner's syndrome (p. 178). Pelvic tumours or aneurysms may involve the lumbosacral plexus, sciatic (p. 383) and obturator nerves (p. 388). Root pain tends to be early and persistent and is followed by weakness and sensory loss which are usually unilateral.

Irradiation

Irradiation for malignant disease in the axilla, supraclavicular region and pelvis may damage the brachial and lumbosacral plexuses leading to progressive weakness and numbness a few years after treatment. Any pain is a late feature. Recurrent tumour must be ruled out by appropriate imaging (plain X-ray, CT, bone scan, myelogram, etc.).

Cervical rib

An extra rib on the 7th cervical vertebra or, more often, a fibrous band extending from an elongated 7th cervical transverse process to the 1st rib, may angulate and compress the C8 and T1 nerve roots, or lower trunk of the brachial plexus. Females are affected more often than males. Although cervical ribs are common, the neurological clinical syndrome is rare.

It usually presents with pain in the shoulder, axilla and down the inner arm to the hand which is worse when carrying heavy weights and with arm elevation. Weakness and wasting of the small hand muscles (particularly the abductor pollicis brevis) occur and any sensory loss extends, unlike in an ulnar nerve lesion (p. 376), above the wrist (C8 dermatome) or is on the inner side of the forearm (T1 dermatome). Median nerve conduction velocity is normal (cf. carpal tunnel syndrome, p. 372); ulnar sensory action potential amplitude is small or absent, and there is denervation on EMG of the small hand muscles. Removal of the rib or fibrous band relieves the symptoms and prevents neurological progression.

If the rib compresses the subclavian artery, there may be additional vascular symptoms in the arm and hand.

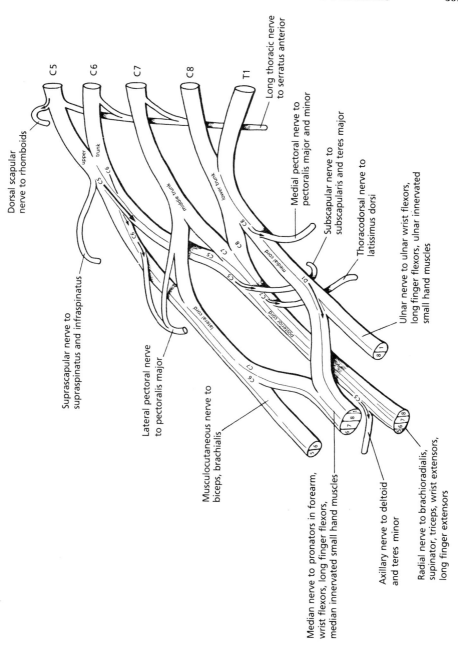

Fig. 14.1 The anatomy of the brachial plexus.

Neuralgic amyotrophy

Neuralgic amyotrophy (brachial neuritis, brachial plexus neuropathy) is quite a common and easily recognizable clinical syndrome of unknown cause. The incidence is about 1.6/100 000 population per annum.

It starts with severe pain, coming on over hours or days, in the shoulder and down the arm and, within a few days, progressive and rapid weakness but rather slight sensory loss appear in the same limb. This is followed by muscle wasting. The neurological deficit suggests that the cervical nerve roots, brachial plexus or nerves arising from the plexus are damaged in a diffuse and patchy kind of way. The axillary, long thoracic and suprascapular nerves seem to be particularly susceptible, as do the C5 and C6 nerve roots. The pain subsides in a week or two and the neurological deficit usually recovers in a few months.

The differential diagnosis includes acute cervical disc prolapse (p. 326) and herpes zoster radiculopathy (p. 524). An identical syndrome can occur with no pain and is difficult to differentiate from other painless causes of cervical root (p. 320) and brachial plexus compression.

Sometimes the condition is bilateral and occasionally it recurs. It can run in families as a dominant feature. Occasionally it complicates serum sickness (p. 448), borrelia (p. 517), herpes simplex type 2 (p. 523), vaccinations and nondescript viral infections. The CSF is normal.

A similar, but much less common, condition can affect the lumbosacral plexus and nerve roots. The differential diagnosis includes prolapsed lumbar disc (p. 326), but straight leg raising, the back and the myelogram are normal.

Indirect trauma

- rucksack straps affecting the C5 and C6 roots and upper trunk of brachial plexus
- forced shoulder abduction during general anaesthesia
- during open chest surgery
- birth trauma

Herpes zoster (p. 523)

Peripheral nerves

Cutting a peripheral nerve produces symptoms and signs characteristic for that nerve and for the position along its course where it is cut. Cutting a motor nerve causes immediate paralysis and wasting within a matter of weeks of the muscles it alone supplies (Table 1.2), and some paralysis (often undetectable) of muscles it shares in supplying. Cutting a sensory nerve causes loss of pain, touch and temperature sensation (and less consistently loss of position sense) over an area of skin which is *smaller* than the nerve's sensory supply; this is because of the considerable overlap between the sensory territories of some adjacent peripheral nerves.

Peripheral nerve injury short of complete section produces only a partial and incomplete expression of this picture. The most obvious loss my be of sensory, motor or both components. Sensory nerve damage causes tingling, pain and numbness in its distribution; sometimes there are severe sensory symptoms but no sensory signs.

Note: Pain in the shoulder, arm or hand may also be due to joint, bone, ligament or muscle disease and to angina.

Causalgia is an unpleasant burning pain with exquisite sensitivity of the skin which occurs after traumatic partial nerve injury, particularly of the median nerve in the forearm. The skin becomes red, shiny and dry and may sweat excessively. The underlying bones become osteoporotic (Sudek's atrophy).

Chronic motor nerve damage can cause muscle wasting and weakness which is unnoticed by the patient who has, over the years, adapted to it.

If a peripheral nerve is involved in a reflex arc (p. 12), the appropriate deep tendon reflex will be depressed or absent.

Nerve conduction studies (p. 55) can be helpful when the clinical features are incomplete or atypical, if differentiation from a root lesion is difficult, and if subclinical involvement is suspected. Both motor and sensory nerve conduction are slowed or blocked at the site of nerve injury and in demyelinating neuropathies, but this is not invariable. The compound muscle action potential is reduced in amplitude when stimulating below compared with above a focal nerve lesion in both axonal and demyelinating neuropathies. Sensory nerve action potentials are small, dispersed and delayed if the lesion is distal to the dorsal root ganglion. The involved muscles show electrical signs of denervation (p. 58).

Sometimes the electrical tests give results inconsistent with the clinical findings; the latter are usually correct.

Causes of individual peripheral nerve lesions

- trauma: penetrating, bone fracture, needles
- acute compression: coma, general anaesthesia, deep sleep, tourniquet, plaster cast, haematoma. Symptoms appear more or less abruptly
- chronic compression (or entrapment neuropathy) where nerves pass through confined spaces (e.g. the carpal tunnel, p. 372, pronator teres, p. 371, cubital tunnel, p. 374, tarsal tunnel, p. 388). The symptoms develop slowly and progressively

● acute ischaemia: collagen vascular disorders (p. 444), diabetes (p. 453), etc.
The symptoms appear more or less abruptly, perhaps with later progression

It is not easy to predict recovery in individual cases. If the nerve is transected or infarcted by acute ischaemia, then any recovery is likely to be slow and incomplete, particularly the more proximal the lesion because the cut axons have to regrow and remyelinate over a long distance (regrowth rate is about 1 mm per day). On the other hand, relief of acute or chronic compression is more likely to be followed by complete recovery in a matter of weeks since the nerve remains in continuity and the axons are less likely to have been damaged than their surrounding myelin.

Mononeuritis multiplex is when there are lesions of several individual peripheral nerves. Causes include:
● collagen vascular disorders (p. 444)
● diabetes mellitus (p. 453)
● leprosy (p. 514)
● borrelia (p. 517)
● AIDS (p. 526)
● sarcoidosis (p. 472)
● paraneoplastic syndrome (p. 476)
● alcohol (p. 544)
● Tangier disease (p. 398)
● familial predisposition to pressure palsies (p. 398)

Note: Some individuals have a particular tendency to pressure palsies of exposed nerves; this may be familial (p. 398), idiopathic or as a result of a peripheral neuropathy due to, for example, diabetes mellitus (p. 453).

Median nerve (C6, C7, C8, T1 root components)

This is a mixed motor and sensory nerve supplying most of the flexor muscles in the forearm, pronators of the forearm and the muscles of the thenar eminence (Fig. 14.2).

Lesions in the arm

Lesions in the arm are caused by:
● penetrating injury
● intravenous injections at the elbow
● fractures of forearm bones
● tumour in the forearm
● haematoma in the forearm
● mononeuritis multiplex (p. 370)

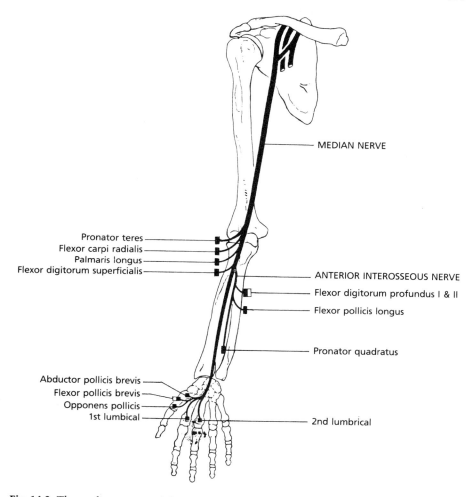

Pronator teres
Flexor carpi radialis
Palmaris longus
Flexor digitorum superficialis

MEDIAN NERVE

ANTERIOR INTEROSSEOUS NERVE
Flexor digitorum profundus I & II
Flexor pollicis longus

Pronator quadratus

Abductor pollicis brevis
Flexor pollicis brevis
Opponens pollicis
1st lumbical

2nd lumbrical

Fig. 14.2 The median nerve and the muscles which it supplies (reproduced with permission from *Aids to the Examination of the Peripheral Nervous System*, Ballière Tindall).

- neuralgic amyotrophy (p. 368)
- entrapment in the pronator teres (p. 378)
- arteriovenous fistula in the forearm (p. 467)

The forearm flexor group of muscles and abductor pollicis brevis waste and the most obvious weakness is of flexion of the distal interphalangeal joint of the forefinger (flexor digitorum profundus) and abduction of the thumb (abductor pollicis brevis). Sensory loss is shown in Fig. 14.3, but it may not be as extensive as this, particularly on the palm. Loss of light touch is more extensive than loss of pain sensation.

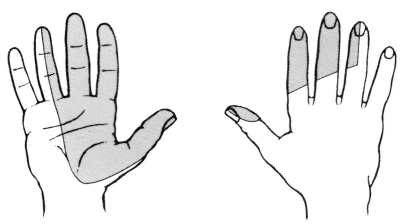

Fig. 14.3 Approximate area in which light touch and pain sensation are reduced in a median nerve lesion. *Note:* root, cord and plexus lesions do not 'split' the ring finger.

The *anterior interosseous nerve* can be traumatized, or compressed between the two heads of pronator teres. The only weakness is flexion of the distal interphalangeal joint of the thumb (flexor pollicis longus), forefinger and perhaps middle finger (flexor digitorum profundus). There is no sensory loss. If no improvement occurs within a couple of months, the nerve should be explored and, if appropriate, decompressed.

Lesions in the wrist

Lesions in the wrist are caused by:
- carpal tunnel syndrome (below)
- penetrating injury
- fracture of the wrist

Carpal tunnel syndrome

This is the most common entrapment neuropathy (incidence 100/100 000 population per annum) and is caused by sustained pressure on, or repetitive trauma to, the median nerve as it passes deep to the flexor retinaculum of the wrist. It is more common in females than males (3:1), presents at almost any age, is commonly bilateral, but tends to occur in the dominant hand first. Often even an asymptomatic contralateral hand is found to be affected on electrical testing. Frequently there is no explanation but possible predisposing causes include:
- obesity
- arthritis of the wrist
- fracture of the wrist in the past

- repetitive wrist movements:
  vibrating tools
  knitting
  piano playing
  wringing out washing
- pregnancy
- hypothyroidism (p. 456)
- acromegaly (p. 458)
- granulomas (TB, p. 512, sarcoid, p. 472, etc.)
- eosinophilic fasciitis
- ganglion
- forearm arteriovenous fistula for dialysis (p. 467)
- amyloid deposits in the wrist (p. 473)
- familial predisposition to pressure palsies (p. 398)
- background peripheral neuropathy, e.g. diabetes (p. 453)

The first symptoms are usually pain, tingling, burning and numbness, worse when the hand is used, in the median innervated area, particularly the index and middle fingers and sometimes across the rest of the hand as well. Characteristically, the pain wakes the patient from sleep and may radiate up the arm even to the shoulder and across the hand to the little finger. It is relieved by hanging the hand out of bed or shaking the wrist. In the morning the fingers often feel swollen, stiff, lifeless and clumsy. At this stage the sensory signs may be absent or slight (e.g. only impaired two point discrimination on the index finger). Eventually the abductor pollicis brevis becomes weak and wasted and more obvious median distribution sensory signs develop. Sharp taps over the median nerve at the wrist, with the wrist extended, may give an electric shock feeling in the fingers, but this can be found in normals and is not particularly useful (Tinel's sign).

The differential diagnosis includes other causes of wasting of the small muscles of the hand (p. 33) and cervical root lesions (p. 319) causing pain, but which is usually felt down rather than up the arm and normally does not waken the patient at night.

Diagnosis. The median sensory nerve action potential from the index finger is reduced in amplitude or is absent and the latency prolonged. Median motor nerve distal latency is prolonged across the wrist and, on EMG, the abductor pollicis brevis may be denervated. Electrical confirmation of the clinical diagnosis is only really needed in uncertain cases or before surgery.

Treatment. Treatment is, if possible, of the underlying condition. A wrist splint (in slight extension) worn at night will stop the nocturnal and even sometimes the day-time pain. Surgical decompression is necessary if:

- conservative measures fail to relieve the sensory symptoms

- the cause cannot be reversed (e.g. obesity) and the sensory symptoms are persisting
- the development and progression of definite sensory *signs*
- weakness of abductor pollicis brevis if it can be caught at an early stage *and* provided nerve conduction studies are diagnostic

Surgery is excellent for relieving the intermittent sensory symptoms immediately, but sensory signs, wasting and weakness take longer to resolve and may not ever recover; they should not, however, become worse after surgery.

Ulnar nerve (C7, C8, T1 root components)

This is a mixed sensory and motor nerve supplying the flexors of the ulnar side of the wrist, the long flexors to the ring and little fingers, and most of the small muscles in the hand (Fig. 14.4). Sensory loss is shown in Fig. 14.5, but it may not be as extensive as this. Loss of light touch is more extensive than loss of pain sensation.

Note: In under 2% of normals the ulnar nerve supplies all the small muscles in the hand.

Lesions at the elbow

Lesions at the elbow are caused by:
- penetrating injury
- fracture/dislocation
- arthritis
- pressure or repetitive trauma to the nerve as it lies unprotected in the ulnar groove of the medial epicondyle, particularly if the groove is shallow:
  during general anaesthesia or coma
  elbow crutches
  driving with elbow on open car window
  cubitus valgus (often secondary to an old fracture at elbow)
- cubital tunnel syndrome (entrapment by the fibrous band between the two heads of flexor carpi ulnaris)
- mononeuritis multiplex (p. 370)
- neuralgic amyotrophy (p. 368)
- arteriovenous fistula in forearm for dialysis (p. 467)

Clinical features

Clinical features are motor, sensory or both. Pain along the inner forearm is common in the cubital tunnel syndrome or at the elbow if the cause is trauma. Numbness and tingling are in the little and ring fingers, sometimes on the ulnar side of the palm as well. Weakness and wasting is most obvious

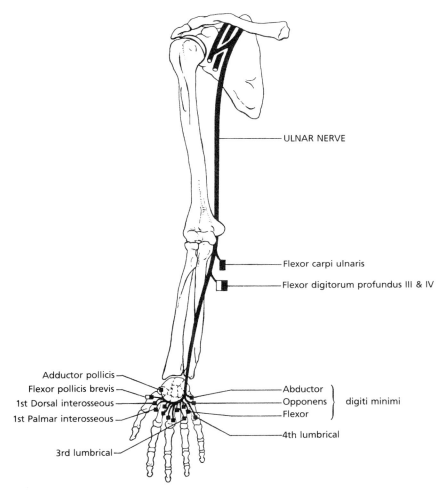

Fig. 14.4 The ulnar nerve and the muscles which it supplies (reproduced with permission from *Aids to the Examination of the Peripheral Nervous System*, Ballière Tindall).

in the ulnar-innervated hand muscles (particularly the first dorsal interosseous and abductor digiti minimi). Weakness can often be detected in flexion of the distal interphalangeal joint of the little finger if the lesion is above the branch to the flexor digitorum profundus.

Differentiating ulnar nerve compression in the ulnar groove from compression in the cubital tunnel is difficult and nerve conduction studies are of no help (p. 377). The cubital tunnel syndrome is likely if the nerve is neither thickened nor tender behind the medial epicondyle; if there has been no past elbow trauma, particularly fracture; and if the elbow carrying angle is normal. If the flexor digitorum profundus to the little finger is weak, then the

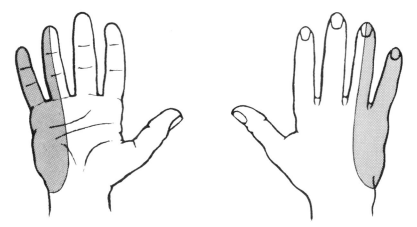

Fig. 14.5 Approximate area in which light touch and pain sensation are reduced in an ulnar nerve lesion. *Note*: root, plexus and cord lesions do not 'split' the ring finger.

lesion must be above the cubital tunnel, but if it is normal it has no localizing value.

Treatment

Treatment is to avoid any abnormal pressure on the nerve and to avoid repetitive flexion and extension of the elbow. Decompression of the trapped nerve in the cubital tunnel may help if, despite conservative treatment, there is definite progression and the site of the lesion is clinically and electrically consistent. Sometimes it is necessary to transpose the nerve anteriorly at the elbow to prevent functional deterioration by repetitive trauma although there is seldom much improvement.

Lesions at the wrist

Lesions at the wrist are caused by:
• penetrating injury
• fracture/dislocation
• ganglion
• arthritis
    The clinical features are as above but without weakness of the flexors of the wrist, little and ring fingers, and sensation on the ulnar side of the palm is normal.

Lesions in the hand

Lesions in the hand are caused by:
• repetitive trauma:

vibrating tools
drop handlebars
weight lifting
lawn mowing
crutch pressure
- arthritis
- ganglion
- penetrating trauma

Only the deep motor branch is involved so that sensation is *normal*. The abductor digiti minimi may be relatively spared.

Note: Some individuals (often on a familial basis, p. 398) and patients with a generalized neuropathy (e.g. diabetes mellitus, p. 453) are predisposed to entrapment neuropathies.

Note: In a T1 root lesion *all* the small muscles of the hand are affected and any sensory loss is on the inner side of the forearm.

Treatment

Treatment of ulnar nerve compression in the wrist and hand is to remove, if possible, the compressing lesion. This relieves pain and prevents progression of sensory signs and motor weakness.

Electrical diagnosis

The ulnar sensory nerve action potential from the little finger is reduced in amplitude and delayed (or absent) unless the nerve is affected in the palm distal to the origin of the sensory branches when it is normal. The motor nerve conduction velocity is often reduced across the lesion or, if not, the compound muscle action potential is reduced in amplitude. The distal motor latency to abductor digiti minimi and/or the first dorsal interosseous muscle is prolonged with lesions in the wrist and palm. The abductor digiti minimi and/or first dorsal interosseous muscles may be denervated.

Radial nerve (C5, C6, C7, C8 root components)

This is a mixed motor and sensory nerve supplying the extensors of the elbow, wrist, fingers and thumb and the brachioradialis (Fig. 14.6). The posterior cutaneous nerves of the arm and forearm arise above the elbow, but even if injured seldom cause sensory loss because of overlap from other cutaneous nerve territories. Any sensory loss is slight and limited to the skin over the first dorsal interosseous muscle (Fig. 14.7).

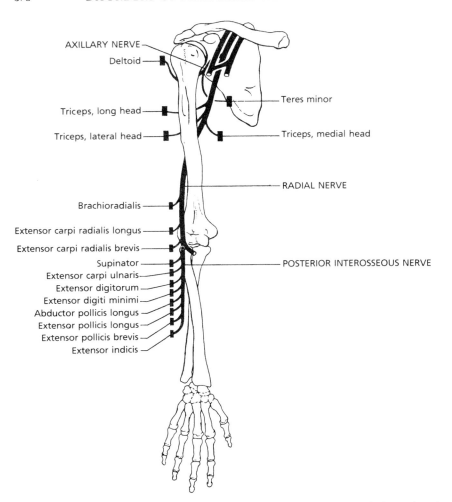

AXILLARY NERVE
Deltoid
Teres minor
Triceps, long head
Triceps, lateral head
Triceps, medial head
RADIAL NERVE
Brachioradialis
Extensor carpi radialis longus
Extensor carpi radialis brevis
Supinator
POSTERIOR INTEROSSEOUS NERVE
Extensor carpi ulnaris
Extensor digitorum
Extensor digiti minimi
Abductor pollicis longus
Extensor pollicis longus
Extensor pollicis brevis
Extensor indicis

Fig. 14.6 The radial and axillary nerves and the muscles which they supply (reproduced with permission from *Aids to the Examination of the Peripheral Nervous System*, Ballière Tindall).

Causes of lesions

- penetrating injury
- fracture of the shaft of the humerus (also sometimes secondary to callus formation)
- pressure in the axilla from crutches or arm hanging over the bed during general anaesthesia
- malignancy in the axilla
- pressure on the radial groove of the humerus from the back of a chair while in a drunken stupor (i.e. Saturday night palsy), tourniquet, etc.

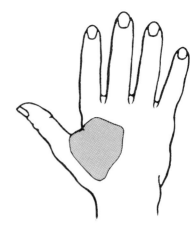

Fig. 14.7 Approximate area in which light touch and pain sensation are reduced in a radial nerve lesion.

- mononeuritis multiplex (p. 370)
- neuralgic amyotrophy (p. 368)

Clinical features

Weakness of the triceps and loss of the triceps tendon reflex occur only with high radial nerve lesions (i.e. in the axilla). The most prominent weakness is in extension of the wrist and at the metacarpophalangeal joints of the fingers and thumb, with wasting of the extensor muscle group in the forearm. Brachioradialis is usually affected, causing loss of the supinator reflex and weakness of elbow flexion in the semiprone position. Tingling and numbness on the back of the hand are slight, if present at all.

Note: The interphalangeal joints of the fingers can still be extended by the lumbricals and interossei.

The *posterior interosseous nerve* can be entrapped in the forearm extensor muscles, causing weakness of only the thumb and finger extensors, often with pain in the forearm. This can happen spontaneously, after vigorous orchestral conducting or using a screwdriver.

Note: A C7 root lesion causes some weakness of shoulder adduction and wrist flexion in *addition* to elbow, wrist, finger and thumb extension. In contrast, a radial nerve lesion affects the brachioradialis whose nerve supply comes from C6 and depresses its reflex (the supinator jerk). Sensory loss may be slight in both cases, but in C7 root lesions any disturbance is over the middle finger, whereas in radial nerve lesions it is on the back of the hand. Finally, the triceps jerk is depressed in a C7 lesion but not in a radial nerve lesion unless it is high, above the origin of the nerve to triceps.

Treatment

A wrist splint is helpful to avoid strain on the wrist joint and to allow the fingers to function normally until the radial nerve recovers. 'Wrist drop' is so disabling because the interossei cannot work properly in this position. *Early exploration and decompression of an entrapped posterior interosseous nerve is worth while.*

Less commonly affected forearm nerves

The musculocutaneous nerve (C5, C6)

This supplies the biceps and brachialis (elbow flexion) and ends as the lateral cutaneous nerve of the forearm. The sensory loss is shown in Fig. 14.8. It is rarely affected except by trauma, the causes of mononeuritis multiplex (p. 370) and neuralgic amyotrophy (p. 368).

The axillary nerve (C5, C6)

This supplies the deltoid (shoulder abduction) and a small area of skin on the lateral part of the upper arm (Fig. 14.9). It is affected by similar conditions to the musculocutaneous nerve above.

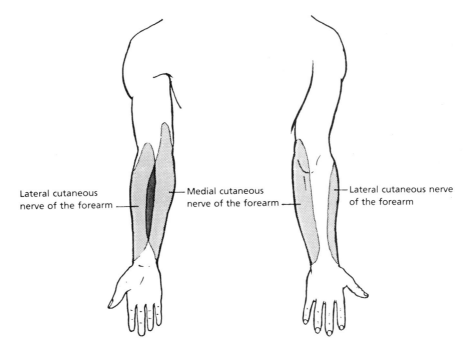

Lateral cutaneous nerve of the forearm

Medial cutaneous nerve of the forearm

Lateral cutaneous nerve of the forearm

Fig. 14.8 Approximate areas in which light touch and pain sensation are reduced in a lesion of the lateral and medial cutaneous nerves of the forearm (the latter arises from the brachial plexus, C8 and T1).

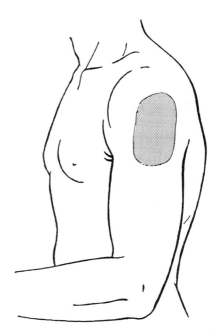

Fig. 14.9 Approximate area in which light touch and pain sensation are reduced in an axillary nerve lesion.

The suprascapular nerve (C5, C6)

This nerve arises from the brachial plexus and supplies the supra- and infra-spinatus muscles. Causes of damage are as the musculocutaneous nerve above. Clinical features are shoulder pain with wasting and weakness of the spinatii muscles.

The long thoracic nerve (C5, C6, C7)

This supplies the serratus anterior which fixes the scapula. Lesions result in winging of the scapula and are caused by trauma, neuralgic amyotrophy (p. 368) and causes of mononeuritis multiplex (p. 370).

Femoral nerve (L2, L3, L4 root components)

This is a mixed motor and sensory nerve supplying the quadriceps (and some of the muscles of hip flexion, Fig. 14.10).

Causes of lesions

- trauma
- femoral artery catheterization
- abdominal tumours and aneurysms

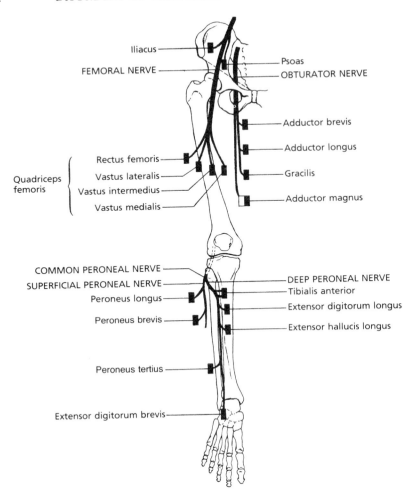

Fig. 14.10 The femoral, obturator and peroneal nerves and the muscles which they supply (reproduced with permission from *Aids to the Examination of the Peripheral Nervous System*, Ballière Tindall).

- abdominal haematoma:
  ruptured aneurysm
  anticoagulants
  haemophilia
- psoas abscess
- femoral hernia
- femoral artery aneurysm
- diabetic amyotrophy (p. 454)

Clinical features

The clinical features are of weakness of knee extension with wasting of the quadriceps and loss of the knee jerk, sometimes with a little weakness of hip flexion. Any sensory loss is slight because of overlap from adjacent nerve territories; on the anterior part of the thigh with perhaps some extension below the knee on the medial side.

An L3/L4 root lesion may appear similar but there is additional weakness of inversion of the ankle and any sensory loss is below the knee.

Sciatic nerve (L4, L5, S1, S2, S3 root components)

This is a large mixed motor and sensory nerve which supplies the muscles of knee flexion, part of the adductor magnus, and all the muscles below the knee (Figs. 14.10 and 14.11). Sensory loss is over the foot and extending up the lateral part of the leg towards the knee (Fig. 14.12). Above the knee the sciatic divides into the common peroneal and tibial nerves.

Causes of lesions

- penetrating injury
- external compression (coma, general anaesthesia, etc.)
- misplaced intramuscular injection
- pelvic tumours and aneurysms
- compression by the pregnant uterus, trauma during difficult delivery
- fracture of the femur and pelvis
- hip surgery, fracture or dislocation

Clinical features

There is wasting and weakness of the hamstrings and all the muscles below the knee with loss of the ankle jerk. The whole foot is anaesthetic (apart from the skin around the medial malleolus supplied by the long saphenous nerve, a branch of the femoral nerve) with some extension up the lateral and posterior lower leg.

Common peroneal (lateral popliteal) nerve (L4, L5, S1 root components)

This is a mixed motor and sensory nerve (Fig. 14.10), arising from the sciatic nerve above the knee and dividing (near the neck of the fibula) into a super-ficial branch which supplies the peroneal muscles and sensation on the dorsolateral part of the foot and lateral lower leg (Fig. 14.13), and a deep branch which supplies the extensors of the foot and toes and a small area of skin between the first and second toes on the dorsum of the foot (Fig. 14.14).

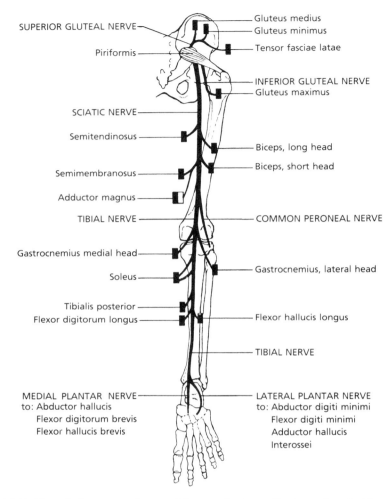

SUPERIOR GLUTEAL NERVE
Piriformis
SCIATIC NERVE
Semitendinosus
Semimembranosus
Adductor magnus
TIBIAL NERVE
Gastrocnemius medial head
Soleus
Tibialis posterior
Flexor digitorum longus
MEDIAL PLANTAR NERVE
to: Abductor hallucis
    Flexor digitorum brevis
    Flexor hallucis brevis

Gluteus medius
Gluteus minimus
Tensor fasciae latae
INFERIOR GLUTEAL NERVE
Gluteus maximus
Biceps, long head
Biceps, short head
COMMON PERONEAL NERVE
Gastrocnemius, lateral head
Flexor hallucis longus
TIBIAL NERVE
LATERAL PLANTAR NERVE
to: Abductor digiti minimi
    Flexor digiti minimi
    Adductor hallucis
    Interossei

Fig. 14.11 The sciatic nerve and some of the muscles it supplies (reproduced with permission from *Aids to the Examination of the Peripheral Nervous System*, Ballière Tindall).

Causes of lesions

- penetrating injury
- fracture/dislocation
- injury or compression of the nerve as it lies exposed at the neck of the fibula:
    prolonged recumbency
    prolonged squatting or kneeling (gardeners)
    plaster cast on leg

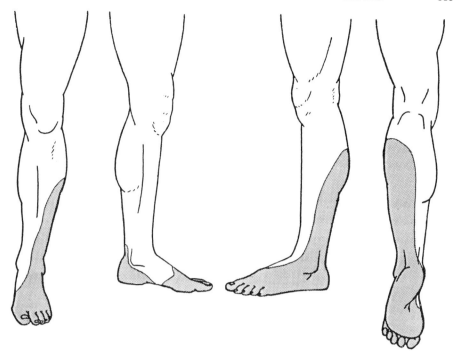

Fig. 14.12 Approximate area in which light touch and pain sensation are reduced in a sciatic nerve lesion.

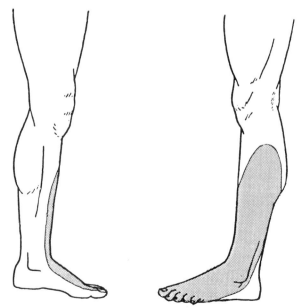

Fig. 14.13 Approximate area in which light touch and pain sensation are reduced in a common peroneal nerve lesion above the origin of the superficial peroneal nerve.

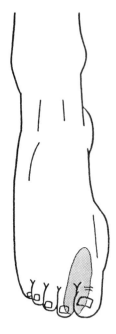

Fig. 14.14 Approximate area in which light touch and pain sensation are reduced in a deep peroneal nerve lesion.

splints or tight bandages
popliteal cyst
- mononeuritis multiplex (p. 370)
- background peripheral neuropathy (e.g. diabetes, p. 453) or familial predisposition to pressure palsies (p. 398)

Clinical features

There is wasting and weakness of the peroneal muscles, causing weakness of ankle eversion, and of the muscles in the anterior tibial compartment, causing weakness of ankle and toe dorsiflexion. The extensor digitorum brevis on the dorsum of the foot is also wasted and weak. Inversion and plantar flexion of the ankle are normal. Sensory loss may be very slight and the *maximum* area is shown in Fig. 14.13. Sometimes only the superficial branch is affected in which case the sensory loss is similar but only ankle eversion is weak. Pressure palsies usually recover spontaneously in a matter of weeks or months.

Note: An L5 root lesion also causes weakness of dorsiflexion of the foot and toes and of ankle eversion. However, dorsiflexion of the ankle is usually less affected than that of the toes and there may be some detectable weakness of the calf muscles, hamstrings and hip abduction. In an L5 root lesion the sensory loss tends to be more obvious and extends up to the knee. In cases of doubt nerve conduction studies are useful.

Note: An L4 root lesion may cause some weakness of ankle dorsiflexion but, unlike a peroneal nerve lesion, there is also weakness of inversion of the ankle and any sensory loss is on the medial side of the lower leg.

Ski boot neuropathy

Pressure from ski boots at the ankle and over the dorsum of the foot can compress small cutaneous nerves, so producing tingling and numbness in their sensory distribution. Any ill-fitting tight footwear will do the same.

Tibial (medial popliteal) nerve (L4, L5, S1, S2 root components)

This is a mixed motor and sensory nerve supplying the muscles which plantar flex the ankle and toes, and invert the ankle (Fig. 14.11). Sensory loss is over the sole of the foot and extending on to its medial and lateral borders (Fig. 14.15). The ankle jerk is lost. It can be injured but is seldom affected by any other pathology.

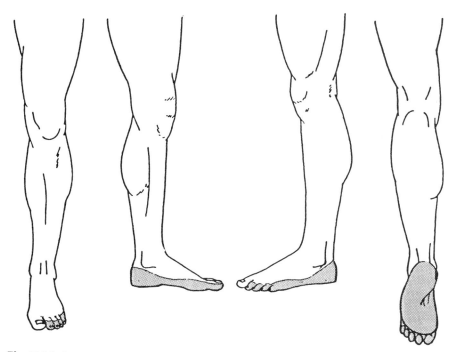

Fig. 14.15 Approximate area in which light touch and pain sensation are reduced in a tibial nerve lesion.

The sural nerve

The sural nerve, a branch of the tibial, is seldom damaged except by biopsy, which leaves an area of numbness just below the lateral malleolus.

The tarsal tunnel syndrome

This is entrapment of the tibial nerve beneath the flexor retinaculum behind and below the medial malleolus. It may be caused by local trauma, ganglion, arthritis of the ankle, diabetes (p. 454) and hypothyroidism (p. 456). The clinical features are pain, burning, tingling and sometimes numbness of the sole of the foot and heel which is aggravated by standing or walking and relieved by rest and foot elevation.

Morton's metatarsalgia

This is pain, burning, paraesthesia and tenderness in the region of one or more metatarsophalangeal joints, usually due to a neuroma on the digital branches of a plantar nerve. Excision of the neuroma or carbamazepine (p. 90) may help.

Lateral cutaneous nerve of the thigh (L2, L3 root components)

This sensory nerve can be entrapped under the lateral end of the inguinal ligament to cause the syndrome of 'meralgia paraesthetica'. There is a combination of pain, burning, tingling and numbness over the anterolateral thigh (Fig. 14.6). There is no weakness and the knee jerk is normal.

This tends to occur in the obese and pregnant, and sometimes as a result of a pelvic tumour or very constricting clothes. Treatment, apart from explanation and weight reduction, is hardly ever necessary.

Obturator nerve (L2, L3, L4 root components)

This arises from the lumbar plexus and leaves the pelvis through the obturator foramen (Fig. 14.10). It can be compressed by a pelvic tumour or pregnant uterus. There is weakness of adduction of the thigh, pain in the medial part of the thigh, but little if any sensory loss on the upper medial thigh.

Genito-femoral nerve (L1, L2 root components)

This can be damaged at operation for inguinal hernia and appendicectomy, leaving the patient with pain, tingling and numbness in the groin and perineum.

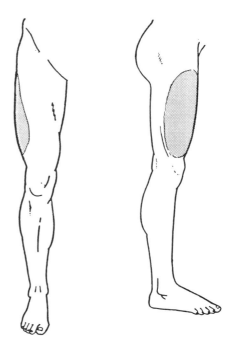

Fig. 14.16 Approximate area in which light touch and pain sensation are reduced in a lateral cutaneous nerve of the thigh lesion.

Peripheral neuropathies

Peripheral neuropathies include all general disorders of the peripheral motor, sensory or autonomic nerves, but exclude single nerve lesions (mononeuropathies) due to entrapment or trauma. If the nerve roots are particularly involved, the term 'polyradiculopathy' is used.

Causes

Hereditary:
- peroneal muscular atrophy (Charcot–Marie–Tooth disease, hereditary motor and sensory neuropathy, type I and type II) (p. 396)
- hypertrophic polyneuropathy (hereditary motor and sensory neuropathy, type III) (p. 396)
- hereditary sensory neuropathy (p. 397)
- hereditary ataxic neuropathy (Refsum's disease) (p. 397)
- familial dysautonomia (Riley–Day syndrome) (p. 397)
- Fabry's disease (p. 397)
- Tangier disease (p. 398)
- porphyria (p. 398)
- familial amyloidosis (p. 473)

- Krabbe's disease (p. 478)
- metachromatic leucodystrophy (p. 478)
- abetalipoproteinaemia (p. 479)
- ataxia telangiectasia (p. 202)
- xeroderma pigmentosum (p. 203)
- chorea-acanthocytosis
- Cockayne syndrome (p. 482)

Metabolic:

- diabetes (p. 453)
- renal failure (p. 465)
- amyloidosis (p. 473)
- hyperthyroidism (p. 456)
- hypothyroidism (p. 456)
- acromegaly (p. 458)
- hypoglycaemia (p. 108)

Infections:

- Guillain–Barré syndrome (p. 398)
- brucellosis (p. 510)
- leprosy (p. 514)
- borrelia (p. 517)
- tetanus (p. 518)
- botulism (p. 520)
- diphtheria (p. 520)
- herpes simplex type 2 (p. 523)
- herpes zoster (p. 523)
- Epstein–Barr (p. 524)
- HIV (p. 526)
- rabies (p. 529)
- gnathostomiasis (p. 537)

Collagen vascular disorders:

- systemic lupus erythematosus (p. 444)
- systemic vasculitis (p. 447)
- hypersensitivity vasculitides (p. 448)
- rheumatoid disease (p. 448)
- Sjögren's syndrome (p. 449)
- giant cell arteritis (p. 450)

Deficiency states:

- vitamin B_1 (thiamine, p. 468)
- vitamin B_{12} (p. 470)
- vitamin B_6 (pyridoxine, p. 470)
- nicotinic acid (pellagra, p. 471)
- vitamin E (p. 471)

Toxins:

- alcohol (p. 542)

- organic solvents (p. 546):
  carbon disulphide
  methyl butyl ketone
  n-hexane
  toluene
- metals:
  lead (p. 547)
  mercury (p. 547)
  arsenic (p. 547)
  tin (p. 547)
  thallium (p. 548)
  gold (p. 548)
  platinum (p. 548)
- organophosphorus compounds (p. 548)
- acrylamide (p. 549)
- chronic cyanide poisoning (p. 549)
- ethylene oxide (p. 550)
- methyl bromide (p. 550)
- nitrous oxide (p. 550)
- pyridylmethyl nitrophenyl urea (p. 550)
- subacute myelo-optico-neuropathy (SMON, p. 550)
- pyridoxine abuse (p. 470)

Drugs (p. 402):
- amiodarone, chloramphenicol, chloroquine, cisplatin, clioquinol, colchicine, corticosteroids, dapsone, disulfiram, ethambutol, ethionamide, griseofulvin, hydralazine, indomethacin, isoniazid, tryptophan, lithium, methaqualone, metronidazole, nitrofurantoin, perhexiline, phenobarbitone, phenytoin, streptomycin, sulphonamides, thalidomide, tricyclic antidepressants, vinblastine, vincristine, vindesine, zimeldine

Malignant disease:
- paraneoplastic syndrome (p. 476)
- multiple myeloma (p. 460)
- solitary plasmacytoma (p. 461)
- Waldenström's macroglobulinaemia (p. 461)
- benign paraproteinaemia (p. 461)
- lymphoma (p. 275)
- direct infiltration of roots or peripheral nerves
- insulinoma and chronic hypoglycaemia (p. 108)

Miscellaneous:
- neuralgic amyotrophy (p. 368)
- ischaemic neuropathy (p. 402)
- hypereosinophilic syndrome (p. 459)
- polycythaemia rubra vera (p. 458)
- migrant sensory neuritis of Wartenberg (p. 402)

- critical illness polyneuropathy (p. 402)
- sarcoidosis (p. 472)

Pathophysiology

Peripheral neuropathies may affect the axon, the myelin sheath or both. In axonal neuropathies motor nerve conduction is normal until late, whereas in demyelinating neuropathies conduction is slowed early. In both situations electrical signs of muscle denervation develop if the axons of motor nerves are affected. The sensory action potentials are small and/or delayed if sensory nerves are affected.

The peripheral nerves may be damaged by acute ischaemia (e.g. polyarteritis nodosa, p. 447); infiltration (e.g. sarcoid, p. 472, amyloid, p. 473, or malignant cells); toxins (e.g. alcohol, p. 542); metabolic derangements (e.g. diabetes, p. 453); inflammation (e.g. Guillain–Barré syndrome, p. 398), etc.

There is almost always damage of both sensory and motor peripheral nerves even if this can only be demonstrated electrically. Neuropathies tending to be predominantly 'motor' are caused by peroneal muscular atrophy (p. 396), diphtheria (p. 547), lead (p. 547), dapsone, porphyria (p. 398), etc.; those tending to be predominantly 'sensory' are caused by carcinoma (p. 476), renal failure (p. 465), hereditary sensory neuropathy (p. 389), vitamin B_{12} deficiency (p. 470), pyridoxine abuse (p. 470), etc.

In any neuropathy there can be involvement of the peripheral autonomic nerves and this is particularly likely in:
- amyloidosis (p. 473)
- diabetes (p. 453)
- Guillain–Barré syndrome (p. 398)
- porphyria (p. 398)
- alcoholism (p. 542)
- AIDS (p. 526)
- pyridylmethyl nitrophenyl urea (p. 550)
- vincristine
- botulism (p. 520)
- familial dysautonomia (p. 397)

Clinical features

Usually there is diffuse and symmetrical involvement of the nerves to the extremities, the feet before the hands. In mononeuritis multiplex (p. 370) the picture is more patchy and asymmetrical, reflecting damage to individual peripheral nerves. Depending on the cause, the onset may be rapid or insidious with gradual recovery, relapses and remissions.

Sensory symptoms

These include tingling, numbness, 'woolliness' and sometimes pain or burning. On the whole they are persistent rather than intermittent (cf. anxiety, overbreathing, entrapment neuropathy). The symptoms tend to start in the toes and feet, spread up the leg and then involve the fingers, spreading up the arms. The symptoms may spread from the limbs to the trunk and sometimes to the face and mouth. The signs may not be obvious, but usually there is distal blunting of cutaneous sensation (light touch and pain) and loss of vibration sense at the ankles. The cutaneous sensory loss is often in a glove and stocking distribution but can, in severe cases, involve the whole body. Sometimes there is hyperalgesia (enhanced pain sensation). Occasionally joint position sense is severely impaired.

Motor symptoms

These include distal muscle weakness and wasting. This spreads proximally and may ultimately involve the muscles of respiration, the face, swallowing, speaking and very rarely the eyes. Proximal muscle weakness is particularly common in the Guillain–Barré syndrome (p. 398), porphyria (p. 398) and diabetic amyotrophy (p. 454).

The deep tendon reflexes are usually depressed or lost early, particularly the ankle jerk, but they can be normal (e.g. in distal sensory neuropathies).

Occasionally there is a postural and action tremor due to neither cerebellar nor postural sensation disturbance, and sometimes restless legs (p. 306).

Autonomic symptoms

These include postural or exercise induced hypotension, impotence, reduced (sometimes increased) sweating, constipation or diarrhoea, urinary hesitancy or retention and various abnormalities of cardiac rhythm (p. 403).

Hypertrophy of peripheral nerves

Hypertrophy of peripheral nerves is best felt, if it is present, over the clavicle and dorsum of the foot. The greater auricular, ulnar and common peroneal nerves are also worth examining. It occurs particularly in:
- leprosy (p. 514)
- neurofibromatosis (p. 277)
- hereditary motor and sensory neuropathy type I (p. 396)
- hypertrophic polyneuropathy (p. 396)
- amyloidosis (p. 473)
- acromegaly (p. 458)

Myokymia

Myokymia (coarse undulating movements of muscle, p. 192) has been described in gold (p. 548) and lead (p. 547) neuropathies and the Guillain–Barré syndrome (p. 398).

Diagnosis

If there is any doubt about the clinical diagnosis, then nerve conduction studies and EMG should be carried out. The main challenge is to identify the cause of the neuropathy, particularly of a treatable one.

In the history it is important to consider the patient's general health, family history, occupation (toxin exposure?), drug and alcohol intake. Other family members should be examined if a hereditary condition is suspected.

Routine investigations must include:
- full blood count and ESR
- urea and electrolytes
- blood glucose
- chest X-ray
- serum B_{12} level

and, if indicated, or in an obscure case:
- organ specific and non-organ specific antibodies
- plasma protein electrophoresis (? myeloma)
- skeletal survey (? myeloma, metastases)
- Bence-Jones proteinuria (? myeloma)
- urine porphyrins
- HIV antibodies
- liver function tests
- thyroid function
- plasma lipids (? abetalipoproteinaemia)
- plasma phytanic acid (? Refsum's disease)
- mammography (? paraneoplastic syndrome)
- barium studies (? paraneoplastic syndrome)

Nerve biopsy (usually the sural or distal radial sensory nerve and always in collaboration with a pathologist) may be useful if the diagnosis has not already been made in other ways. For example in:
- sarcoidosis (p. 472)
- amyloidosis (p. 473)
- leprosy (p. 514)
- polyarteritis nodosa (p. 447) and other vasculitides (p. 448)

Associated clinical features may be helpful diagnostically:

Cerebellar disorder:
- alcohol (p. 542)

- paraneoplastic syndrome (p. 476)
- vitamin E deficiency (p. 471)
- abetalipoproteinaemia (p. 479)
- Refsum's disease (p. 397)

Dementia/confusion:
- metachromatic leucodystrophy (p. 478)
- alcohol (p. 542)
- collagen vascular disorders (p. 444)
- porphyria (p. 398)
- vitamin B_{12} deficiency (p. 470)
- AIDS (p. 526)

Hepatosplenomegaly:
- paraneoplastic syndrome (p. 476)
- lymphoma (p. 275)
- sarcoidosis (p. 472)
- alcoholic cirrhosis (p. 542)
- Tangier disease (p. 398)
- POEMS syndrome (p. 461)

Skin involvement:
- borrelia (p. 517)
- leprosy (p. 514)
- Fabry's disease (p. 397)

Lymphadenopathy:
- paraneoplastic syndrome (p. 476)
- sarcoidosis (p. 472)
- lymphoma (p. 275)
- Tangier disease (p. 398)

Renal failure/proteinuria:
- amyloidosis (p. 473)
- diabetes (p. 453)
- myeloma (p. 460)
- Fabry's disease (p. 397)

Anaemia:
- paraneoplastic syndrome (p. 476)
- vitamin B_{12} deficiency (p. 470)
- hypothyroidism (p. 456)
- renal failure (p. 465)
- nutritional deficiency

Treatment

In many neuropathies treatment of the underlying condition, if possible, will restore neurological function or at least prevent progression. Motor disability must be dealt with on its merits (physiotherapy, aids, adaptations, etc.) and severe cutaneous sensory loss by protecting the vulnerable skin from trauma.

Of great concern is the treatment of neuropathic pain; occasional patients are helped by analgesics, carbamazepine (p. 90), phenytoin (p. 80), tricyclic anti-depressants (amitriptyline, 25–150 mg at night) with or without phenothi-azines, and perhaps mexiletine (150 mg daily, gradually up to 10 mg/kg/day in 3 divided doses), but most are not. Transcutaneous electrical or mechanical stimulation may be effective for some patients.

Hereditary neuropathies

These are recognized by their slowly progressive course, family history and lack of alternative explanation. They are often associated with other neuro-logical lesions and non-neurological disorders.

Peroneal muscular atrophy

Peroneal muscular atrophy (Charcot–Marie–Tooth disease) is usually dom-inantly inherited, but can be recessive, and starts in childhood or adoles-cence. It is slowly progressive, but patients seldom become wheelchair bound. There are two main types:
● Hereditary motor and sensory neuropathy type I (HMSN type I); motor conduction velocities are severely slowed due to segmental demyelination of peripheral nerves which are often thickened. The sensory action potentials are small or absent.
● Hereditary motor and sensory neuropathy type 2 (HMSN type II); motor conduction velocities are more or less normal and there is axonal degenera-tion. Sensory action potentials are small or absent.
    Initially there is distal weakness and wasting and, in type I but not type II, areflexia in the lower limbs. Eventually the distal upper limbs are involved. Sensory symptoms are mild and the only sign may be absent vibration sense at the ankles. The clinical picture can, therefore, be identical to that of spinal muscular atrophy (p. 359), but then not only is motor nerve conduction velocity normal but the sensory action potentials are also normal.
    Other features include:
● pes cavus and scoliosis, particularly in HMSN type I
● tremor and/or ataxia, particularly in HMSN type I
● myotonic (p. 178) or sometimes Argyll Robertson pupils (p. 177)
    It is important not to confuse HMSN type I with chronic inflammatory demyelinating neuropathy, which is treatable (p. 399).

Hypertrophic polyneuropathy

Hypertrophic polyneuropathy (Dejerine–Sottas disease or hereditary motor and sensory neuropathy type III) is a rare, recessive and more severe motor and sensory neuropathy which starts in infancy or childhood. The peripheral nerves are thickened and often the CSF protein is high. Motor nerve conduction velocities are extremely slow and sensory action potentials absent. Other features include:

- pes cavus
- scoliosis
- cerebellar degeneration
- Argyll Robertson pupils possibly (p. 177)

Hereditary sensory neuropathy

This starts in childhood with loss of pain sensation in the feet and hands. Charcot joint deformities (p. 18) of the ankles and neuropathic foot ulcers are common. It may be autosomal dominant or recessive.

Hereditary ataxic neuropathy (Refsum's disease)

Hereditary ataxic neuropathy is a very rare recessive disorder in which there is excessive accumulation of phytanic acid in the body tissues and blood. The onset is in childhood or adolescence with:

- peripheral sensorimotor neuropathy
- cerebellar degeneration
- sensorineural deafness
- retinitis pigmentosa and night blindness
- anosmia
- ichthyosis of the skin
- pes cavus
- scoliosis
- cardiomyopathy
- cataracts

Familial dysautonomia

Familial dysautonomia (Riley–Day syndrome) is another very rare recessive disorder. Features include:

- widespread autonomic neuropathy
- insensitivity to pain

  The onset is in infancy and most patients die in adolescence.

Fabry's disease

This is a rare X-linked disorder with a deficit in lysosomal alpha galactosidase A, leading to accumulation of glycolipid in the walls of blood vessels in peripheral nerve, brain, skin, kidney and lymph nodes. Onset is in childhood with attacks of severe limb pains and a punctate reddish-purple maculopapular rash on the lower trunk, inguinal, scrotal and buttock areas (bathing trunks distribution). Later features include ischaemic stroke, renal failure and corneal opacities. The painful neuropathy is seldom accompanied by any signs. The diagnosis is by demonstrating deficient enzyme activity in leucocytes or skin fibroblasts.

Tangier disease

Tangier disease (hereditary high density lipoprotein deficiency) is a rare autosomal recessive disorder with widespread deposition of cholesterol esters, causing enlargement of the tonsils, liver and spleen along with a generalized peripheral neuropathy or mononeuritis multiplex, lymphadenopathy, corneal opacities, thrombocytopenia, anaemia and cardiomegaly. The neuropathy may be the presenting feature and can sometimes look rather like syringomyelia (p. 334). Plasma cholesterol and particularly HDL cholesterol are very low and skin, nerve or rectal biopsy shows cholesterol-laden cells.

Porphyria

The autosomal dominant varieties of acute intermittent porphyria, variegate porphyria and hereditary coproporphyria may be complicated by acute attacks of psychosis, seizures, encephalopathy, confusion (along with abdominal pain, constipation and tachycardia) and an evolving, sometimes subacutely, severe predominantly proximal motor neuropathy (cf. Guillain–Barré syndrome, p. 398). The latter two types may also be complicated by photosensitivity. The diagnosis is made by finding increased urine and faecal porphyrins. Attacks may be precipitated by pregnancy, alcohol, barbiturates, sulphonamides, sulphonylureas, griseofulvin, oral contraceptives and many other drugs.

Familial predisposition to pressure palsies

Some families run a dominant tendency to develop entrapment neuropathies (carpal tunnel syndrome, etc.).

Guillain–Barré syndrome

This is a subacute, inflammatory, demyelinating polyneuropathy and polyradiculopathy which affects motor more than sensory nerves. Probably it is due to an abnormal immune response to a preceding infection; about half the patients have a respiratory infection or diarrhoeal illness a few days or weeks before the onset of neurological symptoms. Antecedent infections include influenza (p. 526), cytomegalovirus (p. 525), Epstein–Barr (p. 524), herpes zoster (p. 523), non-A non-B hepatitis, mycoplasma (p. 521), campylobacter (p. 511), toxoplasmosis (p. 536) and immunization. Epidural anaesthesia, surgery and pregnancy have been implicated in occasional cases.

It affects any age group, males somewhat more than females. The incidence is about 2/100 000 population per annum.

The neurological symptoms develop over days or a few weeks, stabilize for a matter of weeks, and at the nadir there may be anything from mild disability to paralysis of all voluntary muscles. There is no malaise or fever. Recovery occurs slowly over several weeks or months and is complete in about 80% of patients. Five percent die in the acute stage. About 5% of cases recur and a few patients pursue a much more slowly progressive and chronic course, sometimes with relapses and remissions (chronic inflammatory demyelinating neuropathy, CIDP).

A poor outcome is most likely if patients are elderly, become unable to walk in a few days from onset, or require mechanical ventilation.

Clinical features

These are dominated by motor disability and sensory symptoms. There is flaccid weakness and later wasting of proximal and/or distal limb muscles which is always bilateral but often somewhat asymmetrical. Tendon reflexes are lost early. The weakness spreads to involve more of the limb muscles and very often the facial muscles. It can then spread further to the muscles of respiration, swallowing, speaking and exceptionally the extraocular muscles. There are no upper motor neurone features. Myokymia of facial muscles may occur and, particularly during recovery, a postural and action tremor may develop in the arms.

Sensory symptoms of numbness, pins and needles, burning and pain are usually prominent, but signs are not obvious except in fairly severe cases. Sometimes there is severe back pain and even impaired straight leg raising due to radicular inflammation.

There may be more ataxia than might be predicted from the weakness and any loss of joint position sense. The sphincters are seldom affected.

Electrical tests can be normal in the first week or so, but then usually reveal marked slowing of motor nerve conduction velocities (demyelinating neuropathy), delayed latency of the F waves, diminished compound muscle action potentials and eventually signs of denervation on EMG. Sensory action potentials are diminished or absent.

The CSF protein is normal at first and then usually somewhat raised, but rarely more than 5 g/l, and the cell count is normal.

The *Miller Fisher syndrome* is an unusual variant with initial involvement of eye movements due to 3rd, 4th or 6th cranial nerve palsies, cerebellar ataxia of the limbs and areflexia. More typical Guillain–Barré motor and sensory features in the limbs then develop to a greater or lesser extent.

Other causes of a subacute polyneuropathy must be excluded:
- toxins and drugs (p. 391)
- paraneoplastic syndrome (p. 476)
- botulism (p. 520)
- AIDS (p. 526)
- borrelia (p. 517)
- critical illness polyneuropathy (p. 402)
- collagen vascular disorders (p. 444)
- diphtheria (p. 520)
- porphyria (p. 398)
- serum sickness

and other disorders which may present with subacute flaccid weakness:
- myasthenia gravis (Chapter 15)
- polymyositis and other myopathies (Chapter 16)
- acute spinal cord lesion (p. 322)
- paralytic polio (p. 522)
- 'dumb' rabies (p. 529)
- hypokalaemia (p. 431)
- snake bite (p. 551)
- pelagic paralysis (p. 552)

Complications

- venous thromboembolism
- cardiac arrhythmias, sinus tachycardia and sinus bradycardia often precipitated by endotracheal suction; labile blood pressure; postural hypotension; excessive sweating and pupillary abnormalities due to autonomic neuropathy
- pneumonia due to respiratory failure and/or aspiration
- pressure sores, skin infection and septicaemia
- hyponatraemia, sometimes due to inappropriate ADH secretion
- papilloedema and raised intracranial pressure, perhaps due to the high CSF protein blocking CSF absorption at the arachnoid villi
- anxiety and depression

Management

Management is concentrated on supporting the patient, psychologically as well as physically, until natural recovery occurs. This must include good nursing, feeding, fluid balance, attention to any swallowing difficulty and sometimes mechanical ventilation. Physiotherapy is crucial at all stages. Pain may be relieved with non-steroidal anti-inflammatory drugs or opiates (from skin pressure, joint immobility, neuropathic) and corticosteroids may help the severe radicular back and leg pain which some patients experience. Low dose subcutaneous heparin (5000 units twice daily) should be given for venous thromboembolism prophylaxis until the patient is starting to walk again.

Patients with anything more than mild disease must be admitted to hospital and forced vital capacity (FVC) monitored every few hours. If there is facial weakness, the lips must be held around the mouthpiece. If the FVC is falling fast, it must be measured every hour, the patient intubated (orally or transnasally) when it reaches 1000 cm^3 and preparations made to ventilate if it drops any further. If the FVC is drifting slowly downwards, it should be measured every few hours and tracheal intubation can perhaps wait until the FVC is a little less than 1000 cm^3 (approximately equivalent to 15 cm^3 per kg body weight). Tracheostomy is necessary if ventilation is required for more than a few days; sedation, except perhaps at night, is seldom necessary if the nursing and medical care is sympathetic.

Note: Monitoring the peak flow or blood gases is *no* substitute for the FVC in respiratory neuromuscular weakness.

In severe cases it is wise to monitor continuously the heart rhythm, rate and blood pressure so that autonomic instability can be detected early and treated on its merits.

No medical treatment is needed for the mild acute case which stabilizes in a week or two. However, for a severe case with rapidly increasing paralysis and incipient or actual respiratory failure, plasma exchange will hasten recovery. The usual regimen is to remove 50 ml per kg of plasma once a day, or on alternate days, on about five occasions. The replacement fluid is 5% albumin and normal saline (50/50 ratio), although it is still somewhat unclear what the best replacement fluid is; variations in practice, which may have an effect on efficacy, include fresh frozen or stored plasma and purified protein fraction. An alternative is infusions of human immunoglobulin; 0.4 g/kg/day for 5 days.

Complications of plasma exchange are unusual but include:
• chills, skin rash, fever
• volume overload or depletion
• infection (hepatitis, AIDS)
• hypoproteinaemia
• septicaemia
• hypocoagulability

For the patient who slowly becomes worse over several weeks (i.e. chronic inflammatory demyelinating polyneuropathy), corticosteroids often induce remission and can be slowly tailed off as the patient recovers (starting dose 80 mg daily, oral, prednisolone). A few patients relapse after steroid withdrawal and some become dependent on steroids. Patients who do not remit on corticosteroids may respond to azathioprine or infusions of human immunoglobulin. Plasma exchange has a limited role in acute relapses.

Useful address

Guillain–Barré Support Group
'Foxley'
Holdingham
Sleaford
Lincs: NG34 8NR
Tel: 0529 304615

Drug-induced neuropathies

These are usually rather rare adverse effects of many different drugs (p. 391). If a patient is on *any* drug and develops a peripheral neuropathy, particularly axonal in type, then the role of that drug should be questioned. It is quite possible of course that the neuropathy is actually due to the disease being treated by the suspect drug. If in doubt, and if possible, the drug should be withdrawn and usually, but not always, the neuropathy recovers if the drug is responsible. Drug-induced neuropathies are more likely if the patient cannot metabolize the drug adequately, e.g. isoniazid neuropathy in slow acetylators and nitrofurantoin neuropathy in renal failure.

Ischaemic neuropathy

Acute ischaemia usually causes infarction of not just nerve but muscle and skin, leading to gangrene and obvious ischaemia of a limb. Occasionally, however, acute temporary limb ischaemia may cause an acute distal painful neuropathy with no other particular features apart perhaps from absent pulses. It occurs as a result of atherothrombosis, embolism or a vascular surgical procedure in the limb.

Migrant sensory neuritis of Wartenberg

The clinical manifestations are sudden and brief superficial pains, often immediately followed by sensory loss, in the distribution of a cutaneous nerve such as the digital, sural, ulnar, terminal radial and patellar plexus. This recovers in a few weeks but relapses and remissions are common in various parts of the body. It tends to be precipitated by stretch of the appropriate nerve (e.g. by kneeling, turning a handle) and can be confused with multiple sclerosis.

Critical illness polyneuropathy

Patients who are severely ill with multiple organ failure and sepsis, and who are usually in intensive care units as a consequence, may develop an insidious polyneuropathy which is recognized when they begin to recover from their underlying illness and are slow to mobilize or difficult to wean from mechanical ventilation. Clinically, it is similar to the Guillain–Barré syndrome (p. 398) but the neuropathy is axonal with normal or mildly reduced motor conduction velocities, and the CSF is normal. Causes such as drugs, toxins, nutritional deficiency and any underlying disease must be excluded. Slow but complete recovery is usual.

Autonomic failure

The autonomic nervous system is concerned with the control of blood pressure, heart rate, sphincters, sweating, lacrimation, the gut, the pupil, and erection and ejaculation in males. The neural pathways may be disrupted anywhere from the brainstem and spinal cord to the peripheral sympathetic and parasympathetic nerves to cause a variety of restricted (e.g. Horner's syndrome, p. 178) or generalized clinical consequences.

Causes of generalized autonomic failure

- central autonomic failure:
  Shy–Drager syndrome (multisystem atrophy, p. 291)
  Parkinson's disease (p. 280)
  acute spinal cord lesion, e.g. trauma, transverse myelitis (p. 322)
  tabes dorsalis (p. 515)
- peripheral autonomic failure:
  drugs which block sympathetic or parasympathetic peripheral transmission, e.g. hypotensive drugs, atropine
  peripheral neuropathies (p. 392)
  epidural anaesthesia (p. 44)
  bilateral lumbar sympathectomy
- idiopathic pure orthostatic hypotension (p. 404)

Clinical features

- Cardiovascular: postural hypotension (p. 102) is by far the most common clinical manifestation and the easiest to measure (usually defined as a fall in systolic blood pressure of at least 30 mmHg or to less than 80 mmHg on, or within a minute or two of, standing up). However, such falls can occur in the normal asymptomatic elderly, cardiac failure, Addison's disease, etc. (*Note*: individuals vary considerably in whether they become symptomatic with postural hypotension.) Impaired heart rate response to respiration, standing, Valsalva manoeuvre, mental arithmetic. Tachycardia at rest. Sometimes paroxysmal hypertension or tachycardia (e.g. in spinal cord injury, Guillain–Barré syndrome, p. 398).

- Bladder: frequency, urgency, retention and incontinence of urine. This is best analysed by cystometrography (p. 30).
- Bowels: constipation, diarrhoea.
- Impotence and/or failure of ejaculation.
- Lacrimation: dry eyes, rarely excessive lacrimation. Quantified by Schirmer's tear test.
- Salivation: dry mouth, occasionally hypersalivation.
- Sweating: usually loss of, but occasionally excessive, sweating (e.g. gustatory facial sweating in diabetics), tested by Quinizarin on the skin which turns blue with sweat or with Alizarin Red which turns red.
- Pupils: Horner's syndrome (p. 178), pupillary dilatation or constriction and impaired pupil light response.
- Impaired control of body temperature is rare.

Diagnosis

The suspicion of autonomic failure is based on the symptoms (usually postural hypotension or sphincter problems) and often on the context (a patient with a peripheral neuropathy). The diagnosis is confirmed by the demonstration of autonomic failure, usually by documenting postural hypotension or impaired beat-to-beat heart rate variation in response to respiration.

The causes of autonomic failure may be an obvious peripheral neuropathy (e.g. diabetes, p. 453), associated central nervous system disorder (e.g. Shy–Drager syndrome, p. 291) or due to drugs. In a few patients there is pure autonomic failure, usually manifest as postural hypotension sometimes with a Holmes–Aidie pupil (p. 178), but no other neurological signs, which is the result of loss of sympathetic neurones in the spinal cord and/or a peripheral autonomic neuropathy.

Treatment

The aims of treatment are to remove the underlying cause of the autonomic failure if possible, and to relieve symptoms of which symptomatic postural hypotension is the most problematic (for treatment of sphincter disturbance, see p. 353).

Conservative measures such as avoiding sudden standing, particularly on waking in the morning, after hot baths, heavy meals; keep feet propped up during the day as far as possible; sleep with the head as propped up as possible and tolerable at night; elasticated stockings; abdominal binder.

Drugs
- fludrocortisone: oral, 0.1 mg daily, increasing to 0.2 mg twice daily as necessary, but this may be limited by peripheral oedema, hypokalaemia, cardiac failure and supine hypertension

- ephedrine: oral, 15 mg 3 times daily, increasing to 60 mg 3 times daily as necessary, but this may be limited by supine hypertension which itself may respond to beta-blockade
- indomethacin: oral, 25–50 mg 3 times daily, but this is seldom effective and may cause headache

Atrial tachypacing may help in patients who do not have a tachycardia on standing up.

15   Myasthenia gravis

Myasthenia gravis is a rare autoimmune disease. The prevalence is about 5/100 000 population; females are affected more often than males, 2:1. It may start at any age and the peak age of onset is 20–30 years with a smaller peak at 50–60 years.

It is caused by circulating IgG antibodies to acetylcholine (ACh) receptors on the postsynaptic membrane of neuromuscular junctions on skeletal muscle which block the action of ACh released from motor nerve terminals. This results in weakness and, the hallmark of the disease, excessive fatiguability relieved by rest.

Clinical features

Muscle weakness and painless excessive fatiguability may start in, or spread to, any group of muscles and can sometimes be remarkably focal. The disease may be mild, with no more than unilateral ptosis, or severe, causing respiratory and bulbar paralysis.

The onset is usually insidious but can sometimes be subacute. The weakness is variable from hour to hour, and day to day, tending to be least on waking and most after physical activity. Exacerbations may occur as a result of emotion, pregnancy, infection, surgery, hyperthyroidism, excessive heat and certain drugs (see p. 410).

Extraocular muscles

These are often involved early and almost always eventually. Binocular diplopia, due to weakness of various combinations of eye muscles, tends to be more obvious in the evening. Occasionally, nystagmus-like jerks are present and also what can look very like an internuclear ophthalmoplegia (p. 180). Ptosis, which is usually bilateral, but can be asymmetrical and even unilateral on occasion, is characteristic; eye lid closure is almost always weak as well. On prolonged upward gaze the ptosis becomes more obvious due to muscle fatigue. The pupil responses are normal (cf. third cranial nerve palsy, p. 182).

Facial weakness

Facial weakness is common and usually bilateral. Weakness of eye lid closure, lip closure and the myasthenic 'snarl' are characteristic.

Bulbar involvement

This causes difficulty chewing and swallowing, usually worse as the meal proceeds, and dysarthria with particular difficulty towards the end of sentences or after talking for a while.

Weakness of neck flexion is common (cf. polymyositis, motor neurone disease, etc., p. 417).

Limb weakness

This tends to be variable, usually bilateral but not always, and is both proximal and distal. The tendon reflexes and sensation are normal. Muscle wasting occurs only rarely in advanced cases. There may be no weakness if the patient is examined after rest, or it can be intermittent during the examination, so making the diagnosis of 'hysteria' a common mistake.

Respiratory and truncal weakness

This occurs in advanced cases leading to respiratory failure and pneumonia.

Associated conditions

About 10% of cases are associated with thymoma and in about 60% there is thymic hyperplasia. Thymoma is rare under the age of 30. Occasionally myasthenia develops after a thymoma has been removed.

Sometimes other autoimmune diseases are present, e.g. hyperthyroidism, thyroiditis, systemic lupus erythematosus, rheumatoid disease.

Lambert–Eaton myasthenic syndrome

This syndrome is very rare. It has many of the features of myasthenia gravis, also being an autoimmune disorder of neuromuscular transmission, but at the presynaptic level. There are no circulating anti-ACh receptor antibodies. The age of onset is rather later than myasthenia gravis with a peak at 50–60 years, and if anything males are more often affected than females. Presentation is usually with leg weakness (proximal more than distal) and this affects almost all patients eventually. Often the weakness is *improved* temporarily after a short muscular contraction but excessive fatiguability follows. Aching in the limbs is common. The tendon reflexes are depressed but increase after exercise of the relevant muscles. Extraocular muscle and bulbar weakness are unusual although mild ptosis is quite common. Autonomic features are common: dry mouth, impotence, constipation, impaired sweating, dry eyes, etc.

There is a specific association with small cell carcinoma of the lung in 60% of cases, the neurological symptoms typically preceding the diagnosis of cancer by 1–2 years, occasionally 5. There may be a personal or family history of organ-specific autoimmune disease.

Neonatal myasthenia

This occurs in about 10% of children born to myasthenic mothers. It is due to placental transfer of circulating maternal anti-ACh receptor antibodies. The baby is floppy, sucks poorly, has a weak cry and may need ventilatory support but recovers in a few weeks.

Congenital myasthenia

Congenital myasthenia is a rare group of heterogeneous disorders which develops in infancy with extraocular muscle weakness. Relatively mild generalized weakness follows some years later. There are no anti-ACh receptor antibodies and there is a poor response to immunosuppression.

Note: Certain drugs exacerbate myasthenia in some patients, therefore caution should be exercised:
- neuromuscular blocking drugs used in general anaesthesia may cause severe weakness for several days, so the patient cannot be taken off the ventilator at the end of the anaesthetic
- aminoglycosides, polymyxins, tetracyclines, ampicillin, lincomycin, clindamycin, erythromycin
- membrane stabilizers, e.g. quinine, quinidine, procainamide, lignocaine, phenytoin, and perhaps beta-blockers
- lithium
- chlorpromazine
- CNS depressants, e.g. morphine, barbiturates
- timolol eye drops
- intravenous iodinated contrast agents
- enemas may cause sudden deterioration and even death
    Some drugs actually *cause* a myasthenia-like syndrome which remits after the drug is withdrawn, e.g. penicillamine, beta-blockers very rarely.

Diagnosis

The diagnosis is not difficult once it is considered. Unfortunately the average time from clinical onset to diagnosis is 2 years and the usual problems are the mistaken diagnosis of:
- hysteria, if there is only limb weakness or 'fatigue' (p. 38)
- motor neurone disease if there is mostly bulbar weakness (Chapter 13)
- ocular muscular dystrophy if there is only ocular weakness (p. 424)
    It is important to emphasize that in myasthenia there is no muscle wasting (except late) and the reflexes, tone and sensation are normal; indeed, there is often no weakness at all unless the patient exerts the affected muscle.

'Tensilon' test

Edrophonium (Tensilon) is an anticholinesterase which, when given i.v., prolongs the action of ACh at the neuromuscular junction for a few minutes.

A test dose of 2 mg is given and, if after 30 seconds all is well, followed up with 8 mg. Within 30–60 seconds there should be an *obvious* improvement in the power of weak muscles which wears off in another minute or two. It is best to test at least two weak muscle groups since the response can be different. In a very sick patient it is essential to test bulbar and respiratory muscles (the latter by vital capacity), which are the most important for vital functions. If there is any possibility of the response being exaggerated by an hysterical patient (or optimistic doctor), the test should be conducted double-blind with saline control.

In an untreated patient this test can be used for diagnosis in the outpatient clinic, with the patient lying supine, *provided* an assistant and full resuscitation facilities are available. Occasionally, bradycardia and hypotension occur but can be reversed by atropine (0.6 mg i.v.), and probably avoided altogether if this is given before the Tensilon. Other muscarinic adverse effects are common but trivial: lacrimation, salivation, sweating, small pupils, and pallor; vomiting is unusual. Fasciculation of eye lid muscles and facial flushing can occur.

In the Lambert–Eaton syndrome the test is not necessarily positive. Also, it may be equivocal in polymyositis (p. 435) and motor neurone disease (Chapter 13).

EMG

EMG is often helpful but can be misleading if the patient is taking anticholinesterases. Muscles, which are not necessarily weak, show a decremental response in the evoked compound muscle action potential during repetitive motor nerve stimulation. In the Lambert–Eaton syndrome there is an *incremental* response, which can also be seen after a sustained voluntary contraction. In both there is increased 'jitter' on single fibre EMG.

Anti-acetylcholine receptor (AChR) antibodies

These antibodies (>0.5 nanomoles/l), provide the best diagnostic test and are found in the serum of more than 85% of myasthenic patients and are almost specific to this disease. To some extent their level correlates with clinical severity. Patients with clinical myasthenia gravis and persistently negative antibodies tend to have mild or early disease or ocular muscle weakness only, or they may have congenital myasthenia (p. 410) or the Lambert–Eaton syndrome (p. 409).

AChR antibodies without overt myasthenia are occasionally detected in first degree relatives of myasthenia gravis patients; non-myasthenic thymoma patients; during penicillamine treatment and in patients with other organ-specific antibodies, particularly thyroid. A low titre may occur in motor neurone disease (p. 362).

Other serum antibodies may also be found, particularly directed against skeletal muscle when a thymoma is present. Sometimes there is a raised titre of antinuclear factor, antithyroid and antigastric antibodies.

Chest X-ray and mediastinal tomography

These, or better a CT scan, should be performed to search for a thymoma.

Treatment

Myasthenia gravis occasionally remits spontaneously for months or years but usually there is permanent and often progressive disability. There are two aims in treatment: to support the patient and to induce remission.

Patient support

In very weak patients nursing care, physiotherapy and sometimes mechanical ventilation are important. Muscle strength can be improved with oral anti-cholinesterases but seldom to normal. In the late stages weak and wasted muscles become unresponsive to medication.

Pyridostigmine

Pyridostigmine has a 2–8 hour action and can be started in an oral dose of 30 mg 4-hourly, working up to 120 mg 3-hourly, depending on the patient's requirements.

Neostigmine

This has a quicker onset but only a 2–6 hour duration of action. It is started at 7.5 mg 3 times daily, oral, and worked up to 45 mg 2-hourly as necessary.

If the patient cannot swallow, these drugs should be given by nasogastric tube, although neostigmine can be given i.m. (1 mg i.m. equivalent to 15 mg oral).

Anticholinesterases tend to cause intestinal colic, increased salivation, nausea, diarrhoea and belching. If necessary, oral atropine (0.6 mg twice or 3 times daily) will reduce these muscarinic adverse effects. Particular caution is needed in patients with cardiac conduction problems or a recent myocardial infarction because of occasional bradycardia and hypotension.

Too much anticholinesterase will result in 'cholinergic crisis' when the patient becomes weak due to cholinergic block at the neuromuscular junction. This may affect some muscle groups and not others in an unpredictable way. In cases of doubt, particularly in a very sick patient, all anticholinesterases should be stopped and, if necessary, the patient ventilated for a few days before reintroducing them. Alternatively, a 'Tensilon' test is done (but only 2 mg i.v.) as an inpatient with ventilation facilities to hand; a patient in 'cholinergic' crisis will temporarily worsen, whereas if the weakness is due to the myasthenia and too little anticholinesterase the patient should improve. In crises like this it is *essential* to monitor the vital capacity since the respiratory muscles may be in 'cholinergic' block when other muscles are still responding to anticholinesterases.

Plasma exchange

Plasma exchange often produces a fairly quick (within days) but temporary improvement in a very weak patient while more permanent measures are being organized. The usual regimen is to replace 50 ml per kg body weight of plasma daily for 5 days with a mixture of 50% plasma protein fraction and 50% dextrose/saline. Possible adverse effects include septicaemia from catheter infection (see also p. 401).

Induction of remission

In mild cases, particularly those confined to the eye muscles, only anticholinesterases are necessary, although prolonged use over many years may perhaps damage the neuromuscular junction and make weakness worse. For more severe cases there are three options:

Thymectomy

This is usually the first step for those with onset under the age of 45. A sternal split allows all the thymus, and any aberrant thymic tissue, to be removed. About 70% of patients improve or remit in 6–12 months. Improvement is most likely in young patients, those with a short history, and those with thymic hyperplasia. Patients with thymomas are less likely to improve but thymectomy usually has to be performed in any case to reduce the risk of local malignant spread.

Corticosteroids

Corticosteroids may induce remission in a matter of weeks or months. They are helpful in the elderly, those with mild disease, patients who are too sick for thymectomy, if thymectomy fails, and following thymectomy to induce remission while that induced by the thymectomy is taking time to develop. Patients should be admitted to hospital because there is often an increase in weakness for a few days after starting at a dose of 100 mg on alternate days. To avoid this, treatment can start in out-patients with 10 mg on alternate days building up at the rate of 10 mg per week to the full dose. Once in remission, and this may take some months to become maximal, the dose can be slowly reduced (by 5 mg per month) until a maintenance dose is achieved (usually 20–40 mg on alternate days). The alternate day regime can be both effective and remarkably free of adverse effects. However, sometimes a high daily dose is necessary in which case the adverse effects may be severe. Eventually it is occasionally possible to stop treatment altogether.

Azathioprine

Azathioprine is used in combination with, or instead of, corticosteroids. In combination, the prednisolone can often be slowly reduced and perhaps even stopped. This drug may take up to 12 months to have any effect and the usual dose is 50 mg per day building up in 3 weeks to 2.5 mg/kg/day with regular checks on the white cell count, platelet count and liver function. Adverse effects are quite often a problem: acutely — abdominal pain, vomiting, diarrhoea, rash; longer term — thrombocytopenia, leucopenia, infections, hepatitis and possibly lymphoma. The risk of fetal abnormality is small.

Cyclophosphamide, cyclosporin and intravenous gammaglobulin may have some useful effect.

The Lambert–Eaton myasthenic syndrome

This responds poorly, or not at all, to anticholinesterases. However, the neuromuscular block can to some extent be diminished by:
- 3–4 diaminopyridine: 30–100 mg, oral, daily in 2–4 divided doses. Adverse effects: paraesthesia, seizures (available from the Pharmacy, Radcliffe Infirmary, Oxford OX2 6HE).
- guanidine: 20–50 mg/kg/day oral in 3 divided doses. Adverse effects: liver, marrow, renal failure.

These drugs may potentate the effects of the anticholinesterases.

Apart from thymectomy, which is ineffective, the same treatment regimen used in myasthenia gravis can induce remission in some non-cancer cases, and plasma exchange may provide short-term benefit. Survival in the cancer-associated cases is very poor, so that treatment of the myasthenic syndrome may have little to offer unless the patient is likely to survive 6 months or more.

Measuring the effect of treatment in myasthenia is best done clinically, rather than by measuring anti-ACh receptor antibodies which do not accurately reflect the clinical state. There are no particular scales, so bedside tests of muscle strength and endurance (arm elevations and squats), vital capacity, speaking, swallowing and walking are probably best.

Useful address

British Association of Myasthenics
Keynes House
Central Office
77 Nottingham Road
Derby DE1 3QS
Tel: 0332-290219

16 Muscle disorders (myopathies)

A myopathy is any structural, electrical or biochemical disorder in voluntary muscle fibres or interstitial tissue.

Clinical features and diagnosis

Weakness is usually proximal rather than distal and is more or less symmetrical. The age of onset and rate of progression of weakness are important clues to the diagnosis.

Neonates present with floppiness and feeding difficulties. Causes of hypotonia in neonates who are otherwise well and alert include:

- mental retardation
- spinal cord:
  injury
  spinal muscular atrophy (p. 358)
  tumours (p. 321)
  myelodysplasia
  paralytic polio (p. 522)
- neonatal myasthenia (p. 410)
- myopathies:
  neonatal myotonic dystrophy (p. 425)
  congenital muscular dystrophy (p. 424)
  acid maltase deficiency (p. 427)
  specific congenital myopathies (p. 426)

Motor milestones may be delayed and typically a child has difficulty standing up from sitting on the floor.

In adults, the usual difficulties are lifting the arms above the head to comb the hair or hang out washing due to shoulder girdle weakness, and climbing stairs, getting on buses and trains, and getting out of a chair due to pelvic musculature weakness. The gait may be 'waddling' and unexpected falls occur due to quadriceps weakness. Muscle power in the lower limbs must be tested by standing and squatting as well as on the bed.

Wasting usually occurs in the progressively weakening muscles. Selective wasting of individual muscles suggests a muscular dystrophy.

Distal weakness and wasting occur in:
- myotonic dystrophy quite commonly (p. 424)
- distal muscular dystrophy (p. 424)
- inclusion body myositis (p. 436)
- myasthenia gravis, but very rarely (Chapter 15)

The *facial and ocular muscles* are often affected early in:
- myotonic dystrophy (p. 424)

* ocular dystrophies (p. 424)
* facioscapulohumeral dystrophy (p. 423)
* mitochondrial cytopathies (p. 429)
* myasthenia gravis (Chapter 15)

Weakness of neck flexion tends to be particularly prominent in:
* polymyositis (p. 434)
* myasthenia gravis (Chapter 15)
* myotonic dystrophy
* acid maltase deficiency (p. 427)
* motor neurone disease (Chapter 13)

Respiratory failure may be a prominent feature of:
* acid maltase deficiency (p. 427)
* polymyositis (p. 434)
* myasthenia gravis (Chapter 15)
* nemaline myopathy (p. 427)
* motor neurone disease (Chapter 13), Guillain–Barré syndrome

In neuromuscular respiratory failure the respiratory rate may be raised and the accessory muscles in use, breathlessness is not always present, the diaphragm may be weak, the vital capacity reduced and eventually blood gases are disturbed. Diaphragmatic weakness is particularly likely to cause orthopnoea, paradoxical abdominal wall motion (inward rather than the normal outward movement on inspiration), a marked fall in vital capacity on lying down and therefore respiratory failure at night, and consequent headache on wakening.

Intermittent paralysis occurs in:
* hypokalaemic periodic paralysis (p. 431)
* hyperkalaemic periodic paralysis (p. 432)
* hyperthyroidism (p. 437)

Differential diagnosis of intermittent weakness includes myasthenia gravis (Chapter 15) and porphyria (p. 398).

Muscle pseudo-hypertrophy with normal or reduced strength occurs in:
* Duchenne dystrophy (p. 422)
* Becker dystrophy (p. 423)
* myotonia congenita (p. 425)
* peripheral neuropathies very rarely (p. 389)

Muscle pain at rest may occur in:
* inflammatory myopathies (the muscles may also be tender) (p. 433)
* metabolic bone disease myopathies (p. 438)
* acute myoglobinuric myopathies (p. 432)
* some drug-induced myopathies (p. 439)

- myxoedematous myopathy (p. 438)
- Addison's disease (p. 455)
- Cushing's syndrome (p. 455)
- polymyalgia rheumatica (p. 451)

The differential diagnosis is of neuropathic pain (p. 393), arthritis, skeletal pain, nerve root pain (p. 319), sickle cell crisis (p. 460), parkinsonism (p. 280) and cramp (p. 418).

Pain during or after exercise of a particular muscle tends to occur in polymyositis (p. 434) and myopathies due to a defect in energy metabolism:

- myophosphorylase deficiency (McArdle's disease) (p. 428)
- phosphofructokinase deficiency (p. 428)
- carnitine palmityl transferase deficiency (p. 429)
- myoadenylate deficiency (p. 429)

Differential diagnosis includes muscle claudication and claudication of the cauda equina (p. 328).

Myotonia, i.e. delayed relaxation after cessation of voluntary effort, occurs in:

- myotonic dystrophy (p. 424)
- myotonia congenita (p. 425)
- paramyotonia congenita (p. 426)
- hyperkalaemic periodic paralysis (p. 432)

Usually it is painless. The patient may not notice anything or may complain that the muscles are stiff, that there is difficulty walking and manipulating objects. To demonstrate myotonia the patient is asked to grip the examiner's hand tightly and then relax quickly, or an affected muscle is tapped sharply with a tendon hammer and the slow relaxation is observed; often a dimple appears and subsides in a few seconds. Myotonia of the tongue can be tested by tapping it against a spatula held over the lower teeth.

Myotonia tends to be worse in cold weather and less obvious after repeated use of the muscle. The EMG is characteristic (p. 58).

Tendon reflexes are usually preserved until the relevant muscle is very weak and wasted. In the dystrophies, however, the reflexes tend to be depressed or absent as soon as a muscle is weak.

Cramps are sudden powerful, involuntary, and painful muscle contractions which last from seconds to minutes, occasionally longer. The cramped muscle is electrically active. Cramp should be distinguished from dystonia (p. 302), tetany, and muscle pain or stiffness at rest (p. 417). It can be caused by:

- unaccustomed exertion
- dehydration and sodium depletion
- hypomagnesaemia (p. 465)
- renal failure (p. 466)
- renal dialysis (p. 467)
- Addison's disease (p. 455)

- hypothyroid myopathy (p. 437)
- hypocalcaemic (p. 457)
- motor neurone disease (Chapter 13)
- tetanus (p. 518)
- stiff man syndrome (p. 439)
- Ehlers–Danlos syndrome (p. 484)
- drugs:
    bumetanide
    cimetadine
    danazol
    lithium
    metolazone
    phenothiazines
    salbutamol
    vincristine

The usual treatment is quinine sulphate: 125–300 mg at bedtime or up to 3 times daily. Adverse effects (p. 535). Nifedipine is a possible alternative.

Family history. It is particularly important to document inherited conditions. Enquiries should be made about parental consanguinity. It may be relevant to examine relatives even if they are said to be unaffected.

Past medical history. It is important to note developmental milestones, sporting abilities at school, etc.

Drug exposure. A careful history of exposure to drugs and toxins is essential.

Investigations

Unless the cause is obvious the screening tests should include:
- full blood count
- erythrocyte sedimentation rate
- blood urea, electrolytes and glucose
- liver function
- blood calcium, phosphate and alkaline phosphatase
- thyroid function
- serum proteins and electrophoresis
- urine examination
- chest X-ray
- ECG
- urine myoglobin
- plasma lactate

and, if further indicated:
- organ specific antibodies
- antinuclear factor

- plasma cortisol
- faecal occult blood (? cancer)
- mammography (? cancer)
- acetylcholine receptor antibodies (? myasthenia gravis)

Muscle enzymes

These leak from damaged muscle fibres. There may be elevation of serum aldolase, AST and LDH, but the most useful is the creatine kinase level (CK). The normal resting CK level is <200 iu/l.

There is a *marked* elevation of CK (1000–10 000 iu/l) in:
- Duchenne dystrophy (early stages) (p. 422)
- Becker dystrophy (early stages) (p. 423)
- inflammatory myopathies (p. 433)
- acute myoglobinuric myopathies (p. 432)

There is moderate elevation of CK (200–1000 iu/l) in most other myopathies. However, it may be normal.

Note: The CK can be elevated under other circumstances:
- occasionally in spinal muscular atrophy (p. 358)
- occasionally in motor neurone disease (p. 362)
- sometimes after vigorous exercise
- intramuscular injection, particularly with irritant drugs, e.g. chloroquine, chlorpromazine, diazepam, digoxin, lignocaine, opiates, paraldehyde
- after EMG needling
- after tonic-clonic seizures (p. 82)
- after muscle biopsy
- acute myocardial infarction

CK levels tend to fall during pregnancy.

EMG

EMG and nerve conduction studies help differentiate muscle weakness due to denervation, myasthenia and myopathy. However, the EMG can be normal even when there is obvious wasting and weakness, presumably because myopathic processes can spare many muscle fibres in a clinically affected muscle.

In myopathies the motor unit action potentials are polyphasic and reduced in amplitude and duration. At rest the muscle is electrically silent except in polymyositis. Nerve conduction is normal (see also p. 58).

Muscle biopsy

Muscle biopsy is often helpful. It is best to sample a moderately weak muscle, but not one which has been previously sampled with an EMG needle, usually the deltoid or quadriceps in practice. The biopsy may be open (under local or rarely general anaesthesia), with the advantage of a large sample but the disadvantage of a scar, and it cannot be repeated often. Needle biopsy under local anaesthesia can be repeated, is quick, and several sites can be sampled, but the samples are small and may be distorted and difficult to orientate. In all cases the pathologist should be consulted and will usually be present at the time of biopsy to ensure that tissue is collected correctly and put into the appropriate fixatives. The biopsied muscle should be examined by routine histology (haematoxylin and eosin, fat stains, glycogen stains, etc.), histochemistry, and sometimes electronmicroscopy and biochemical analysis. It may be normal if the myopathy is patchy in distribution, in the periodic paralyses, and in several metabolic myopathies.

In the dystrophies the muscle fibres are different sizes and shapes with fibre splitting, regeneration and central nuclei. The muscle fibres become necrotic and are replaced by fatty and then fibrous tissue. In denervation due to a primary neural disease (e.g. motor neurone disease, neuropathies) there is atrophy of groups of fibres supplied by a single motor unit (neurogenic changes).

Unless it is absolutely certain what the diagnosis is clinically, a muscle biopsy must be done to avoid the mistake of leaving a treatable myopathy diagnosed as an untreatable 'dystrophy'.

Ischaemic lactate test

This test is undertaken if a deficiency of one of the glycolytic enzymes is suspected, e.g. myophosphorylase (p. 428), phosphofructokinase (p. 428), debranching enzyme (p. 428).

Antecubital venous blood is taken for lactate level which in the normal resting state should be 0.5–1.5 mmol/l. Then a sphygmomanometer cuff is inflated around the upper arm to occlude arterial blood flow. The hand is exercised by gripping an object intermittently until limited by pain, usually approximately one minute. If muscle cannot degrade glycogen to lactic acid, there is no rise in the venous lactate taken from the ipsilateral antecubital fossa. Blood should be taken 30 seconds, 1, 2 and 4 minutes after cuff release to allow any lactate formed in the exercising arm muscle to reach the venous sampling site. The normal rise in level is 3–5 times. Within about 25 minutes the lactate levels should have returned to normal. Muscle lactate may also fail to rise in hypothyroid (p. 438) and alcoholic (p. 544) myopathy.

Exercise lactate test

An abnormal rise (to >10 mmol/l) after aerobic exercise on a bicycle to double the resting heart rate for 15 minutes suggests a mitochondrial cytopathy (p. 429).

Nuclear magnetic resonance

Nuclear magnetic resonance of forearm muscles shows characteristic features in McArdle's disease (p. 428). Measurement can be made non-invasively of muscle pH, phosphocreatine, ATP, ADP and inorganic phosphate.

Note: In patients with progressive proximal muscle weakness, a normal or mildly elevated CK, and a normal or non-specifically abnormal muscle biopsy without any evidence of denervation one must consider:
- metabolic myopathy (particularly acid maltase deficiency, mitochondrial cytopathy, p. 427)
- endocrine myopathy or metabolic bone disease (p. 437)
- drug or toxin induced myopathy (p. 439)
- chronic polymyositis (p. 434)
- limb girdle dystrophy (p. 423)
- myasthenia gravis/Lambert–Eaton syndrome (Chapter 15)

Muscular dystrophies

These are inherited disorders characterized by muscle fibre degeneration. The course is progressive. Since there is no treatment, it is essential to consider other muscle disorders which can masquerade as dystrophies, particularly if there is no family history (i.e. if the 'dystrophy' appears to be recessive or sporadic). All patients should have muscle biopsy, EMG and muscle enzyme levels.

The differential diagnosis includes:
- chronic polymyositis (p. 434)
- metabolic bone disease (p. 438)
- congenital myopathies (p. 426)
- hyperthyroid myopathy (p. 436)
- metabolic myopathies (p. 427)
- motor neurone disease (Chapter 13)
- spinal muscular atrophy (p. 358)
- disease of the hip joints

In dystrophies the muscle wasting and weakness have a characteristic pattern, the tendon reflexes associated with weak muscles are depressed, there is no sensory loss and no fasciculation.

Duchenne muscular dystrophy

This is the most common dystrophy but is still a rare disease; 30/100 000 live male births. It is X-linked recessive, the abnormal gene is located at the Xp21 region of the X-chromosome, and the missing gene product is a muscle protein named 'dystrophin'. It occurs mainly in boys, and very rarely in girls due to autosomal translocation or if there is only one X-chromosome (e.g. Turner's syndrome). About a third of cases are new mutations; their mothers are not carriers.

The symptoms start as the child is learning to walk. There is delay in walking, frequent falls, difficulty standing from sitting on the floor and a waddling gait due to pelvic muscle weakness. Enlarged but weak calf muscles are characteristic (pseudo-hypertrophy); this is due to excess fat and connective tissue plus large but ineffective muscle fibres. Eventually the weakness spreads to all muscle groups with development of muscle contractures and thoracic deformities. The boys are in wheelchairs by adolescence and usually dead by the age of 20.

There is always a cardiomyopathy and non-progressive mental retardation is common. Smooth muscle can be affected, causing paralytic ileus, gastric dilatation and atony of the bladder wall.

Genetic counselling is important for all families with an affected male. In female carriers there may be some mild muscle weakness and the CK level is raised in about 70%; however, DNA analysis is now more accurate. Prenatal diagnosis is possible, but not perfect, by DNA analysis of chorion villus biopsy material.

Becker muscular dystrophy

This is very similar to the Duchenne type but starts rather later (about the age of 10), is more benign, and cardiac and intellectual involvement is rare. It is also sex-linked recessive and is due to low levels, or abnormality of, muscle dystrophin.

Limb-girdle dystrophy

This type is autosomal recessive in both sexes and is very rare; about 7/100 000 live births. Weakness of the pelvic, thigh and shoulder girdle muscles appears at about the age of 20 and progresses slowly to death at about the age of 50. The intellect is normal, cranial muscles are spared, and the heart is seldom involved. It is clinically more or less indistinguishable from chronic spinal muscular atrophy (p. 358) and is often confused with acid maltase deficiency (p. 427), chronic polymyositis (p. 434) and even myasthenia gravis (Chapter 15). Muscle biopsy is always required along with appropriate biochemical tests and exclusion of endocrine and drug-induced myopathies.

Facioscapulohumeral dystrophy

This is autosomal dominant in either sex and is relatively benign. Weakness of the shoulder girdle muscles is noticed at about the age of 20 and is followed by weakness of the face and pelvic girdle. Anterior tibial muscles may be affected early.

Scapuloperoneal dystrophy

Scapuloperoneal dystrophy is autosomal dominant or X-linked recessive. Anterior tibial and peroneal muscle weakness starts at about the age of 20 and the course is benign. Scapular and other proximal limb muscle involvement occurs eventually.

Ocular and oculopharyngeal dystrophies

Various types have been described, the simplest of which is merely mild extraocular weakness with ptosis. Usually there is no significant diplopia. In addition, dysphagia, facial, sternomastoid and limb muscle weakness sometimes occurs. The onset is at any age and some cases show dominant inheritance. The main differential diagnoses are myasthenia gravis (Chapter 15) and mitochondrial cytopathies (p. 429).

Distal muscular dystrophy

Distal muscular dystrophy (of Wellander) is extremely rare in the UK. It is autosomal dominant, with onset in middle age of weakness and wasting of the small muscles of the hand. It is benign but there is some spread of weakness to the arms and lower legs.

Congenital muscular dystrophy

This is present at birth and seldom progresses. It is recessive and the baby may be only hypotonic or, at worst, severely weak.

Useful address

Muscular Dystrophy Association
Nattrass House
35 Macaulay Road
London SW4 0QP
Tel: 071-720-8055

Myotonic disorders

Myotonic dystrophy

Myotonic dystrophy (dystrophia myotonica) is an autosomal dominant disorder affecting several organs as well as muscle. It occurs in about 14/100 000 live births. It starts in young adult life, is slowly progressive, and is of very variable severity; there is no stereotype.

Clinical features

- Distal weakness and wasting in the limbs (particularly of the hands) with myotonia of affected muscles. Falls and difficulty walking are common.
- Weakness and wasting of facial, jaw, temporalis and sternomastoid muscles.
- Dysarthria due to myotonia of the tongue and facial weakness.
- Dysphagia due to oropharyngeal involvement.
- Ptosis and, occasionally, extraocular muscle weakness.
- Frontal baldness.
- Cataracts.
- Cardiac conduction defects which are rarely symptomatic, asymptomatic mitral leaflet prolapse, and occasionally cardiac failure.
- Gonadal atrophy, impotence, loss of libido.
- Mental apathy, low intellect and perhaps progressive dementia. The patients may lack insight into their condition and genetic counselling may be ignored.
- Somnolence (usually due to obstructive sleep apnoea, p. 116).
- Pulmonary hypoventilation.
- Endocrine abnormalities; hypothyroidism, impaired glucose tolerance.
- Obstetric complications.
- Serum IgG reduced.
- Skull hyperostosis, small pituitary fossa.
- Malignant hyperpyrexia (p. 430).

Note: These patients tend to tolerate general anaesthetics badly.

The EMG is characteristic (p. 58) and, if the clinical picture is typical, muscle biopsy is unnecessary.

Usually the myotonia itself is not a serious enough problem to require any treatment (see below). Referral for genetic counselling and DNA storage is important.

Neonatal myotonia

This may occur in children born to myotonic mothers, seldom to myotonic fathers. The infant is floppy with facial weakness, feeding and respiratory difficulties but has no myotonia. Often this weakness improves during childhood only to deteriorate as an adult.

Myotonia congenita

This type presents in infancy (autosomal dominant, Thomsen's disease) or childhood (autosomal recessive, Becker type), with generalized myotonia which is very obviously worse in the cold and relieved by warmth or exercise. There is often diffuse muscle hypertrophy and little if any weakness.

Paramyotonia congenita

This is autosomal dominant with attacks of myotonia and flaccid weakness. These are usually precipitated by cold but also by hyperkalaemia and beta-blockers. The myotonia is relieved by hypokalaemia or acetazolamide. There is overlap with the periodic paralyses (p. 431) since in some patients the weakness is associated with hyper- or hypokalaemia.

Chondrodystrophic myotonia

Chondrodystrophic myotonia is a rare recessive condition with myotonia, skeletal deformities and short stature.

Treatment of myotonia

- procainamide 250–500 mg 4 times daily, oral
- phenytoin 100–200 mg twice daily, oral (adverse effects, p. 88)
- disopyramide 100–200 mg 3 times daily, oral
  These drugs may worsen any cardiac condition defect that is already present and also cause cardiac failure. Procainamide may cause nausea, diarrhoea, skin rash, confusion, an SLE-like syndrome and agranulocytosis. Disopyramide has anticholinergic adverse effects.
- nifedipine 10–20 mg 3 times daily, oral, may help and does not affect cardiac conduction
- sometimes a short course of prednisolone is helpful in particularly severe cases

Note: Some drugs may cause or exacerbate myotonia:
- 20, 25 diazacholesterol (lipid lowering agent)
- triparanol (lipid lowering agent)
- beta-blockers
- depolarizing muscle relaxants (e.g. succinylcholine)

Any improvement in myotonia is not necessarily of functional benefit since many patients' muscular problems are more to do with weakness than myotonia.

Specific congenital myopathies with structural changes in the muscle fibres

These rare disorders usually present in infancy with hypotonia, proximal muscle weakness and delayed physical milestones. The diagnosis depends on the muscle biopsy and the conditions vary in severity.

Central core disease

Muscle fibres have central cores of tightly packed myofilaments and are lacking in oxidative enzymes. It is autosomal dominant. There is a susceptibility to malignant hyperpyrexia (p. 430). It tends to be mild and non-progressive. Skeletal deformities and muscle contractures are common.

Nemaline myopathy

Autosomal dominant. Muscle fibres contain small rod-shaped bodies. Often there are skeletal anomalies such as scoliosis, high arched palate and arachnodactyly. The tendon reflexes are depressed.

Centronuclear myopathy

Chains of central nuclei occur in muscle fibres. This affects eye muscles as well as face, limb and trunk muscles.

Fibre-type disproportion

The type I fibres are small.

Rigid spine syndrome

This is rare, usually in males, starts in childhood and has a rather benign course. There is mild muscle weakness but marked limitation of spinal flexion, scoliosis and joint contractures.

Metabolic myopathies

These are rare inherited myopathies in which the biochemical disorder has frequently been identified. The diagnosis depends on histochemistry or biochemical assay of muscle biopsy material.

Disorders of glycogen metabolism

Acid maltase deficiency

This is autosomal recessive. It results in impaired lysosomal conversion of glycogen to glucose so that glycogen accumulates in the liver, heart, central nervous system and muscle. Death occurs in infancy. In adolescents and adults a milder form exists which presents with slowly progressive weakness and wasting of proximal limb, trunk and respiratory muscles, particularly the diaphragm. It may not come to medical attention until the onset of respiratory failure. CK levels are slightly raised and the EMG is non-specifically myopathic. The muscle biopsy features are not always specific and the diagnosis must be made by enzyme assay in muscle or cultured skin fibroblasts.

Myophosphorylase deficiency (McArdle's disease)

This results in impaired conversion of glycogen to glucose-1-phosphate in muscle. It is autosomal recessive but males are affected more than females (4:1).

It starts in children or adolescents with fatigue, weakness, stiffness and muscle pain induced by exercise and relieved by rest. Usually it is not progressive and there is no wasting. Vigorous exercise may cause an electrically silent and painful contracture in the exercised muscle (cf. cramp, p. 418).

The CK level is raised after exercise and occasionally there is myoglobinuria. Venous lactate levels do not rise after ischaemic forearm exercise, and muscle histochemistry or biochemistry reveals the enzymatic defect.

Phosphofructokinase deficiency

This deficiency results in impaired conversion of fructose-6-phosphate to fructose-1,6-diphosphate in muscle and consequently a failure of venous lactate to rise after ischaemic exercise. It is autosomal recessive and clinically similar to myophosphorylase deficiency. Sometimes there is a mild haemolytic tendency.

Debranching enzyme system deficiency

This results in impaired hydrolysis of glycogen to glucose-1-phosphate. It is autosomal recessive. Patients usually present in infancy with growth retardation, fasting hypoglycaemia, ketonuria, seizures, hepatomegaly and a mild myopathy. This tends to improve after puberty so that adults may have only mild weakness of the legs and hands. Cardiomyopathy is a late complication. CK levels are raised, the ischaemic lactate test is positive, and the muscles contain excess glycogen.

Branching enzyme deficiency

This type results in defective synthesis of glycogen. It is autosomal recessive and presents in infancy with hepatosplenomegaly, failure to thrive and sometimes muscle weakness.

Disorders of lipid metabolism

Long chain fatty acids are a major source of muscle energy and are consumed during muscular activity. There are at least two rare but recognized disorders affecting muscle which can be diagnosed by muscle biochemistry:

Muscle carnitine deficiency

Carnitine is involved in the transport of free fatty acids into mitochondria. In *systemic* deficiency there is a low blood level and multi-organ involvement; clinical features include recurrent episodes of metabolic acidosis and encephalopathy, renal failure, hepatic failure, hypoglycaemia, hyperammonaemia and later progressive muscular weakness. In the *myopathic* form the blood level is normal and a myopathy develops in infants or children. Lipids accumulate in muscle which is deficient in carnitine. CK level may be raised.

Carnitine palmityl transferase (CPT) deficiency

This causes impairment of the transport of free fatty acids in to mitochondria. Most patients are male and present with episodes of weakness and muscle pain in adolescence. Following these episodes there is often a raised CK level and sometimes myoglobinuria. The attacks are provoked by sustained exercise, fasting, or a high fat diet.

Biopsy at the time of an attack may show lipid accumulation and little CPT activity.

Myoadenylate deaminase deficiency

This is said to cause weakness and pain during exercise, starting in childhood. CK levels are raised after exercise. However, the enzyme may be absent in many other different conditions without muscle involvement and its absence may, therefore, be of no consequence in the painful myopathies.

Mitochondrial cytopathies

There is an increasing number of syndromes (all rare) which are caused by various biochemical defects in the mitochondrial respiratory chain. The mitochondria are often structurally abnormal on electronmicroscopy. Usually the muscle mitochondria are involved (hence the original name of mitochondrial myopathy), but it is now clear that many other organs can be involved as well (clinically or subclinically). On light microscopy the abnormal muscle mitochondria gives the appearance of 'ragged red fibres' when stained with Gomori's trichrome.

The clinical picture is variable in both extent and severity and the many syndromes described overlap. The onset is usually in childhood or adolescence but can be in middle age. Males and females are affected equally and there may be a family history. At least three clinical varieties exist:

● Progressive external ophthalmoplegia over many years without diplopia. There is almost always ptosis as well as the extraocular muscle weakness (this is the Kearns–Sayre syndrome).

● Myopathic weakness of the limbs, face and neck with prominent fatigue and exercise intolerance (cf. myasthenia gravis, Chapter 15). Sometimes breathlessness occurs as a result of cardiac failure and metabolic lactic acidosis.

● Mitochondrial cytopathy with cerebral features:
  partial and primarily generalized seizures
  stroke-like episodes with hypodensity on CT but not necessarily in any
    specific arterial distribution
  headache with vomiting similar to migraine
  myoclonus
  ataxia
  dementia
  spongy degeneration of the brain
  pyramidal signs
   Other associated features include:
● retinitis pigmentosa
● deafness
● mild mental handicap
● heart block
● short stature
● hypoparathyroidism
● calcification of the basal ganglia on CT

e.g. MELAS syndrome: mitochondrial myopathy, encephalopathy, lactic acidosis and stroke-like episodes

e.g. MERRF syndrome: myoclonic epilepsy with ragged red fibres

The diagnosis is made by finding a raised plasma lactate and/or an excessive rise in response to exercise (p. 421), along with muscle biopsy. The EMG is merely 'myopathic' and CK levels are not necessarily raised.

Malignant hyperpyrexia

This is a serious and often fatal condition which is precipitated by a number of drugs, particularly anaesthetics:

- cyclopropane
- diethylether
- enflurane
- halothane
- ketamine
- methoxyflurane
- monoamine oxidase inhibitors
- succinylcholine
- tricyclic antidepressants

There is a rapid onset of muscular rigidity, rhabdomyolysis, myoglobin-uria, hyperpyrexia, metabolic acidosis, tachycardia, tachypnoea and hyper-kalaemia. CK levels are very high. Clinically it is similar to the neuroleptic malignant syndrome (p. 289).

It is mainly of dominant inheritance and affected individuals may have a subclinical myopathy with mildly raised CK levels. It is essential to screen relatives of patients known to be affected by muscle biopsy; abnormal muscle contracture *in vitro* is induced by caffeine or halothane.

Apart from circulatory and respiratory support, the specific treatment to relieve the muscle rigidity is dantrolene up to 1 mg/kg i.v. repeated every few minutes, to a cumulative maximum of 10 mg/kg.

A similar syndrome occurs in:
- myotonia congenita (p. 425)
- myotonic dystrophy (p. 424)
- Duchenne dystrophy (p. 422)
- central core disease (p. 427)
- osteogenesis imperfecta

The periodic paralyses

These are characterized by attacks of muscular weakness of the limbs and trunk which tend to occur after exercise and may last from minutes to days. Sometimes the weakness is focal in one limb. During the weakness the re-flexes are depressed and the muscles cannot be electrically excited. In some patients permanent muscle weakness eventually develops.

Hypokalaemic periodic paralysis

This is an autosomal dominant condition starting in childhood or adoles-cence. During the attacks the serum potassium usually is low (<3.0 mmol/l) and the urine excretion of potassium also low. Attacks tend to be provoked by a high carbohydrate meal, glucose load, high salt meal and emotion.

Similar attacks can occur in hyperthyroidism (p. 437) and occasionally if there is hypokalaemia from any cause. Normally, however, hypokalaemia causes an enduring flaccid muscular weakness.

Hyperkalaemic periodic paralysis

This is an autosomal dominant condition which usually starts in childhood. In the attacks the serum potassium is often raised (>5.0 mmol/l), as is the urine excretion of potassium and the CK level. Attacks tend to be provoked by cold, fasting, pregnancy and potassium loading.

In some patients there is myotonia, particularly of the eyelids, tongue, thumb and forearm muscles. The condition seems to overlap with paramyotonia congenita (p. 426).

In conditions causing a very high plasma potassium there can be a form of periodic paralysis.

Normokalaemic periodic paralysis

This is an autosomal dominant condition starting in childhood. It is provoked by cold, alcohol and potassium loads.

Myoglobinuric myopathies

Myoglobin is found in muscle and if there is severe and acute muscle injury it is released into the blood (myoglobinaemia) and appears in the urine (myoglobinuria). The urine is coloured brown in severe cases and reacts to benzidine; if there is neither haematuria nor haemoglobinaemia a positive test strongly suggests myoglobinuria. More specific tests are also available.

The muscle enzymes are always raised and the muscles are tender, weak and sometimes swollen. In severe cases acute renal failure occurs.

There are many causes:

metabolic:
- myophosphorylase deficiency (p. 428)
- phosphofructokinase deficiency (p. 428)
- carnitine palmityl transferase deficiency (p. 429)
- neuroleptic malignant syndrome (p. 289)
- malignant hyperpyrexia (p. 421)
- status epilepticus (p. 82)
- excessive exercise
drugs (p. 439)

ischaemia:
- severe burn injury of muscle
- crush injury of muscle
- heat stroke (p. 485)
- sickle cell crisis (p. 460)

inflammatory myopathies, if acute, and fulminating (below)
snake bite (p. 551)

Inflammatory myopathies

Classification

- idiopathic polymyositis/dermatomyositis (p. 434)
- polymyositis/dermatomyositis complicating (p. 434):
  systemic vasculitis (p. 447)
  rheumatoid disease (p. 448)
  systemic lupus erythematosus (p. 444)
  mixed connective tissue disease (p. 447)
  systemic sclerosis (p. 447)
  Sjögren's syndrome (p. 449)
  paraneoplastic syndrome (p. 434)
  hypereosinophilic syndrome (p. 459)
- inclusion body myositis (p. 436)
- viral myositis (p. 436):
  coxsackie (p. 522)
  influenza (p. 526)
  HIV (p. 526)
- parasitic myositis:
  trichinosis (p. 537)
  cysticercosis (p. 538)
- tropical myositis (p. 436)
- sarcoid myositis (p. 437)
- drugs:
  cimetidine
  hydralazine
  L-tryptophan
  penicillamine
  penicillin
  phenytoin (p. 88)
  procainamide
  sulphacetamide
  zidovudine

Polymyositis/dermatomyositis

This is a rare group of autoimmune disorders affecting voluntary muscle at any age and in both sexes; incidence 0.5/100000 population per annum. About 30% of cases have skin involvement (and are called dermatomyositis). Maybe 25% of cases have either an underlying malignancy (usually carcinoma of the bronchus or breast) or a collagen vascular disorder (usually systemic vasculitis, p. 447); however, the association with malignancy has been exaggerated and may be small or non-existent.

Clinical features

The onset is acute with malaise and fever, subacute, or insidious over many months or even years. The cardinal symptom is diffuse muscle weakness which is usually symmetrical and proximal in the limbs. The neck muscles are often weak as well. Distal limb muscles and bulbar muscles are occasionally, and respiratory and extraocular muscles rarely, affected.

In acute but not chronic cases the affected muscles can be painful and tender, particularly with exercise. The reflexes are preserved until weakness is severe and any wasting is late. Contractures occur in chronic cases.

The skin rash is typically an erythematous/violaceous rash around the eyes, cheeks, forehead, upper trunk and extensor surfaces of the limbs. Induration and scaling may occur. Any subcutaneous oedema is usually periorbital but is sometimes widespread. Arthralgia, Raynaud's phenomenon, pulmonary fibrosis and myocarditis are occasional features.

Investigations

In most cases the ESR is raised and in acute cases there may be myoglobinuria. For a secure diagnosis the clinical picture and three specific investigations (muscle enzymes, EMG and muscle biopsy) must be characteristic.

Muscle enzymes, particularly the CK, are usually raised and can be very high. However, in chronic or quiescent cases the CK may well be normal.

EMG is myopathic with fibrillation potentials (p. 58). It can be normal if an uninvolved part of a muscle is sampled.

Muscle biopsy should come from a moderately weak muscle (usually proximal limb) and preferably from a tender area. Characteristically it shows muscle fibre necrosis with chronic inflammatory cells around blood vessels and between muscle fibres, and eventually fibrosis. Intensive inflammatory changes around small arteries affected by fibrinoid necrosis are characteristic of polyarteritis nodosa (p. 447). Because polymyositis affects muscles patchily, biopsy can be normal; if it is, and the patient does not respond to treatment, it should probably be repeated and other causes of proximal myopathies and weakness re-considered (p. 422).

If all these investigations are carried out, it is unlikely that the diagnosis will be confused with:

- chronic spinal muscular atrophy (p. 358)
- limb girdle and other dystrophies (p. 423)
- motor neurone disease (Chapter 13)
- metabolic myopathies (p. 427)
- toxic and drug-induced painful myopathies (p. 439)
- polymyalgia rheumatica (p. 450)

Note: The Tensilon test (p. 410) may sometimes be slightly positive.

Once the diagnosis of polymyositis is made, it is important to consider possible associated conditions (p. 434):

- full blood count; often a mild normochromic, normocytic anaemia
- eosinophil count (? polyarteritis nodosa)
- plasma proteins and electrophoresis (? paraproteinaemia)
- urine analysis (? polyarteritis nodosa, systemic lupus erythematosus)
- ANF, DNA binding (? systemic lupus erythematosus)
- rheumatoid factor (? rheumatoid arthritis)
- chest X-ray (? malignancy)
- mammography (? malignancy)
- faecal occult bloods? (? malignancy)
- Australia antigen (? polyarteritis nodosa)
- renal angiogram (? polyarteritis nodosa) is very seldom helpful, even when polyarteritis nodosa is actually present
- HIV antibodies (? AIDS)

It is not fruitful to pursue extensive and uncomfortable investigations in the search for an underlying malignancy unless there is a clinical clue (e.g. positive faecal occult bloods may lead to barium studies).

Treatment

Prednisolone is usually tried first, 80 mg daily. It can take some weeks before there is any response in muscle weakness or CK, after which the dose should be very slowly (5–10 mg per month) reduced to a maintenance dose of about 20 mg daily depending on any tendency for the weakness or CK to relapse. An alternate day regimen may be possible at that stage in some patients. Complete withdrawal should be tried every year or so and can eventually be successful.

Corticosteroids may need to be continued for years although in children the prognosis is better than in adults.

Often such high doses of prednisolone are needed for so long that adverse effects are problematic; it is particularly important to consider steroid-induced proximal muscle weakness as a cause for 'a lack of response' to treatment. Biopsy can help in the distinction but is not conclusive. If the CK level is normal or near normal, and there is no inflammation on repeat biopsy, then probably steroids should be reduced or stopped and the effect on muscle weakness observed.

Additional means of immunosuppression may be required if corticosteroids are ineffective or adverse effects are intolerable. The following have been suggested: azathioprine (dose, p. 414), methotrexate, cyclophosphamide, cyclosporin, thymectomy and whole body low-dose irradiation. However, data on which to base sensible guidelines about which treatment to use, when, and for how long are profoundly lacking. Plasma exchange may help in the acute situation.

The effect of treatment can be monitored by objective tests of muscle strength (dynamometer if possible), walking time over a standard distance, squats, and to some extent by the ESR and CK levels.

Inclusion body myositis

This is a relatively benign, chronic myopathy which affects distal as well as proximal muscles. Onset is usually over the age 50. CK levels are normal or moderately raised. There are no associated diseases. Muscle fibres contain eosinophilic inclusions and on EM there are tubular filaments in the cytoplasm and nuclei. The response to corticosteroids and immunosuppressive agents is poor.

Viral myositis

General, or occasionally focal, myositis with pain and tenderness, but rarely weakness, can sometimes complicate coxsackie (p. 522), influenza (p. 526), HIV (p. 526) and exceptionally other viral infections. Rhabdomyolysis is extraordinarily unusual. Coxsackie B viruses have a tendency to cause epidemics of focal myositis affecting the chest, back, abdominal and shoulder muscles (Bornholm disease). The CK may be raised. Recovery takes days or weeks.

After almost any viral infection there can be a prolonged period of muscle fatigue, subjective but no objective muscle weakness, muscle aching and general malaise lasting months: the so-called 'post-viral fatigue syndrome'. It is perhaps particularly associated with influenza (p. 526), infectious mononucleosis (p. 524) and enterovirus infections (p. 522).

Tropical myositis

This occurs in natives of, or occasionally travellers to, the tropics. Often only one muscle or limb is affected and there is pain, tenderness, firmness and swelling of the involved muscles due to suppuration. If the iliopsoas is affected, it may mimic appendicitis. The cause is unknown but muscle suppuration is usually due to secondary staphylococcal aureus infection. Fever, septicaemia and arthralgia are common.

Sarcoidosis (also p. 472)

Although muscle granulomas are common in sarcoidosis, muscle weakness is rare and if present there is almost always evidence of sarcoidosis elsewhere.
   Muscle granulomas may also occur in:
- miliary tuberculosis (p. 512)
- toxoplasmosis (p. 536)
- tertiary syphilis (p. 515)
- fungal infections (p. 531)
- myasthenia gravis (Chapter 15)
- rheumatoid disease (p. 448)
- thymoma
- polymyositis (p. 434)
- Crohn's disease (p. 463)

Endocrine myopathies and metabolic bone disease

Hyperthyroidism

Hyperthyroidism (p. 456) may be associated with the following:
- Myopathy is common. Muscle weakness and some wasting are proximal, reflexes normal or brisk, and sometimes there is fasciculation (cf. motor neurone disease, Chapter 13). Occasionally only bulbar muscles are affected (cf. myasthenia, Chapter 15). CK is normal and the EMG myopathic. The hyperthyroidism may be relatively mild. The myopathy resolves with the euthyroid state.
- Periodic paralysis (p. 431) is very rare and is seen in Orientals in particular. Usually the plasma potassium is low but it can be normal.
- Dysthyroid eye disease (exophthalmic ophthalmoplegia). There is diplopia (usually with difficulty of up-gaze to begin with), lid retraction, exophthalmos, conjunctival and lid oedema, exposure keratopathy, often ptosis but little pain (grittiness or fullness). It can be very asymmetrical. Eventually raised intraocular pressure and blindness may occur. The patient is usually but not necessarily thyrotoxic; thyroid antibodies are often positive and the response to thyrotrophin releasing hormone is abnormal. CT of the orbit shows the enlarged extraocular muscles. Treatment is to ensure the patient is euthyroid and, if necessary, surgical correction of diplopia and tarsor-

rhaphy to protect the cornea. In severe cases, high doses of corticosteroids are used, perhaps cyclosporin, or even orbital decompression to save sight.

Hypothyroidism

Hypothyroidism (p. 456) may cause:
- aching and painful muscles
- cramps
- slowing of reflexes (often)
- weakness (very rare)
- increase in muscle bulk
- myoedema (ridging of muscle on percussion)
- CK raised sometimes

Acromegaly

Acromegaly (p. 458) may cause:
- increased muscle bulk
- improved strength at first but wasting and weakness later
- CK elevation sometimes

Cushing's syndrome (p. 455)

About 70% of patients have muscle weakness which is usually proximal, sometimes painful, legs before the arms, and wasting is late. CK is normal.

The same picture occurs with corticosteroid treatment, particularly with fluorinated steroids such as dexamethasone and triamcinolone. The dose required to do this varies between individuals.

Primary hyperaldosteronism (p. 455)

Addison's disease (p. 455)

Hypoparathyroidism (p. 457)

Metabolic bone disease

In primary hyperparathyroidism, but more often in osteomalacia, both conditions in which calcium is removed from bone, there can be a proximal limb and often very painful myopathy. There is very little wasting, the tendon reflexes are normal, and CK levels are often normal. Bone pain and tenderness are common. The plasma calcium can be normal, but the serum alkaline phosphatase is raised. The EMG and muscle biopsy can also be normal.

Stiff man syndrome

This is a rare and poorly understood syndrome in which adults, usually male, develop progressive stiffness and muscle rigidity, with painful muscle spasms of the trunk and spine precipitated by emotion, startle or movement. On EMG there is continuous motor activity at rest. It has been associated with hyperthyroidism and pituitary failure.

Toxic and drug-induced myopathies

The muscle involvement is usually symmetrical, proximal rather than distal, with normal tendon reflexes and sparing of the cranial musculature. Often the same drugs cause both myopathy and neuropathy in which circumstance the tendon reflexes are depressed. Usually the myopathy recovers when the offending drug is withdrawn.

Acute or subacute painful proximal myopathy can be caused by:
- alcoholic binge in chronic alcoholics (p. 544)
- amphetamines (p. 551)
- amphotericin
- barbiturates
- beta-blockers
- bezafibrate
- bumetanide
- carbenoxolone
- chloroquine
- cimetidine
- clofibrate
- cocaine
- colchicine
- danazol
- diamorphine (heroin)
- diazepam
- dimethylsulphoxide
- emetine
- epsilon-amino-caproic acid
- hydralazine
- ipecac (contains emetine)
- isoetharine
- isoniazid
- isotretinoin
- L-tryptophan

- labetalol
- lithium
- lovastatin
- meprobamate
- mercaptopropionyl glycine
- methadone
- metolazone
- nicotinic acid
- penicillamine
- penicillin
- phencyclidine
- phenytoin (p. 88)
- procainamide
- quinine (p. 535)
- rifampicin (p. 514)
- salbutamol
- theophylline
- vincristine
- zidovudine (p. 529)

The muscles are weak, painful and often tender. Sometimes the illness can be extremely severe with raised muscle enzymes, muscle necrosis, muscle swelling, myoglobinuria and acute renal failure (cf. polymyositis, p. 434).

Chronic painless myopathy can be caused by:
- amiodarone
- corticosteroids (p. 455)
- chloroquine (p. 535)
- chronic alcoholism (p. 544)
- drugs causing hypokalaemia (sometimes this is painful)
- diamorphine (heroin)
- hydroxychloroquine
- perhexiline
- thyroxine
  Usually the CK is normal.

Other effects on muscles are caused by:
- drugs exacerbating myasthenia (p. 410)
- neuromuscular blocking agents
- drugs exacerbating myotonia (p. 427)
- drugs to relieve spasticity (p. 352)
- drugs causing inflammatory myopathies (p. 433)
- drugs causing malignant hyperpyrexia (p. 431)

Cancer

Patients with cancer (usually metastatic carcinoma) may develop muscle weakness for the following reasons:
- cachexia
- polymyositis/dermatomyositis (p. 434)
- Lambert–Eaton myasthenic syndrome (p. 409)
- neuropathic muscle wasting (p. 476)
- secondary endocrinopathies (e.g. Cushing's syndrome, p. 455)
- malignant muscle infiltration (very rare)
- secondary amyloidosis (p. 473)

17   Neurological complications of systemic disorders

Collagen vascular disorders

- systemic lupus erythematosus (p. 444)
- progressive systemic sclerosis (p. 447)
- systemic vasculitis (polyarteritis nodosa, Churg–Strauss syndrome, Wegener's granulomatosis) (p. 447)
- hypersensitivity vasculitides (p. 448)
- rheumatoid disease (p. 448)
- Sjögren's syndrome (p. 449)
- relapsing polychondritis (p. 449)
- Behçet's syndrome (p. 449)
- malignant atrophic papulosis (Degos' disease, p. 450)
- isolated granulomatous angiitis of the nervous system (p. 450)
- ankylosing spondylitis (p. 450)
- giant cell arteritis (p. 450)
- Takayasu's disease (p. 453)

Note: The cerebral angiographic findings occasionally found in cerebral vasculitic disorders (focal narrowing, dilatation and beading of small arteries, sometimes with aneurysms) are far from specific; similar changes occur in malignant meningitis (p. 277), meningovascular syphilis (p. 515), chronic meningeal infection (p. 497), drug abuse vasculitis (p. 551), malignant hypertension (p. 214) and after subarachnoid haemorrhage (p. 228).

Systemic lupus erythematosus (SLE)

SLE occasionally presents with neurological symptoms but usually they occur along with obvious features of multisystem disease (fever, arthralgia, skin rash, nephritis, pericarditis, livedo reticularis, etc.) or in patients with an established diagnosis of SLE. Neurological complications are common at some stage in the disease, patients may have more than one, and they tend to relapse and remit:

Generalized encephalopathy

This is the most common with symptoms ranging from anxiety, agitation and headache to depression, paranoia, catatonia, visual hallucinations, seizures, dementia and coma. The EEG may be diffusely slow and the CSF is normal or contains a mild excess of protein and lymphocytes, perhaps with excess immunoglobulin and oligocloncal bands (p. 349). At postmortem there is intimal proliferation of small arterioles and capillaries with rather unimpressive microinfarcts, but no vasculitis.

Chorea

Chorea may be an isolated and transient feature (for days or weeks) or part of a generalized encephalopathy. It is rare and usually generalized rather than focal.

Seizures

Seizures, partial and generalized tonic-clonic, are common as a chronic problem separate from the encephalopathy.

Note: some anticonvulsants *cause* an SLE-like syndrome which can be difficult to distinguish from primary SLE (p. 88).

Stroke

Stroke is due to intracereberal small vessel intimal proliferation (and rarely extracranial large vessel disease) often associated with a circulating lupus anticoagulant and/or anticardiolipin antibody; embolism from Libman-Sacks endocarditis usually affecting the mitral valve is rare; intracranial haemorrhage due to thrombocytopenia or hypertension; intracranial venous thrombosis.

Aseptic meningitis

Aseptic meningitis, acute or chronic, is rare with headache, fever and excess lymphocytes or polymorphs in the CSF but a normal glucose; the CSF protein is slightly raised or normal.

Cranial neuropathies

Cranial neuropathies, particularly involving the nerves to the extraocular muscles and sensory divisions of the trigeminal nerve, are rare as is ischaemic optic neuropathy (p. 175) which seldom recovers.

Spinal cord infarction (p. 333)

This may cause a persistent or relapsing paraplegia somewhat similar to multiple sclerosis.

Polymyositis (p. 434)

Polymyositis is rare.

Peripheral neuropathy

This is also rare. It is usually chronic, symmetrical and sensorimotor. Mononeuritis multiplex and subacute generalized neuropathy, similar to the Guillain–Barré syndrome, are both most unusual.

Opportunistic infections

Opportunistic infections as a consequence of SLE or immunosuppressive treatment (p. 490)

Neurological complications of the general effects of SLE

- renal failure (p. 465)
- hypertension (p. 213)
- thrombocytopenia (p. 462)
- thrombotic thrombocytopenic purpura (p. 462)
- corticosteroids:
  myopathy (p. 438)
  hypomania
  depression
  benign intracranial hypertension (p. 264)

Myasthenia gravis (Chapter 15) is an occasional association.

Sneddon's syndrome is probably a variant of SLE with a particular emphasis on transient ischaemic attacks and strokes, widespread livedo reticularis, maybe with circulating lupus anticoagulant and anticardiolipin antibodies.

Diagnosis

The background SLE may already be obvious and the main issue is to be sure that any neurological problem is not due to a complication of treatment or an opportunistic infection. The neurological complications correlate rather poorly with the activity of the SLE, the ESR and the other blood abnormalities, i.e. leucopenia, antinuclear factor, anti-DNA antibodies, lupus anticoagulant (usually screened by finding a prolonged activated partial thromboplastin time which does not correct with normal plasma), anticardiolipin antibodies, etc.

Note: Lupus anticoagulant and anticardiolipin antibodies are also found in other collagen vascular disorders, AIDS (p. 526), malignancy, malaria (p. 534), drugs (phenothiazines, procainamide, Fansidar).

Occasionally SLE mimics multiple sclerosis (Chapter 12) with multifocal CNS lesions, optic neuropathy and CSF oligoclonal bands being present in both.

Treatment

Treatment is that of the underlying SLE with an emphasis on corticosteroids if the neurological complication is severe, persistent and progressive. Spontaneous remission is common, so that mild complications are probably best left untreated except symptomatically.

Progressive systemic sclerosis

This is rarely complicated by neurological disorders unless it is part of the overlap syndrome with systemic lupus erythematosus and polymyositis (*mixed connective tissue disease*) and their associated neurological problems. Otherwise, the only at all common complication is trigeminal sensory neuropathy (p. 187). Arteritis of cerebral, extracranial and spinal arteries is almost unheard of and any association with peripheral neuropathy is uncertain.

Systemic vasculitis (polyarteritis nodosa, Churg–Strauss syndrome, Wegener's granulomatosis)

This group of related disorders is characterized by a necrotizing vasculitis affecting medium and small arteries, usually involving several organs. Vasculitic lesions with infarction, aneurysm formation and haemorrhage are the cause of most of the neurological features which usually occur in the context of established disease although they can be a presenting feature, or even isolated:

Peripheral neuropathy

Peripheral neuropathy, which is usually a mononeuropathy (p. 368) or mononeuritis multiplex (p. 370), is the most common. It is often painful, subacute in onset and may persist. Nerve roots may also be involved. Distal symmetrical sensorimotor neuropathy is less common.

Encephalopathy

Encephalopathy with subacute onset of headache, confusion, seizures, hallucinations, dementia and coma. The CSF may have raised cells (lymphocytes and/or polymorphs) and protein.

Stroke

Stroke (Chapter 8) due to cerebral infarction, intracerebral or subarachnoid haemorrhage.

Spinal cord infarction

Spinal cord infarction (p. 333) or spinal subarachnoid haemorrhage (p. 336).

Cranial neuropathies

These are unusual; in Wegener's granulomatosis there may be direct inflammatory invasion from the skull base.

Polymyositis

Polymyositis (p. 434) is rare.

Eye

Retinal infarction (p. 175), exudates and haemorrhages; ischaemic optic neuropathy (p. 175).

Plus the neurological complications of hypertension (p. 213), renal failure (p. 465) and the treatment of the underlying disease.

Diagnosis

This is made in the setting of the systemic disease, usually backed up by histological confirmation from biopsy of affected tissue (peripheral nerve, muscle, kidney, etc.). Blood eosinophilia is common. The cholesterol embolization syndrome (p. 213) and the *L.* tryptophan induced eosinophilia-myalgia syndrome can look very similar, and multiple CNS lesions can mimic multiple sclerosis (Chapter 12).

Treatment

This is with high doses of corticosteroids. If there is no response within a matter of days or weeks, then cyclophosphamide or perhaps azathioprine should be added.

Hypersensitivity vasculitides

Neurological complications are unusual except in serum sickness; encephalopathy with seizures and coma, peripheral neuropathy (p. 389), neuralgic amyotrophy (p. 368).

Rheumatoid disease

Neurological complications arise as a result of:
- entrapment neuropathy in the wrist, at the elbow, etc., due to local inflammation or arthritis.

- systemic vasculitis, particularly peripheral neuropathy (p. 447).
- cervical spinal cord disease. Atlantoaxial dislocation may cause high cervical cord compression (p. 320) and occasionally vertebral artery compression with brainstem stroke/transient ischaemic attack. Vertical subluxation of the odontoid peg, causing brainstem compression, is much less common.

Treatment is based on corticosteroids and/or immunosuppression for vasculitic complications and surgical decompression/stabilization for the mechanical complications.

Sjögren's syndrome

This syndrome of dry eyes, dry mouth and parotid swelling due to chronic inflammation and destruction of the lacrimal and salivary glands may occur alone or in combination with systemic lupus erythematosus (p. 444), rheumatoid disease (p. 448), systemic sclerosis (p. 447) and myositis (p. 434). These associated diseases have neurological complications of their own; isolated Sjögren's syndrome may have much the same complications, e.g. systemic vasculitis (p. 447), aseptic meningitis, peripheral neuropathy.

Relapsing polychondritis

This rare disorder consists of recurrent inflammatory episodes involving cartilage, particularly of the ear, nose, trachea and larynx, and often accompanied by inflammation of the eyes and joints, deafness and vertigo, fever, anaemia and high ESR. Neurological complications include a generalized encephalopathy with headache, confusion, dementia, seizures and ataxia; cranial nerve palsies; ischaemic optic neuropathy (p. 175); occasionally stroke-like episodes. The CSF may contain excess cells (lymphocytes or polymorphs) and protein.

Behçet's syndrome

This rare syndrome tends to affect young adults, males more than females. Neurological complications are common, usually occurring in relapses and remissions at the same time as flare-ups of the muco-cutaneo-ocular symptoms. Vasculitis affects the brain, rarely the spinal cord, and exceptionally the peripheral nerves.

Clinical features are a combination of:
- encephalopathy with confusion, headache, seizures, dementia
- stroke and transient ischaemic attack-like episodes tending to affect the brainstem more than the cerebral hemispheres
- benign intracranial hypertension due to dural sinus thrombosis (p. 224)
- recurrent aseptic meningitis, perhaps with cranial nerve palsies

In all forms the CSF often contains excess cells (polymorphs as well as lymphocytes) and protein. Treatment is with corticosteroids.

Malignant atrophic papulosis (Degos' disease)

This is a very rare syndrome characterized by crops of painless pinkish papules on the trunk and limbs with distinctive central porcelain-white atrophy. It may be complicated by ischaemic gut lesions (causing abdominal pain, vomiting, ulceration, haemorrhage and perforation) and multiple infarcts in the brain and spinal cord (causing stroke-like episodes, cranial nerve palsies, myelopathy). There is endothelial proliferation of small arteries with little if any inflammation.

Isolated granulomatous angiitis of the nervous system

This rare disorder affects intracerebral, leptomeningeal and occasionally spinal cord blood vessels and occurs at any age. Histologically it is similar to sarcoid angiitis (p. 472), but there is seldom pathological, and almost never clinical, evidence of involvement of other organs. It can occur after herpes zoster (p. 524) or in patients with lymphoma (p. 276), but most cases have no cause.

The course is progressive, usually to death, over weeks or months, with confusion, headache, vomiting, mental impairment, stroke-like episodes due mostly to cerebral infarction rather than haemorrhage, myelopathy and seizures. The ESR, CSF protein and lymphocytes may be normal or modestly raised. Chronic meningeal infection or malignant meningitis must be excluded (p. 497), if necessary by brain or meningeal biopsy.

Corticosteroids and immunosuppression may help.

Ankylosing spondylitis

Neurological complications are surprisingly rare. The spinal cord may be damaged by traumatic fracture of the rigid cervical spine, or at other levels, and the cauda equina may be involved in an inflammatory arachnoiditis. Nerve root compression is rare and any root involvement is much more likely to be due to local inflammatory lesions (e.g. of the sacroiliac joints).

Giant cell arteritis (cranial or temporal arteritis)

This is a disorder of the elderly, being rare under the age of 55 and exceptional under the age of 40. The walls of medium and large arteries are infiltrated with mononuclear inflammatory and giant cells with obliterative fibrosis and secondary thrombosis. The branches of the external carotid artery are the most often affected but others can be involved such as the ophthalmic, vertebral, coronary and aorta (renal involvement being very rare).

This condition overlaps with polymyalgia rheumatica.

Clinical features

These are related to arterial inflammation, occlusion and sometimes ischaemia:

- Headache, scalp tenderness, nodular thickening and tender swellings over the branches of the superficial temporal and occipital arteries. Their pulses may be lost.
- Pain in the face if facial arteries involved.
- Jaw pain and claudication if facial and maxillary arteries involved.
- Amaurosis fugax or blindness, usually due to ischaemic optic neuropathy (p. 175), rather than retinal artery occlusion (p. 175), caused by posterior ciliary and ophthalmic artery involvement respectively.
- TIA and stroke (more often due to vertebral than to carotid involvement) and sometimes dementia, psychosis and personality change.
- Diplopia due to ischaemia of the orbital muscles or their nerve supply.
- Peripheral neuropathy, mononeuritis multiplex and isolated mono-neuropathy.
- Myocardial infarction and angina if coronary arteries involved.
- Mesenteric ischaemia.
- Ischaemia of the arm due to subclavian involvement and sometimes claudication in the legs due to femoral artery involvement.
- Aortic aneurysm which may rupture.
- Bruits, symptomatic or asymptomatic, are common and may be heard over the involved medium and large arteries.

General symptoms shared with polymyalgia rheumatica include:
- pain and stiffness (particularly on waking) in muscles of the neck, shoulders, buttocks and thighs. There is no muscle weakness but pain may prevent maximum effort
- anorexia and weight loss
- malaise and fatigue
- depression
- low grade fever, night sweats
- raised ESR

Other features on investigation include:
- mild normochromic normocytic anaemia often
- neutrophil leucocytosis occasionally
- raised plasma alpha 2-globulin and fibrinogen often
- mildly abnormal liver function tests commonly; hepatic granulomas can be found
- normal CK level
- normal muscle biopsy
- normal EMG

Note: Usually the onset is subacute and insidious, but it can be rather sudden (e.g. waking one morning with stiffness). Often the diagnosis is missed for weeks or months. It should be considered in *any* patient over the age of 60 with an ESR greater than 50, even more so if greater than 100, but no evidence of a paraproteinaemia, and in elderly patients with recent onset of headache or facial pain.

Management

The clinical features are often so characteristic that the patient should be started on oral prednisolone (40 mg twice daily) as soon as blood has been taken for an ESR, which is usually above 50 mm in the first hour, although it can very occasionally be normal (in the elderly an ESR of 40 is not exceptional).

Note: Once the symptoms and elevated ESR are suppressed, the risk of serious complications is negligible.

With treatment, the headache and general symptoms should resolve in less than 48 hours. If not, the diagnosis is wrong. The ESR becomes normal in about 2–4 weeks, but neurological and ocular complications may not improve.

In most patients, particularly if the clinical picture is uncertain, a temporal artery biopsy should be carried out (taking about one centimetre of a tender section of artery if possible) under local anaesthesia. If there is local facial or occipital artery tenderness, it is better to biopsy that artery. The diagnostic microscopical changes will not have resolved if biopsy is performed within a day or two of starting corticosteroids, and are present in about 60% of cases. A negative biopsy does *not* exclude the diagnosis since arterial lesions can be 'patchy' or not affect the biopsied artery at all. However, a positive biopsy, even in a clinically obvious case, is reassuring when some months later it is proving difficult to withdraw steroids or adverse effects are a problem.

Long-term treatment

Prednisolone, in a maintenance dosage of about 10 mg daily, which can be achieved within a month or two of starting treatment, is required from one to more than 10 years depending on how long the disease takes to 'burn out'. Attempts to reduce the dose very slowly should be made annually. The correct dose is monitored by *both* recurrence of symptoms *and* increase in the ESR, which may occur together or separately. Some patients can be controlled on alternate day corticosteroids with fewer adverse effects.

Takayasu's disease

This is a chronic vasculitis, histologically identical to giant cell arteritis (p. 450), but preferentially affecting large arteries (aorta and the large arteries arising from it), particularly in young Asian women. Systemic features are common and usually precede the effects of arterial occlusion: malaise, fever, anorexia, weight loss, arthralgia, myalgia, anaemia, raised ESR. Chronic ischaemia then develops in the kidneys (to cause hypertension); arms but rarely the legs (to cause ischaemic symptoms in the arms and hands); external carotid artery distribution (jaw claudication, alopecia, ulceration and necrosis of the nasal septum, palate and lips); eye (ischaemic oculopathy, p. 175); and brain (syncope, confusion, non-specific dizziness, headache, seizures, boundary zone infarction, p. 217, but rather rarely focal strokes or transient ischaemic attacks).

Corticosteroids are not very helpful; vascular reconstructive surgery may be technically feasible.

Note: Other causes of an *aortic arch syndrome* are:
• giant cell arteritis (p. 450)
• atheroma (p. 211)
• syphilis (p. 515)
• dissection (atheroma, Marfan's syndrome, p. 484, Ehlers–Danlos syndrome, p. 484, pseudoxanthoma elasticum, p. 484)

Diabetes

Neurological complications are common, particularly a mild, mainly sensory distal symmetrical neuropathy. They develop unpredictably, either as a presenting feature or more frequently as a complication in established disease which is not necessarily severe. In diabetics it is important to consider non-diabetic causes of the various neurological syndromes before necessarily concluding that the diabetes is responsible.

Peripheral neuropathy

• A distal and generalized sensory, or sensorimotor, neuropathy may be subclinical, mild, or severe with painless foot ulcers, Charcot joints (p. 18) and neuropathic pain. Usually it is an axonal neuropathy, although in some cases there is segmental demyelination. The onset is insidious with slow progression but can be subacute. Improving diabetic control helps some but not all patients.
• Autonomic neuropathy (p. 403) may accompany the above with impotence, postural hypotension, resting tachycardia, diarrhoea, gustatory sweating and occasionally Argyll Robertson pupils (p. 177).

- Mononeuritis multiplex (p. 370) which tends to be acute and recover in weeks or months with long periods between individual nerve lesions.
- Radiculopathy is acute or subacute with pain and segmental motor involvement but rather few sensory signs. The onset may be at a time of marked weight loss. Recovery occurs in weeks or months. The most common roots involved are high lumbar and thoracic. Usually onset is unilateral, but later other roots may be involved on the same or the other side.
- Entrapment neuropathies are common (p. 369).

Note: *Diabetic amyotrophy* refers to the subacute onset of pain in the thigh with wasting and weakness of the quadriceps muscle and depression of the knee jerk. It is due either to a femoral mononeuropathy or lumbar radiculopathy.

Cranial neuropathies

Acute and subacute single, multiple or recurrent cranial nerve palsies are quite frequent and are probably due to nerve ischaemia. Recovery in a few months is usual. The most common nerves affected are the 3rd (often painful and pupil-sparing, p. 182), 4th, 6th (p. 183) and 7th (p. 189).

Focal (partial) motor seizures

These seizures, usually frequent and without any interictal focal deficit, are a particular complication of non-ketotic hyperglycaemia and may be the presenting feature. Anticonvulsants are unnecessary since restoring normoglycaemia abolishes the seizures.

Coma

Coma is usually due to drug-induced hypoglycaemia or spontaneous hyperglycaemia.

Premature vascular disease

Premature vascular disease due to atheroma (p. 211) (e.g. cerebral ischaemia and infarction, ischaemic optic neuropathy, etc.).

Mucormycosis (p. 533)

Hypoglycaemia

Hypoglycaemia (drug-induced) may cause coma, confusion, behavioural disturbances, motor neuropathy, seizures, hemiplegia, etc. (p. 108).

Associated disorders

Myotonic dystrophy (p. 424)
Friedreich's ataxia (p. 336)

On balance, the better the diabetic control, the less likely are the neurological complications to be a problem.

Endocrine disorders

The adrenal gland

Addison's disease

Addison's disease and other forms of hypoadrenalism may be complicated by:
- muscle cramps, fatigue, proximal weakness, myalgia and sometimes
flexion contractures in the legs which are often painful
- hypoglycaemia (p. 108)
- postural hypotension (p. 102)
- lassitude
- hyponatraemia (p. 464)
- confusional state, stupor and coma
    It occurs as one component of adrenoleucodystrophy (p. 456).

Cushing's syndrome

Cushing's syndrome may be complicated by:
- proximal muscle weakness (p. 438)
- osteoporosis, vertebral body collapse and spinal cord/root compression
(p. 320)
- hypertension and stroke (p. 213)
- diabetes (p. 453)
- irritability, euphoria, insomnia, depression, dementia, confusional state
- hypokalaemic muscle weakness (p. 431)
- spinal cord/root compression (p. 320) due to excessive epidural fat

Primary hyperaldosteronism

Primary hyperaldosteronism may be complicated by hypokalaemic muscle
weakness (p. 431) and the complications of hypertension (p. 213).

Phaeochromocytoma (p. 109)

Adrenoleucodystrophy

Adrenoleucodystrophy is an X-linked recessive disorder in which there is excessive deposition of unbranched very long chain fatty acids in many organs with demyelination in the brain and spinal cord along with adrenal failure. At neurological presentation hypoadrenalism may be subclinical or even absent.

Boys develop progressive dementia, cortical blindness, deafness, hyperreflexia, ataxia and occasionally seizures.

Adult males tend to develop a spinal cord syndrome (adrenomyeloneuropathy) with spastic paraparesis, sphincter involvement and perhaps mild sensory loss. Dementia, cerebellar ataxia and peripheral neuropathy are unusual.

Heterozygote adult females may have a very slowly progressive spastic paraparesis with mild sphincter and sensory involvement.

Diagnosis is by demonstrating excessive very long chain fatty acids in skin fibroblasts or plasma (a ketogenic diet can cause raised levels in normals). Brain CT may show widespread periventricular low density, particularly posteriorly.

The thyroid gland

Hyperthyroidism

Hyperthyroidism (thyrotoxicosis) may be complicated by, or present with:
- proximal myopathy, which is common (p. 437)
- dysthyroid eye disease (p. 437)
- tremor (p. 294)
- atrial fibrillation and embolic stroke (p. 218)
- confusional state, mania, nervousness, irritability, anxiety
- generalized seizures
- chorea
- peripheral neuropathy is very rare indeed
- corticospinal tract dysfunction, causing a progressive spastic paraparesis, is very rare

Associated disorders are:
- myasthenia gravis (Chapter 15)
- hyperthyroid periodic paralysis (p. 432) similar to hypokalaemic periodic paralysis, particularly in Orientals

Hypothyroidism

Hypothyroidism (myxoedema) is commonly associated with neurological complications which are often the presenting feature:

Central nervous system:
- mental retardation (cretinism)

- dementia
- headache
- psychosis, hallucinations, delusions, confusional states (i.e. myxoedema madness)
- excessive day-time sleepiness (p. 116)
- drowsiness and coma
- cerebellar ataxia

Peripheral nerve:

- entrapment neuropathy (p. 369) (particularly carpal tunnel syndrome, p. 372)
- peripheral neuropathy

Muscle (see p. 438)

Others:

- deafness
- raised CSF protein
- benign intracranial hypertension (p. 264)
- chiasmal compression (p. 168) (pituitary enlargement in primary hypothyroidism)
- dysthyroid eye disease (p. 437)
- hypothermia (p. 486)

Associated disorders:

- myasthenia gravis (Chapter 15)
- hypopituitarism in secondary hypothyroidism
- hypoglycaemia (p. 108)
- POEMS syndrome (p. 461)
- hyponatraemia (p. 464)

Parathyroid and calcium metabolism

Hypoparathyroidism

Hypoparathyroidism (primary, secondary, pseudo) causes hypocalcaemia which leads to tetany; paraesthesia around the mouth, fingers and toes; muscle cramps, fatigue and possibly weakness; generalized seizures; irritability; confusional states with delusions, hallucinations and psychosis; dementia and mental retardation. It may be associated with benign intracranial hypertension (p. 264), basal ganglia calcification (p. 293), chorea (p. 296), dystonia (p. 302) and parkinsonism (p. 280).

Hyperparathyroidism

Hyperparathyroidism and other causes of hypercalcaemia are complicated by mood disturbance, confusion and coma. Proximal myopathy, often painful, is rare (p. 438).

Osteomalacia

This is associated with a proximal and often painful myopathy (p. 437).

Acromegaly/gigantism

Neurological complications are common:
- entrapment neuropathy (p. 369), particularly the carpal tunnel syndrome (p. 372)
- peripheral sensorimotor neuropathy, sometimes with enlarged nerves
- non-specific headache
- myopathy (p. 437)
- pituitary enlargement may cause visual field defects (p. 168) and hypo-pituitarism
- obstructive sleep apnoea (p. 116)

plus neurological complications of any associated diabetes (p. 453) or hypertension (p. 213).

Blood disorders

- polycythaemia (p. 458)
- essential thrombocythaemia (p. 459)
- leukaemia (p. 459)
- lymphoma (p. 275)
- hypereosinophilic syndrome (p. 459)
- sickle cell disease/trait (p. 460)
- iron deficiency anaemia (p. 460)
- paraproteinaemias (p. 460)
- extramedullary haematopoiesis (p. 461)
- paroxysmal nocturnal haemoglobinuria (p. 462)
- thrombotic thrombocytopenic purpura (p. 462)
- disseminated intravascular coagulation (p. 462)
- haemostatic failure (p. 462)
- hypercoagulability (p. 462)

Polycythaemia

In polycythaemia the haematocrit is greater than 50 in males and 47 in females.

Polycythaemia rubra vera (primary polycythaemia) may be complicated by:
- non-specific neurological symptoms such as headache, non-specific dizziness, poor concentration, visual disturbance, tinnitus, paraesthesia and limb pains
- occlusive cerebrovascular disease, e.g. cerebral infarction (p. 222), transient ischaemic attack (p. 219), intracranial venous thrombosis (p. 224)

- intracranial haemorrhage (p. 225) due to the associated platelet defect and haemostatic failure is rare
- chorea is rare
- mild sensory peripheral neuropathy

Relative polycythaemia is due to a reduced plasma volume (e.g. as a result of diuretics, hypertension, alcohol, dehydration, obesity) and *secondary polycythaemia* is due to a raised red cell mass (as a result of anoxia, smoking, cerebellar haemangioblastoma, p. 272, renal tumour). Both are modest risk factors for cerebral infarction (haematocrit in high normal range of 45–55).

Essential thrombocythaemia

Essential thrombocythaemia should be suspected if the platelet count is greater than 500 000 per ml.

This rare disorder can be complicated by cerebral infarction/transient ischaemic attack and sometimes by intracranial haemorrhage due to the associated defect in platelet function. Headache and paraesthesia are common.

Leukaemia

The leukaemias may affect the nervous system in several direct and indirect ways:
- leukaemic malignant meningitis (p. 277)
- spinal cord/root compression (p. 320) by leukaemic deposits
- intracerebral leukaemic deposits (focal deficit, seizures)
- orbital leukaemic deposits (p. 174)
- opportunistic infection (fungi, progressive multifocal leucoencephalopathy, herpes simplex, herpes zoster, cytomegalovirus, etc., p. 490)
- intracranial haemorrhage (p. 225) due to thrombocytopenia (subdural, intracerebral or subarachnoid) and possibly L-asparaginase
- cerebral infarction (p. 222) due to endocarditis (infective or marantic), increased whole blood viscosity and possibly L-asparaginase
- hyperviscosity syndrome (p. 461)
- drug-induced complications, e.g. peripheral neuropathies
- irradiation induced complications (p. 486). *Note:* Low doses of cranial irradiation and intrathecal chemotherapy (particularly with methotrexate) may cause an acute necrotizing leucoencephalopathy with seizures, dementia, ataxia and depressed consciousness
- disseminated intravascular coagulation (p. 462)

Hypereosinophilic syndrome

This is a very rare disorder in which there is eosinophilic infiltration of many organs (lung, heart, skin, brain, etc.) and a persistent blood eosinophilia without any evidence of parasitic, allergic, leukaemic or malignant disease, and no exposure to L-tryptophan. There is no vasculitis. Males are much more affected than females. The onset is in middle age and both progression and severity are variable. Neurological complications include confusion, dementia and coma with excess eosinophils in the CSF; focal neurological signs, probably due to embolism from the associated cardiomyopathy; cranial nerve palsies; distal sensorimotor neuropathy or less often mononeuritis multiplex; myopathy with aching and cramps and perhaps myositis.

Sickle cell disease/trait

This may be complicated by:
- cerebral infarction or transient ischaemic attack due to large and/or small vessel occlusion (p. 207)
- intracranial haemorrhage occasionally (p. 225)
- intracranial venous thrombosis (p. 224)
- seizures (p. 66)
- pains in the limbs or back which can be severe
- infarction of vertebrae with spinal cord and root compression (p. 320)
- rhabdomyolysis (p. 432)
- pneumococcal meningitis (p. 507)

Iron deficiency anaemia (or any other anaemia)

If severe (haemoglobin less than 9 g/dl), anaemia can cause non-specific neurological symptoms: faintness, giddiness, tiredness, generalized weakness, poor concentration, restless legs (p. 306) and, very occasionally, focal transient ischaemic attack-like episodes (p. 219). Loss of consciousness is exceptional and is explained partly by postural hypotension (p. 102) and partly by cerebral anoxia. Benign intracranial hypertension (p. 265) is a possible association. HIV infection (p. 526) may complicate therapeutic blood transfusion.

Paraproteinaemias

Multiple myeloma may be complicated by the following:
- progressive and generalized sensorimotor neuropathy (p. 389). This is common, at least subclinically, and is found more often in osteosclerotic than osteolytic cases. Occasionally respiratory muscles and cranial nerves are also involved. Usually the CSF protein is raised
- spinal cord/nerve root compression (p. 320) due to vertebral collapse or extradural myelomatous deposits
- compression of individual peripheral nerves, cranial nerves and nerve plexus by myelomatous deposits
- orbital myelomatous deposits (p. 174)

- 'hyperviscosity syndrome' with headache, poor concentration, drowsiness, non-specific dizziness, visual blurring, retinal venous dilatation and haemorrhages
- neurological complications of renal failure (p. 465)
- neurological complications of amyloidosis are very unusual (p. 473)
- hypercalcaemic neurological complications (p. 457)
- haemostatic defect due to thrombocytopenia, renal failure and hyperviscosity causing intracranial haemorrhage (p. 225)
- arterial or venous intracranial thrombosis (p. 224), probably due to hyperviscosity

Solitary plasmacytoma, particularly in males, may be complicated by a similar peripheral neuropathy to multiple myeloma. It slowly improves if the plasmacytoma is treated.

Waldenström's macroglobulinaemia has similar complications to multiple myeloma, particularly hyperviscosity and peripheral neuropathy.

Benign paraproteinaemia (or monoclonal gammopathy) with raised blood IgM or IgG levels is found in some normal people, but probably more often in otherwise obscure peripheral neuropathies. Neurological progression is slow, treatment of the paraproteinaemia is seldom rewarding, and eventually a few patients develop multiple myeloma, Waldenström's macroglobulinaemia, amyloidosis (p. 473) or lymphoma (p. 275).

Note: The Crow-Fukase or POEMS syndrome (polyneuropathy, organomegaly, endocrinopathy, M-protein, skin changes) is an association between a paraproteinaemia with peripheral neuropathy; thickening, hyperpigmentation and hypertrichosis of the skin; enlargement of the liver, spleen and lymph nodes; endocrine disturbance with impotence, gynaecomastia, amenorrhoea and occasionally diabetes or hypothyroidism; finger clubbing; mild fever; excessive sweating; oedema of the peripheries, ascites, pleural effusion; and papilloedema.

Note: Since in some paraproteinaemias the neuropathy is caused by binding of serum monoclonal antibody to the peripheral nerves, immunosuppression may be useful (i.e. corticosteroids, azathioprine, plasma exchange).

Extramedullary haematopoiesis

This is a compensatory mechanism when the function of normal bone marrow is disturbed by thalassaemia, myelofibrosis, etc. Haematopoietic tissue masses may cause:
- spinal cord/root compression by an epidural mass (p. 320)
- brain compression from a skull vault mass to cause seizures and focal neurological deficits

Paroxysmal nocturnal haemoglobinuria

This is a rare cause of haemolytic anaemia which can be complicated by intracranial venous or arterial thrombosis. Headache is a common symptom.

Thrombotic thrombocytopenic purpura (TTP)

This is a rare acute or subacute disease, usually of adults, similar to the haemolytic uraemic syndrome in children. Neurological complications are common and probably due to widespread vascular occlusion in the brain:
- seizures, headache
- generalized encephalopathy and coma
- stroke-like episodes
- disseminated intravascular coagulation is unusual

Disseminated intravascular coagulation

Neurological complications of disseminated intravascular coagulation (DIC) are usually lost in the features of the underlying serious illness but include an encephalopathy due to widespread haemorrhagic infarcts; intracranial haemorrhages leading to headache, confusion and coma; and sometimes stroke-like episodes.

Haemostatic failure

Abnormal bleeding may be caused by a defect in blood coagulation (e.g. haemophilia, anticoagulation, fibrinolytic drugs), thrombocytopenia (e.g. aplastic anaemia, leukaemia, idiopathic thrombocytopenic purpura) or a defect in platelet function (e.g. polycythaemia rubra vera, essential thrombocythaemia, renal failure, aspirin therapy).

This may result in:
- intracerebral haemorrhage (p. 227)
- subarachnoid haemorrhage (p. 228)
- subdural haematoma (p. 235)
- spinal cord, root, or nerve compression by haematoma (p. 320)
- haematomyelia (p. 335)
- intraneural haematoma causing a mononeuropathy (p. 368)
- HIV infection (p. 526) from blood transfusion

Hypercoagulability

True hypercoagulable states are very rare: inherited antithrombin III, protein C and protein S deficiencies and widespread carcinoma. These cause peripheral venous and intracranial venous thrombosis (p. 224) but very seldom arterial thrombosis.

Gastrointestinal disorders

Gastrointestinal disorders may be complicated by neurological disease in several ways:

- acute or chronic malabsorption of vitamins (e.g. B_{12}, p. 470; E, p. 471) and drugs (e.g. anticonvulsants)
- stroke associated with inflammatory bowel disease (p. 463)
- gastric restriction surgery (p. 464)
- Whipple's disease (p. 463)
- adverse effects of drugs, e.g. cimetidine and ranitidine, causing confusion, carbenoxolone, causing hypokalaemia, corticosteroids, etc.
- metastases to brain and vertebrae from carcinoma of colon, stomach, pancreas, etc.
- carcinoid syndrome (p. 110)
- coeliac disease (p. 463)

Whipple's disease

This may affect the nervous system and usually the gastrointestinal and other features are prominent. PAS-positive intracellular inclusions, with or without bacteria, are found in the cerebrum, hypothalamus and brainstem.

The main clinical features are progressive apathy and dementia; myoclonus and tonic-clonic seizures; and supranuclear gaze palsies perhaps with nystagmus. Other presentations or features include a hypothalamic syndrome (sleep, drinking, eating disturbances), ataxia and chronic meningitis. Peripheral neuropathy, myopathy and papilloedema are rare. The CSF is normal or contains excess white cells and protein. The EEG is non-specific. The brain CT scan is normal or shows low density areas which may enhance.

Diagnosis is made by demonstrating PAS-positive cells in the CSF or in a jejunal biopsy, but both may be normal. If so, brain biopsy is indicated since antibiotic treatment may arrest progression if the diagnosis is confirmed.

Coeliac disease

This can occasionally be complicated by a progressive cerebellar syndrome, mild dementia, seizures, myelopathy, myopathy and peripheral neuropathy. Malabsorption and definite vitamin deficiency (e.g. of B_1, B_{12}, folic acid, E) cannot always be found and treatment of the coeliac disease does not usually prevent progression.

Inflammatory bowel disease

Inflammatory bowel disease, both ulcerative colitis and Crohn's disease, may be complicated by ischaemic stroke as well as retinal arterial and venous occlusions usually during active, but sometimes during controlled, periods of disease activity. The possible mechanisms are cerebral vasculitis, 'hypercoagulability', paradoxical embolism from the legs and intracranial venous thrombosis perhaps due to dehydration.

Gastric restriction surgery

This surgery for morbid obesity may be followed some months later by:
- peripheral neuropathy
- confusional states similar to metabolic encephalopathy (p. 124)
- Wernicke–Korsakoff's syndrome (p. 468)
- progressive myelopathy
- optic atrophy

These complications appear to be due to loss of weight and persistent vomiting, but there is not always a recognizable nutritional deficiency (e.g. of vitamin B_1, B_{12}, E, folate, etc.).

Electrolyte imbalance

Hyponatraemia

Hyponatraemia may occur acutely (excessive i.v. dextrose, alcoholic binge, acute brain damage, oxytocin infusion, psychogenic polydypsia, etc.) or chronically (diuretics, Addison's disease, renal disease, hypothyroidism, etc.). The former may cause symptoms as the plasma sodium falls below 120 mmol/l but in the latter the sodium level has to fall further.

At first there is headache, nausea, postural hypotension and confusion and then, if the hyponatraemia is not corrected, vomiting, drowsiness, tremor, ataxia, asterixis, rigidity, seizures and ultimately coma. Focal signs are unusual. These neurological complications are due to cerebral oedema.

Chronic hyponatraemia must *not* be treated aggressively but by the removal of the cause along with water restriction if appropriate. Acute hyponatraemia should be similarly treated if it is mildly symptomatic (e.g. confusion and headache only) but otherwise requires i.v. 5% saline (0.05 ml/kg/min) to raise the plasma sodium to about 125 mmol/l, or until severe symptoms (e.g. coma, seizures) have resolved, but not by more than about 2 mmol/l/hour. Hourly electrolyte monitoring is crucial to avoid over-rapid correction or hypernatraemia which may cause central pontine myelinolysis (p. 465), coma and even death.

Hypernatraemia

Hypernatraemia is less common and rarely leads to neurological complications: lethargy, drowsiness and coma. Intracranial venous thrombosis can occur (p. 224).

Hypomagnesaemia

This causes tremor, tetany, delirium, muscle cramps and twitching, hallucinations and generalized seizures, but these effects are difficult to disentangle from those of the underlying cause (e.g. diabetes, hypocalcaemia, renal failure).

Central pontine myelinolysis

This is a rare but serious condition arising in the context of patients already very ill: usually vomiting or comatose alcoholics but sometimes in cachexia and malnutrition. Hyponatraemia is very commonly, but not always, present and its over-rapid correction is probably the cause of the demyelination in the centre of the pons and occasionally in other parts of the brain as well. The clinical picture is of a subacute tetraparesis (spastic or hypotonic), upgoing plantar responses and a pseudobulbar palsy which may progress to the 'locked-in' syndrome (p. 29). It is often confused by features of the underlying cause (e.g. alcoholic coma, seizures, Wernicke's encephalopathy, p. 468, etc.). The CSF is normal and CT (or better MRI) may show central pontine hypodensity.

The disorder is often fatal but recovery is possible. There is no specific treatment.

Hypo and hyperkalaemia (pp. 431 and 432)

Hypo and hypercalcaemia (p. 457)

Renal failure

Neurological complications of renal failure

Peripheral neuropathy

This is the most common. It is distal, symmetrical and more sensory (burning, numbness, paraesthesia, etc.) than motor. The severity is variable, response to dialysis uncertain, but it is relieved by renal transplantation.

Uraemic encephalopathy

This develops in acute uraemia, seldom when the blood urea is stable but high. Symptoms vary and to begin with there may just be lethargy, poor concentration and sleepiness. Then confusion, hallucinations, asterixis, postural and action limb tremors, dysarthria, ataxia, tetany and myoclonus develop. Later generalized and sometimes focal seizures, stupor and coma occur.

This may be exacerbated by infections, cardiac failure and sedative drugs and is relieved by lowering the blood urea. Usually the CSF is normal and the EEG diffusely slowed.

Muscle cramps and restless legs (p. 306)

The latter sometimes due to peripheral neuropathy, are common.

Uraemic myopathy

This is poorly characterized and unusual.

Bleeding complications

These complications are due to the uraemic haemostatic defect, anticoagulants and diffuse intravascular coagulation, e.g. primary intracerebral haemorrhage (p. 227), subdural haematoma (p. 235).

Hyperlipidaemia

An excess risk of coronary artery disease and ischaemic stroke is a consequence of hyperlipidaemia. This is not reduced by dialysis but probably is by renal transplantation.

Neurological complications of other consequences of renal failure

- hypertension (stroke, encephalopathy, p. 213)
- water intoxication and hyponatraemia (p. 464)
- hypomagnesaemia (p. 465)
- cardiac failure and hypoxia
- excessive drug effects due to impaired excretion (sedatives, penicillin, anticonvulsants, etc.)
- hyperparathyroidism (p. 457) and osteomalacia (p. 458)

Neurological complications of the underlying cause of the renal failure

- hypertension (p. 213)
- systemic vasculitis (p. 447)
- systemic lupus erythematosus (p. 444)

Renal dialysis

Renal dialysis may be complicated by:
- acute disequilibrium syndrome during and after dialysis. This is a

transient and usually mild form of uraemic encephalopathy; headache, muscle cramps and confusion are the most common features

- Wernicke's encephalopathy (p. 468) if no thiamine supplementation
- muscle cramps during dialysis (p. 418)
- ulnar (p. 374) or median nerve (p. 370) palsy in the arm containing an arteriovenous fistula due to vascular engorgement causing nerve entrapment. The tendon reflexes may be brisker in the arm with the fistula
- dialysis dementia is rare now that aluminium has been removed from the dialysate. At first it is intermittent, occurring during and just after dialysis but it then becomes persistent and progressive with speech disturbance (stammering, dysarthria, dyspraxia, dysphasia), myoclonus, seizures, confusion, agitation, motor apraxia, tremor, twitching, global dementia and leading to death within a few months. The CSF is normal but the EEG is diffusely slow with paroxysmal high voltage delta waves, often with generalized epileptic discharges
- septicaemia, bacterial endocarditis and embolic stroke
- subdural haematoma due to coagulation defects (p. 235)

Renal transplantation

Renal transplantation may be complicated by:
- opportunistic infections (p. 490)
- lymphoma (p. 275)
- cyclosporin toxicity; transient burning sensation in hands and feet for a few days, seizures, tremor, ataxia, confusion, visual hallucinations, coma
- rejection encephalopathy. Acute graft rejection may be associated with headache, confusion, seizures, irritability, raised intracranial pressure and slowing of the EEG which resolve when the rejection is controlled
- complications of corticosteroids (p. 455), azathioprine (p. 354)

Liver disease

Hepatic encephalopathy may occur in acute liver failure (due to hepatitis, toxins, etc.), intermittently and/or progressively in cirrhosis (due to alcohol, etc.) or as a result of a portacaval shunt. In all these situations the liver fails to detoxify chemicals arising from the gut.

At first there is only mild restlessness, irritability ad perhaps dysarthria. This progresses to drowsiness, ataxia, constructional apraxia, confusion and asterixis and then to coma with bilateral extensor plantars. Early on the EEG is slowed and later it becomes dominated by generalized high amplitude slow or triphasic waves before flattening in late coma. These neurological features may be complicated by others due to accompanying electrolyte disturbance (p. 464), renal failure (p. 465), hypoglycaemia (p. 108), hypotension due to gastrointestinal bleeding (boundary zone infarction, etc., p. 217), alcoholism (p. 542) and haemostatic failure (p. 462).

Normally there are obvious signs of liver disease (e.g. jaundice, enlarged liver, ascites) along with raised liver enzymes and hyperammonaemia. The CSF is normal.

Liver transplantation may be complicated within the first few weeks by an encephalopathy (seizures, confusion, headache, cortical blindness, coma) due to cyclosporin (p. 467), electrolyte imbalance (p. 464), air embolism, intracerebral haemorrhage (p. 227), hypotension (p. 216), hypocalcaemia (p. 457) and hypomagnesaemia (p. 465). Later, opportunistic infections may occur (p. 490).

Drug metabolism and protein binding are frequently disturbed in liver disease and drugs should be either avoided or used with extreme caution (particularly sedatives, phenytoin, valproate, phenobarbitone, dantrolene).

For other causes of hyperammonaemia, see p. 124.

Vitamin deficiency and excess

- vitamin A (p. 265)
- vitamin B_1 (p. 468)
- vitamin B_6 (p. 470)
- vitamin B_{12} (p. 470)
- folic acid (p. 470)
- vitamin D and hypocalcaemia (p. 457)
- nicotinic acid (p. 471)
- vitamin E (p. 471)

Vitamin B_1 (thiamine) deficiency

Vitamin B_1 deficiency is usually the result of malnutrition and causes:
- peripheral neuropathy (dry beri-beri)
- cardiac failure (wet beri-beri)
- Wernicke–Korsakoff syndrome (see below)

Wernicke–Korsakoff syndrome (Wernicke's encephalopathy)

This seems to be an idiosyncratic response in adults to severe vitamin B_1 deficiency as a result of:
- chronic alcoholism and malnutrition (p. 542)
- intractable vomiting:
  pregnancy
  gastric restriction surgery (p. 464)
  pyloric stenosis
- deliberate starvation:
  anorexia nervosa

hunger strike

obesity treatment

- prolonged intravenous feeding
- renal dialysis (p. 466)

There is a symmetrical vasculopathy with petechial haemorrhages around the aqueduct, 3rd and 4th ventricles, and in the mamillary bodies.

Clinical features

The clinical features are subacute, coming on over hours or days, and consist of a very variable combination of:

- ophthalmoplegia; lateral rectus palsies, supranuclear horizontal and/ or vertical gaze palsies sometimes with impaired doll's eye and caloric responses, internuclear ophthalmoplegia, horizontal and/or vertical nystagmus and often diplopia
- cerebellar ataxia of the limbs, trunk and gait
- mental disturbance: apathy, disorientation, confusion, poor memory, drowsiness and even coma. The combination of severe short-term memory loss with confabulation is referred to as *Korsakoff's syndrome* but is seldom seen; the same features are found in bilateral medial thalamic or temporal lobe damage as a result of ischaemia, trauma, tumours, etc. (p. 26)

Other occasional features include hypothermia, hypotension, pupil abnormalities, ptosis, retinal haemorrhages and papilloedema. In alcoholics, there is often a background of peripheral neuropathy, cerebellar ataxia, dementia, disturbed liver function and macrocytosis.

Diagnosis

The diagnosis is based on clinical suspicion and even fragmentary features of the syndrome or coma in at-risk patients, exclusion of other disorders, and response to thiamine. Red blood cell transketolase level may be low. CSF changes (mildly raised protein in some) and the EEG (normal or generalized slow waves) are non-specific.

Treatment

The treatment comprises i.v. 10 ml Parentrovite forte (contains 250 mg thiamine) followed by oral vitamins providing 10–25 mg thiamine daily until patient no longer at risk. The ophthalmoplegia resolves in a few hours but other features often persist longer; coma and Korsakoff's syndrome may be irreversible.

Prevention

- At-risk patients should be given vitamin supplements.
- Comatose patients should be treated with Parentrovite, particularly if

there is no obvious cause and their at-risk status is possible or uncertain.
• At-risk patients must *never* be glucose loaded (nasogastric feeding, intravenous dextrose, etc.) without vitamin supplements for fear of precipitating the syndrome.

Vitamin B$_6$ (pyridoxine)

In adults pyridoxine deficiency is seen as an isolated deficiency in patients taking isoniazid (p. 514), when a peripheral neuropathy can occur, and as part of a general nutritional deficiency in starvation, when any neuropathy has several causes (e.g. vitamin B$_{12}$ deficiency, vitamin B$_1$ deficiency, etc.). In infancy and neonates there is a rare form of epilepsy which responds to large doses of pyridoxine (p. 94). Excessive pyridoxine (50–300 mg daily) can cause a peripheral neuropathy with Lhermitte's symptom together with headache, irritability and tiredness.

Vitamin B$_{12}$ deficiency

Deficiency of vitamin B$_{12}$ commonly causes some combination of progressive peripheral neuropathy, dementia, subacute combined degeneration of the spinal cord and optic neuropathy. The peripheral neuropathy is the most common complication; it is generalized and distal, usually beginning with paraesthesia and numbness in the feet. Although depression is common, organic mental change with memory loss and a confusional state is rare. The degeneration in the spinal cord affects mainly the posterior and lateral columns to give a spastic paraparesis and loss of vibration and joint position sense in the feet; usually it is accompanied by the peripheral neuropathy. Progressive optic atrophy, with bilateral centrocaecal scotomas and visual failure, is rare.

Almost always the patient is anaemic with a raised MCV and a megaloblastic bone marrow. Very occasionally the peripheral blood is normal even though the serum vitamin B$_{12}$ level is low.

Treatment, if given early enough, reverses the symptoms except for the optic atrophy and sometimes the paraesthesia in the feet: i.m. hydroxycobalamin, 1 mg daily for 3 weeks and then every 3 months until any underlying cause is removed.

Note: Macrocytosis can also be due to hypothyroidism (p. 456), alcoholism (p. 542) and inborn errors of cobalamin metabolism causing homocystinuria and methylmalonic aciduria (p. 481).

Folic acid deficiency

Folic acid deficiency causes a megaloblastic anaemia with low serum and red cell folate levels. The existence of neurological complications similar to those of vitamin B_{12} deficiency (see above) is controversial since any relationship is not as clearcut and so often chronic neurological disorders (e.g. dementia, paraplegia, etc.) may *cause* dietary folate deficiency. If there is a relationship, then the blood picture (anaemia and macrocytosis) is *usually* but not always present. In obscure cases of progressive dementia or myelopathy it is therefore sensible to measure serum and red cell folate even if the blood film is normal.

Note: Long-term phenobarbitone (p. 92), mysoline (p. 93) and phenytoin (p. 88) may cause folate deficiency which if corrected does not lead to loss of seizure control.

Replacement therapy is folic acid, oral, 5–15 mg daily until any cause is reversed.

Nicotinic acid deficiency

Nicotinic acid deficiency is usually due to malnutrition, and occasionally to isoniazid, so that pellagra is the manifestion of more than just the lack of a single nutrient. The features are:
- neurological: depression, insomnia, paranoid psychosis, hallucinations (cf. schizophrenia), confusion, dementia and occasionally peripheral neuropathy and spastic paraparesis
- gastrointestinal: indigestion, diarrhoea, sore mouth
- skin: light, heat, pressure, and friction-sensitive dermatitis with marginated dusky brown erythema and later flaking and fissuring of the skin

Vitamin E (tocopherol) deficiency

Vitamin E deficiency is usually the result of severe and prolonged fat malabsorption (cystic fibrosis, biliary atresia, abetalipoproteinaemia, p. 479, etc.) and very rarely occurs alone. Neurological complications can appear at any age and are mainly due to degeneration of the dorsal columns of the spinal cord and peripheral sensory nerves causing progressive:
- areflexia
- impaired joint position sense and vibration sense, legs more than arms
- sensory ataxia of limbs and gait

Less constant features are limb weakness, dysarthria, supranuclear ophthalmoplegia, extensor plantar responses, impaired touch and pain sensation, retinitis pigmentosa and myopathy.

The differential diagnosis includes Friedreich's ataxia (p. 336) and obscure progressive ataxic syndromes (p. 200), particularly those with absent tendon reflexes. Supplementation with vitamin E may arrest or even improve some cases.

Sarcoidosis

Non-caseating granulomas are found in various organs and tissues; in the nervous system they occur in the meninges, brain, spinal cord, optic nerve, muscle, pituitary gland and perhaps peripheral nerves. The disease may present neurologically and even appear clinically isolated to the nervous system, but usually other organs are involved, albeit sometimes subclinically.

Neurological manifestations

• Cranial neuropathies, probably due to chronic meningitis (see below); isolated facial nerve palsy (recurrent and often sequentially bilateral) is the most common complication and can appear identical to Bell's palsy (p. 191). Other cranial nerves may be involved, e.g. olfactory, optic (see below), trigeminal, and those to bulbar muscles, but seldom the 3rd, 4th and 6th.
• Chronic sarcoid meningitis may cause cranial nerve palsies, obstructive hydrocephalus, raised intracranial pressure, infiltration of the optic chiasm and optic nerve (see below), deafness, tinnitus, etc.
• Peripheral nerve; spinal nerves are often involved causing segmental pain and sensory loss, particularly on the trunk. Mononeuritis multiplex (p. 370) and less often a symmetrical subacute and chronic polyneuropathy (p. 399) occur.
• Optic nerve and chiasm may be infiltrated or compressed by granulomas, causing subacute or progressive visual loss, often with papilloedema, but rarely a clinical picture which could be confused with optic neuritis (p. 343) due to multiple sclerosis.
• Orbital sarcoid granulomas have similar consequences to those of other orbital tumours (p. 174).
• Spinal cord may be infiltrated or compressed (p. 320) by granulomas to cause spastic paraparesis or a cauda equina syndrome. Rarely sarcoid vasculitis causes cord infarction (p. 333).
• Granuloma (single or multiple) in the brain may present as a space occupying lesion, seizures, mild mental changes, hypothalamic dysfunction or a brainstem disturbance.
• Sarcoid angiitis in the brain can cause intracerebral haemorrhage (p. 227), cerebral infarction (p. 222) or transient ischaemic attacks.
• Muscle granulomas are common, but a clinically evident myopathy with or without nodules is very rare (p. 437).
• Cerebral embolism from sarcoid cardiomyopathy is exceptional.
• Complications of hypercalcaemia (p. 457).

- Opportunistic infections (e.g. progressive multifocal leucoencephalopathy, cryptococcal meningitis, etc., p. 490).

Diagnosis

A neurological presentation is unusual. Usually there are thoracic, ocular or other features of sarcoidosis either before or at the time of neurological presentation and the main issue is to exclude non-sarcoid neuropathology or an opportunistic infection. Histological confirmation is usually needed, preferably in more than one organ; this can be achieved either at once by biopsy of clinically affected tissue (lymph node, skin, intracranial or intraspinal mass) or by 'blind' biopsy of muscle or conjunctiva, or by a Kveim test which takes some weeks to develop and is not absolutely reliable. Usually the CSF is abnormal with a raised protein, perhaps oligoclonal bands, sometimes an increase in lymphocytes and rarely a low glucose level. Serum angiotensin converting enzyme (ACE) level is often, but not always, raised and is not specific.

Treatment

Spontaneous remission is common, particularly of the cranial neuropathy, and the effectiveness of corticosteroids uncertain. However, the disease can be chronic and progressive. Anything more than trivial neurological dysfunction should be treated with prednisolone (oral, 40–80 mg daily), but if there is no response in a matter of weeks there is no point continuing. Once a response occurs, the dose should be slowly reduced to a maintenance level for months or perhaps years, with regular attempts at slow withdrawal depending on any tendency for neurological or systemic relapse.

Amyloidosis

Systemic and focal deposition of amyloid material is commonly found at postmortem. However, recognizable neurological complications are unusual and occur in cases which are familial (usually dominant inheritance), due to paraproteinaemias (p. 460) or of no known cause, but not in cases secondary to chronic infection or inflammation:
- Peripheral neuropathy, due to amyloid infiltration of nerves, is distal and generalized. The nerves may be thickened. Pain and autonomic features are prominent. The pupils may be involved with a pseudo Argyll Robertson appearance (p. 177) and scalloping of the iris.
- Cranial neuropathies are very unusual.
- Entrapment neuropathy (p. 369), usually the carpal tunnel syndrome, p. 372, due to focal compression by masses of amyloid.

- Myopathy is a very rare complication of amyloid secondary to paraproteinaemias.
- Cerebral and cerebellar complications occur in some familial cases.

There may or may not be other features of systemic amyloidosis such as the nephrotic syndrome, organomegaly, cardiomyopathy, heart block, etc.

Amyloid localized to one organ is usually sporadic. Occasionally focal masses may compress the spinal cord or the median nerve in the carpal tunnel. The most common form is *cerebral amyloidosis*. In this disorder amyloid is mainly deposited in the small cerebral and meningeal blood vessels of the elderly (congophilic angiopathy). Amyloid is also a component of the plaques and tangles seen in Alzheimer's disease (p. 160). Congophilic angiopathy is associated with intracerebral haemorrhage (usually lobar, often multiple and recurrent) and probably with dementia, particularly Alzheimer's disease. A dominantly inherited form in Iceland and Holland causes intracerebral haemorrhage in young adults; in the Icelandic cases, cystatin C is reduced in brain arteries, skin and CSF.

Diagnosis of amyloidosis is by biopsy of the involved organ(s): of the sural nerve in peripheral neuropathy, or of the brain in cerebral amyloid, but only to rule out treatable alternative pathology since amyloid itself is untreatable.

Cancer

Malignant tumours affect the nervous system by direct invasion, a paraneoplastic syndrome, secondary non-metastatic mechanisms and as a complication of treatment:

Direct invasion by malignant primary or secondary tumour:
- intracranial mass (p. 266)
- extradural spinal cord compression (p. 320); intradural/intramedullary spinal cord secondary deposits are rare
- malignant meningitis (p. 277)
- brachial/femoral plexus invasion (p. 366)
- peripheral nerve invasion (rare)
- neoplastic invasion of arterial wall (rare)

Paraneoplastic neurological syndromes:
- limbic encephalomyelitis (p. 475)
- subacute cerebellar ataxia (p. 475)
- polymyositis/dermatomyositis? (p. 434)
- Lambert-Eaton syndrome (p. 409)
- necrotizing myelopathy (p. 476)

- peripheral neuropathy (p. 476)
- opsoclonus-myoclonus-ataxia (p. 476)

Secondary non-metastatic:
- endocrine/metabolic (p. 476)
- opportunistic infections (p. 476)
- nutritional deficiencies (p. 476)
- intracranial haemorrhage (p. 476)
- marantic endocarditis and cerebral embolism (p. 477)
- intracranial venous thrombosis (p. 224)
- muscle weakness (p. 440)

Iatrogenic:
- irradiation (p. 486)
- drug-induced neuropathies (p. 391) and myopathies (p. 439)
- intrathecal methotrexate (p. 459)
- opportunistic infection due to immunosuppression (p. 490)
- corticosteroids (p. 455)

Individual patients may have more than one neurological complication at the same time.

Paraneoplastic syndromes

These are rare and precede (by months or rarely years) or accompany the manifestations of the underlying cancer. Increasingly they are thought to have an immunological basis and treatment with corticosteroids, azathioprine and plasma exchange can help a proportion of cases. The underlying cancers are most often small cell carcinoma of the lung, carcinoma of the breast, carcinoma of the ovary and lymphoma. Treatment of the cancer itself, if possible, may reverse the paraneoplastic syndrome.

Limbic encephalomyelitis

This presents with subacute behavioural disturbance (anxiety, agitation, depression) and increasing memory loss but without cortical features of aphasia, apraxia, etc. Myoclonus, seizures, brainstem signs, sensory ataxia and spinal cord disturbance may occur. The brain, particularly the temporal lobes, shows a scanty infiltrate of chronic inflammatory cells. The CSF cell count and protein are slightly raised.

Subacute cerebellar ataxia

This affects gait, the limbs bilaterally, and causes dysarthria, perhaps with nystagmus, diplopia, vomiting and pyramidal signs.

Necrotizing myelopathy

This presents with a subacute paraparesis, perhaps with spinal myoclonus and spinal muscular atrophy with muscle fasciculations.

Peripheral neuropathies

Peripheral neuropathies of various kinds can occur, subacutely or chronically:
- distal generalized sensory neuropathy
- sensorimotor neuropathy akin to the Guillain–Barré syndrome but with lymphocytes in the CSF
- entrapment and pressure neuropathies (p. 369) due to cachexia
- nutritional neuropathies (see below)

Opsoclonus-myoclonus-ataxia

This is a subacute syndrome of irregular, rapid oscillation of the eyeballs in all directions of gaze, ataxia and myoclonic jerks. It is a rare complication of neuroblastoma in childhood and even rarer in adults with cancer.

Secondary non-metastatic complications

Endocrine/metabolic consequences of cancer may result in neurological complications:
- hypercalcaemia (p. 457)
- inappropriate ADH secretion and hyponatraemia (p. 464)
- adrenal failure due to metastatic tumour in adrenal glands (p. 455)
- Cushing's syndrome due to aberrant ACTH secretion (p. 455)
- hypoglycaemia (p. 108)
- amyloidosis (p. 473)
- 'hyperviscosity' syndrome (p. 461)
- carcinoid syndrome (p. 109)
- renal failure (p. 465)

Opportunistic infections

These (p. 490) are a particular feature of lymphomas as well as immunosuppressive treatment for these and other cancers.

Nutritional deficiencies

Deficiencies, particularly of vitamins B_1 (p. 468), B_{12} (p. 470) and folate (p. 470) occur as a result of anorexia, vomiting, diarrhoea, gastric/intestinal resections and dysphagia.

Intracranial haemorrhage

Intracranial haemorrhage due to thrombocytopenia, diffuse intravascular coagulation, anticoagulation, liver failure with reduced clotting factors and haemorrhagic secondary deposits (p. 268).

Marantic (non-infectious or non-bacterial thrombotic) endocarditis

Non-infected vegetations are sometimes found on cardiac valves, particularly the mitral, in patients dying of cancer. Cerebral embolism is rare but can cause cerebral infarction and transient ischaemic attacks. Usually the patient is cachectic with disseminated cancer and the diagnosis is seldom made during life.

Inborn errors of metabolism

Lysosomal storage diseases

These are very rare, mostly recessive, inborn errors of metabolism which impair lysosomal enzymes, causing accumulation of various metabolites in lysosomes. The diagnosis is usually made by enzyme assay using leucocytes or cultured skin fibroblasts. Some of these disorders have prominent neurological features:

Sphingolipidoses

Sphingolipids accumulate in brain, peripheral nerves and other organs:
- Niemann–Pick disease (p. 478)
- Gaucher's disease (p. 478)
- Krabbe's disease (p. 478)
- metachromatic leucodystrophy (p. 478)
- Fabry's disease (p. 397)
- hexosaminidase deficiency (Tay-Sachs disease, GM_2 gangliosidoses, p. 479)
- GM_1 gangliosidoses (p. 479)

Mucopolysaccharidoses

Carbohydrate polymers accumulate in the brain and other organs:
- Hurler's disease (p. 479)
- Sanfilippo disease (p. 479)

Glycoproteinoses

There is faulty degradation of the oligosaccharide chains of glycoproteins:
- sialidosis (p. 75)

Other related storage disorders include:
- Tangier disease (p. 398)
- abetalipoproteinaemia (p. 479)
- adrenoleucodystrophy (p. 456)
- neuronal ceroid lipofuscinosis (Kufs' disease, etc., p. 480)

Niemann–Pick disease

This has various forms, some of which cause neurological involvement in childhood, rarely later: progressive mental retardation, seizures, macular cherry-red spot. There may also be hepatosplenomegaly and lymphadeno-pathy. The deficient enzyme (syphingomyelinase) is assayed in leucocytes or skin fibroblasts. The diagnosis can also be made by bone marrow aspiration because sphingomyelin accumulates in marrow cells ('sea-blue' histiocytes).

Gaucher's disease

This disease can present in children or adults with hepatosplenomegaly due to accumulation of glucocerebroside which also accumulates in bone mar-row cells and erythrocytes. There is variably progressive mental retardation, dementia, seizures, myoclonus, spasticity and chorea. Serum acid phospha-tase may be extremely raised and the enzyme deficiency (glucocerebrosidase) is detected in leucocytes and skin fibroblasts.

Krabbe's disease

Krabbe's disease presents in infancy with developmental delay, seizures, peripheral neuropathy, optic atrophy and deafness. Assay of serum, leucocytes or skin fibroblasts reveals deficient galactocerebrosidase.

Metachromatic leucodystrophy

This is due to a deficiency of arylsulphatase A (cerebroside sulphatase) which causes an accumulation of cerebroside sulphates in the central and peripheral nervous systems with progressive demyelination in the white matter of the brain, spinal cord and peripheral nerves. In infants the onset tends to be with flaccid paralysis, mental retardation, optic atrophy and a macular cherry-red spot. In childhood and adolescence there is more obvious motor disorder (and at onset rather less intellectual deterioration) with clumsiness, poor gait, dystonia, dysarthria and pyramidal signs. Adolescents and adults may present with a schizophrenic type of psychosis followed by progressive intellectual and motor decline.

    Diagnosis is made by measuring arylsulphatase A in the urine, leuco-cytes, skin fibroblasts and plasma; also, sural nerve biopsy shows segmental demyelination with metachromatic deposits. CT may show low density in periventricular white matter and the urine may contain metachromatic granules. In adults, clinical evidence of neuropathy is unusual but nerve conduction may be slowed.

Hexosaminidase deficiency (GM₂ gangliosidoses)

There are a number of autosomal recessive and very variable clinical syndromes due to hexosaminidase deficiency and excessive storage of GM_2 ganglioside in various organs, including the nervous system. Many patients are Ashkenazi Jews. Onset is in infancy (Tay–Sachs disease) and childhood, occasionally in adults. There is progressive multisystem involvement with various combinations of cerebellar ataxia and dysarthria; dementia; seizures; dystonia; supranuclear ophthalmoplegia; spasticity and neurogenic atrophy (cf. motor neurone disease, p. 359); macular cherry-red spot and progressive blindness.

Diagnosis is made by finding neuronal inclusions on rectal biopsy and deficient enzyme in plasma, leucocytes or skin fibroblasts.

GM₁ gangliosidoses

These are due to a deficiency of beta-galactosidase with accumulation of GM_1 ganglioside. Onset is at birth, or in children, with hepatosplenomegaly, mental and motor deterioration, seizures, retinal degeneration with macular cherry-red spot and skeletal abnormalities.

Hurler's disease

This disease (one cause of gargoylism) causes mental retardation and (by mucopolysaccharide deposition in the meninges) hydrocephalus and spinal cord compression. There is a large number of other features: corneal clouding, deafness, dysmorphic features, dwarfism, stiff straight hair, hepatosplenomegaly. Leucocytes contain mucopolysaccharide inclusion bodies and are deficient in alpha L–iduronidase, as are fibroblasts. Death occurs in childhood, although in the similar Hunter disease survival to middle age is possible.

Sanfilippo disease

This causes severe mental retardation and hyperkinetic behaviour in infants but few somatic features (abundant coarse scalp hair). Death occurs in adolescence.

Abetalipoproteinaemia

Abetalipoproteinaemia is a rare autosomal recessive disorder. Fat malabsorption develops in infancy and there is a striking reduction in plasma low density lipoproteins and cholesterol together with acanthocytosis of the red blood cells. The neurological complications develop in adolescence or before and may be due to malabsorption of vitamin E; progressive limb and gait ataxia, dysarthria, absent tendon reflexes (cf. Friedreich's ataxia, p. 336), retinitis pigmentosa and sometimes ptosis, extra ocular muscle weakness and sensory loss due to peripheral neuropathy.

Neuronal ceroid lipofuscinosis

This is a group of rare disorders with neuronal storage of lipopigment. The metabolic defect is unknown. Lysosomal inclusions are found on brain, rectal, skin or muscle biopsy. There is some combination of progressive dementia, myoclonic epilepsy (p. 75), spasticity, ataxia, retinal degeneration and optic atrophy. The onset may be infantile (Santavuori), late infantile or juvenile (Batten's disease) or adult (Kufs' disease).

Inborn errors of aminoacid and organic acid metabolism and transport

These are due to single enzyme defects in the intermediary metabolism of amino and organic acids which accumulate in blood and urine where they can relatively easily be measured, which is how the diagnosis is made, followed by specific enzyme assay if necessary. Apart from ornithine transcarbamylase deficiency they are all inherited recessively. Many have neurological complications:

- phenylalaninaemia (p. 480)
- ornithine transcarbamylase deficiency (p. 480)
- homocystinaemia (p. 481)
- Hartnup disease (p. 481)
- oculo-cerebral-renal syndrome of Lowe (p. 481)
- branched chain aminoacidaemias

Phenylalaninaemia (phenylketonuria)

Phenylalaninaemia due to reduced or absent phenylalanine hydroxylase causes accumulation of phenylalanine. Psychomotor delay, seizures, microcephaly, dilution of skin, hair and iris pigmentation develop in early childhood.

Ornithine transcarbamylase (OTC) deficiency

This is a rare X-linked disorder of the urea cycle which causes episodic hyperammonaemia, raised liver enzymes and excess urine orotic acid. Males usually die in neonatal life but the clinical manifestations in heterozygote females are very variable. Some remain asymptomatic until challenged with a high protein meal (which they often learn to avoid), general anaesthesia or sodium valproate. Onset is usually in the first two decades with attacks of metabolic encephalopathy (p. 125) lasting some days and consisting of headache, irritability, vomiting and lethargy. More severe attacks are accompanied by confusion, ataxia, dysarthria, ptosis, seizures, coma and sometimes focal neurological deficits. In some patients there is progressive mental retardation and ataxia. The EEG is diffusely slow. The diagnosis is made by finding excess urine orotic acid during attacks (or after a protein load) and deficient OTC in the liver or blood leucocytes.

Note: A similar syndrome with hyperammonaemia can occur as a result of other enzymatic defects in the urea cycle (e.g. argininosuccinic aciduria, citrullinaemia, argininaemia, carbamylphosphate synthetase deficiency) and lysinuric protein intolerance.

Homocystinaemia (homocystinuria)

This is usually due to cystathione synthetase deficiency, causing accumulation of homocysteine and homocystine. The neurological features are very variable with mental retardation, seizures and dystonia. The children are usually 'marfanoid' with a high-arched palate, kyphoscoliosis, arachnodactyly, pectus excavatum, osteoporosis and dislocated lenses. Multiple arterial and venous thromboses are a curious feature along with livido reticularis and malar flush. Heterozygotes may have an increased incidence of premature atherosclerotic vascular disease.

Note: Homocystinuria and/or methylmalonic aciduria may be very rarely due to a failure to form or accumulate methylcobalamin. This is associated with megaloblastic anaemia (unresponsive to vitamin B_{12}) and neurological complications (mental retardation, dementia, myelopathy) in children and adolescents.

Hartnup disease

Hartnup disease is a combination of generalized aminoaciduria, photosensitive skin eruptions, modest mental retardation, behavioural and psychotic disturbances. There can also be intermittent cerebellar ataxia, seizures and impaired consciousness.

Oculo-cerebral-renal syndrome of Lowe

This is the combination of generalized aminoaciduria, mental handicap, hypotonia, cataracts and dysmorphic features. It is sex-linked recessive.

Miscellaneous disorders

Lesch–Nyhan syndrome

This syndrome is inherited as an X-linked recessive disorder. Deficiency of hypoxanthine-guanine phosphoribosyl transferase causes purine overproduction with hyperuricaemia, excess urine uric acid, gout and occasionally megaloblastic anaemia. The earliest manifestations are neurological in early childhood: mental retardation, spasticity, chorea, dystonia with episodes of agitation and self-mutilation. The deficient enzyme can be assayed in red blood cells, leucocytes and fibroblasts.

Menkes' kinky hair syndrome

This is an X-linked recessive disorder of copper metabolism with low serum copper and caeruloplasmin. Infants become mentally retarded, often with frequent seizures. Scalp hair is sparse, stubbly and kinky. Arterial dissection, rupture and thrombosis may occur.

Cockayne syndrome

This is an autosomal inherited leucodystrophy (CT shows white matter hypodensity) with peripheral neuropathy. The infants are dwarfed and microcephalic with mental retardation, calcification of the basal ganglia, ataxia, sensorineural deafness, retinitis pigmentosa, cataract and photosensitive skin rashes.

Leigh's disease (subacute necrotizing encephalomyelopathy)

This autosomal recessive disorder usually presents in childhood, seldom in adult life, with episodes of vomiting, ataxia, abnormal eye movements and disturbed respiratory rate on a background of progressive ataxia, dysarthria, seizures and pyramidal signs. Optic atrophy and peripheral neuropathy are less constant. During the attacks there is usually a metabolic acidosis with raised blood levels of pyruvate, lactate and alanine, but these are not specific, also occurring in mitochondrial cytopathies (p. 430). The CSF protein may be raised. Definite diagnosis during life is impossible. Death occurs in weeks to years.

CT and MRI may show scattered small lesions in the brainstem and basal ganglia. Similar foci are found in other parts of the brain and spinal cord, which histologically consist of spongy necrosis and microvascular proliferation similar to Wernicke's encephalopathy (p. 468).

Rett's syndrome

This is a rare progressive disorder of girls, with onset in childhood. There is mental retardation and dementia, loss of purposeful movements and the development of stereotyped hand movements, autistic behaviour, ataxia, seizures and growth retardation. The cause is unknown.

Reye's syndrome

This is the rare association of an acute encephalopathy (due to cerebral oedema but without inflammation) with fatty infiltration of the liver and other organs in infants, children and rarely adults. No specific metabolic defect has been discovered but some cases may be due to therapeutic aspirin ingestion.

The onset is with an unremarkable 'viral' infection (e.g. upper respiratory, influenza, varicella, diarrhoea) followed a few days later by repeated vomiting and clouding of consciousness. This may recover or progress to delirium and coma accompanied by seizures, hypoglycaemia and sometimes fever. There is no obvious sign of liver damage except sometimes hepatomegaly. Death may follow or the child recovers completely. Recurrence is exceptional.

Liver enzymes, blood ammonia and prothrombin time are raised (but the bilirubin is usually normal) and the CSF normal. Liver biopsy may be needed for diagnosis. The differential diagnosis includes:
- encephalitis (p. 498) and post-infectious encephalomyelitis (p. 502)
- hepatitis
- other metabolic encephalopathies with hyperammonaemia (p. 124)
- toxic encephalopathy (poisoning, drugs, etc., p. 125)
- aminoacid and organic acidurias (p. 480)
- septicaemia

Treatment is supportive, with control of hypoglycaemia, seizures and raised intracranial pressure.

Miscellaneous disorders of bones and ligaments

Paget's disease of bone

This may be rarely complicated by:
- spinal cord/root compression often at multiple sites
- obstruction of foramina in the skull base leading to cranial neuropathies, particularly deafness and optic atrophy
- compression at the foramen magnum causing cerebellar, brainstem or high spinal cord compression and sometimes hydrocephalus

- proptosis
- headache
- enlarged head

Ehlers–Danlos syndrome

This is a group of inherited and rather varied connective tissue disorders with lax joints, hyperextensible skin and easy bruising. Neurological complications include:
- excessive blood vessel fragility leading to arterial dissection (p. 214), aneurysm (p. 231) and carotico-cavernous fistula (p. 189)
- spinal deformity (scoliosis, kyphosis) causing cord and root compression
- muscle cramp
- mitral valve prolapse (cerebral embolism, arrhythmias, bacterial endocarditis)
- congenital cardiac valve and septal defects

Pseudoxanthoma elasticum

This is a rare inherited disorder of elastic tissue, usually autosomal recessive. The skin is lax, redundant and inelastic over the face, axilla, groin and elbow. Arteries show fibrous proliferation and calcification leading to widespread occlusions, rupture, dissection (p. 214), aneurysms (p. 231) and caroticocavernous fistula (p. 189). Angioid streaks in the fundus are characteristic, with retinal haemorrhages and macular degeneration. Other complications are hypertension, gastrointestinal bleeding and there is an association with Paget's disease of the skull and endocrine disturbances.

Marfan's syndrome

Marfan's syndrome is an autosomal dominant condition of variable penetrance. Neurological complications occur as a result of proximal aortic root dissection (cerebral infarction, syncope, etc., p. 214), mitral and occasionally other cardiac valve prolapse (cerebral embolism, arrhythmias, bacterial endocarditis).

Achondroplasia

This is an autosomal dominant cause of short-limbed dwarfism. It can be complicated by bony abnormality of the skull base leading to brainstem and upper cervical cord compression and hydrocephalus. Kyphosis and spinal stenosis may both cause spinal cord/root compression. Obstructive sleep apnoea may occur (p. 116).

Physical extremes

- decompression sickness (p. 485)
- acute mountain sickness (p. 485)
- heat stroke (p. 485)
- hypothermia (p. 486)
- irradiation (p. 486)

Decompression sickness (the bends)

This is seen mostly in divers, occasionally in tunnel workers, and can be precipitated or exacerbated by flying. It is caused by over-hasty return from high to normal atmospheric pressure, when gas bubbles form in the circulation and tissues to cause infarction in the spinal cord white matter and brain. The spinal form begins from minutes to hours after surfacing; pins and needles, numbness, pain and weakness develop in the upper and/or lower limbs. Although usually mild and spontaneously reversible, it may progress to permanent paraparesis.

The cerebral form begins during or within minutes of surfacing. In mild cases there is just headache, nausea and mild confusion. Dysarthria and cognitive dysfunction can occur as well as limb weakness and numbness. These symptoms usually resolve. Coma is much more ominous with a high case fatality.

Treatment is by recompression as soon as possible.

Acute mountain sickness

This begins a few hours after rapid ascent to high altitude (above about 3000 m) in some individuals. Lethargy, headache, anorexia, nausea, light-headedness, disturbed sleep and unsteadiness are early symptoms which usually resolve in a few days even if altitude is maintained. However, the disorder may progress to cerebral and pulmonary oedema; the former causes drowsiness with papilloedema, leading to coma, and the latter causes cough, dyspnoea, tachycardia and tachypnoea. Retinal haemorrhages are common at altitude even in asymptomatic climbers. Treatment is by rapid descent along with dexamethasone. It is best prevented by slow ascent, perhaps with acetazolamide, 250 mg 3 times daily, oral, for a few days.

Heat stroke

Overheating of the body core is caused by a hot environment and is exacerbated by exercise, old age, obesity, poor sweating (often drug-induced, e.g. anticholinergics or an autonomic neuropathy, p. 403) and impaired temperature control (phenothiazines, barbiturates, hypothalamic lesions). Burns are seldom sufficient to raise the core temperature. Irritability, headache and confusion may progress to coma and even death. The skin is hot and dry and the temperature greater than 41°C. Seizures, hyperventilation, tachycardia, leucocytosis, acute renal failure and rhabdomyolysis occur in severe cases. Recovery is usually complete, but patients can be left with a generalized cerebellar syndrome, less often with cerebral damage or flaccid paralysis.

Hypothermia

This occurs as a result of exposure to cold on mountains or in water, and also in the elderly who are particularly susceptible. Hypothyroidism (p. 456) and hypopituitarism are rare causes. There is confusion, drowsiness and then coma with low heart and respiratory rates and hypotension. The differential diagnosis is of other causes of coma (p. 122), particularly hypoglycaemia, alcohol and drug overdose.

Irradiation

The harmful effects of irradiation depend on the total dose given, the number of fractions in which it is given, the amount absorbed by the tissue at risk, the inherent vulnerability of particular tissues and the time since the irradiation. Calculations of risk to the nervous system in individuals can only be approximate.

Brain

Acute reactions occur within days of an excessive dose, sometimes as low as 3000 rads (30 Gray), due to cerebral oedema; there is transient nausea, vomiting, headache and, with higher doses, coma and death.

Early delayed reactions are rare, occurring some weeks after irradiation and are due to demyelination, causing progressive focal neurological deficits which usually recover.

Late delayed reactions are unusual. Some months or years after irradiation focal cerebral necrosis occurs, often with swelling, causing a progressive focal neurological deficit and seizures which may stabilize or deteriorate to severe disability. The optic nerves and chiasm may also be affected; usually a total dose of less than 5000 rads (50 Gray) to the pituitary and hypothalamus is safe.

Late reactions. Years after even low doses of radiotherapy there is an excess risk of intracranial tumours: schwannomas and meningiomas particularly, and gliomas to some extent.

Carotid arteries

Irradiation of the neck or pituitary region may lead to later obstruction of the carotid arteries with thrombosis, embolism and aneurysm formation.

Spinal cord (see p. 334)

Nerve plexuses (see p. 366)

Fat embolism

The syndrome of fat 'embolism' is a rare complication of long bone fracture (or surgery). 12–48 hours post injury the patient develops respiratory distress, fever, tachycardia and a confusional state. A petechial rash appears, particularly on the upper chest, root of the neck and axillae. Coma, seizures, focal neurological features and disseminated intravascular coagulation occur. The brain is swollen and shows intravascular fat accumulation with petechiae. The differential diagnosis includes head injury as well as toxic, metabolic and infective causes of acute confusional states (p. 162). With respiratory support, recovery usually occurs.

Tuberous sclerosis

In early life hamartomas (looking like tubers) develop in various parts of the body, particularly in the skin and brain (and less commonly in the kidney, lung, heart and eye). The disorder is autosomal dominant with very variable expression of severity.

In the brain, multiple small nodular masses of glial cells are scattered through the cortex and around the ventricles; they may calcify and occasionally transform to gliomas or meningiomas. The clinical features are mental retardation, behavioural disorder, and generalized or partial seizures which can be very intractable. Large tuberous masses may occlude the CSF pathways to produce hydrocephalus. Onset is in childhood and progression variable.

The diagnosis is suggested by the skin changes: adenoma sebaceum or angiofibromas, depigmented patches on the trunk, ungual and subungual fibromas, shagreen patches, pigmented naevi, café-au-lait spots. Brain CT shows multiple and often calcified nodules.

Useful address

Tuberous Sclerosis Association of Great Britain
Little Bansley Farm
Milton Road
Catshill
Bromsgrove
Worcestershire B61 0NQ
Tel: 0527-71898

18 Infections of the nervous system

The brain, spinal cord, meninges, peripheral nerves and muscles may be infected, or affected, by a variety of micro-organisms, most often bacteria and viruses. Individual pathogens tend to cause particular patterns of infection (see Table 18.1, p. 499) and the clinical syndrome depends on which part of the nervous system is involved:

- meningitis (p. 491)
- encephalitis (p. 498)
- intracranial abscess, both cerebral and subdural (p. 503)
- spinal epidural abscess (p. 505)
- transverse myelitis (p. 332)
- infection of peripheral nerves including the Guillain–Barré syndrome (p. 398)
- myositis (p. 433)

Certain and sometimes unusual infections are likely in patients who are immunocompromised by AIDS (p. 526), cytotoxic drugs, corticosteroids (p. 455), lymphoma (p. 275), leukaemia (p. 459), sarcoidosis (p. 472), collagen vascular disorders (p. 444), etc. Such *opportunistic infections* are caused by:

- fungi and yeasts (p. 531)
- toxoplasmosis (p. 536)
- herpes zoster (p. 523)
- cytomegalovirus (p. 525)
- papovavirus (p. 530)
- listeria (p. 511)
- nocardia (p. 512)

Furthermore, 'normal' infections are often severe and difficult to eradicate (e.g. herpes zoster, pneumococcal meningitis).

Note: After splenectomy certain bacterial infections appear to be more severe and fulminating, particularly pneumococcal.

In *all* patients the possible reasons for infection of the nervous system should be considered:

- infection of the paranasal sinuses, ears, mastoids and teeth
- fractured skull, CSF rhinorrhoea, recent neurosurgery, intraventricular shunt
- septicaemia, endocarditis, focal sepsis outside the nervous system
- spinal dysraphism (p. 329)
- pulmonary infection
- immunosuppression (see above)
- occupation, hobbies and activities
- illness in contacts, epidemics
- foreign travel
- contact with animals

- insect bites
- vaccination
- splenectomy

Meningitis

Infection of the leptomeninges (pia and arachnoid membranes) and spread of the infection through the subarachnoid space and ventricular system (ventriculitis) is known as meningitis. Often there is some degree of inflammation or infection of the underlying brain as well (i.e. encephalitis, p. 498).

Bacterial (or pyogenic) meningitis

This is caused by haematogenous spread (from septicaemia or lung suppuration) or local spread (from pyogenic infection of the paranasal sinuses, middle ear, teeth, dermal sinus; penetrating head injury or neurosurgical procedures; intraventricular shunt; and exceptionally by lumbar puncture or epidural anaesthesia). The majority of cases are due to the meningococcus (p. 506), pneumococcus (p. 507) and, in small children, haemophilus bacilli (p. 506). *Viral meningitis* is almost always secondary to viraemia.

Note: A broader definition of 'meningitis' includes non-infectious causes of meningeal inflammation manifest by an increased number of white cells in the CSF (CSF pleocytosis), sometimes referred to as sterile or aseptic meningitis:

- malignant meningitis (p. 277)
- chronic granulomatous conditions, e.g. sarcoidosis (p. 472)
- collagen vascular disorders (p. 444)
- 'chemical' meningitis as a result of myelography with oil-based contrast media; discharge of material from cholesteatomas (p. 274), pituitary tumours (p. 273) and craniopharyngiomas (p. 274); introduction of drugs into the CSF. This may be followed by arachnoiditis and fibrosis (p. 335)
- Mollaret's meningitis is a benign recurrent non-infectious meningitis with fever, malaise and CSF pleocytosis (lymphocytes, neutrophils and endothelial cells). The cause is unknown. It may respond to colchicine, corticosteroids or phenylbutazone

Excessive cells in the CSF may be found in many other conditions, e.g. multiple sclerosis (p. 348), cerebral infarction (p. 244), severe complicated migraine (p. 138), intracranial abscess (p. 503).

Infectious meningitis

Clinical features

It is usually an acute febrile illness with headache, meningism and photophobia developing over a day or two. Bacterial meningitis is severe, with toxaemia, whereas viral meningitis is milder and self-limiting. Tuberculous (p. 512) and fungal (p. 532) meningitis are usually subacute or chronic. The clinical features include:

- headache, usually generalized
- photophobia
- fever, malaise, myalgia, anorexia, tachycardia, vomiting
- irritability and confusion
- meningism, which is painful resistance to passive or voluntary neck flexion because of cervical meningeal inflammation. Kernig's sign is rather unhelpful since it is seldom present without meningism; with the hip flexed, passive extension of the knee causes pain in the back and leg and resistance is felt in the hamstrings. This is due to inflammation or blood around the lumbosacral roots (or to lumbar root entrapment). Meningism is also a feature of subarachnoid haemorrhage (p. 228), a posterior fossa mass (p. 257) and cerebellar tonsillar coning (p. 259). Obviously extrapyramidal rigidity and traumatic or arthritic lesions of the neck are other possibilities
- skin rash. Purpura is almost diagnostic of meningococcal infection (p. 506). Non-specific rashes occur in several viral infections and as a result of anti-biotic hypersensitivity

Focal neurological signs do not occur unless meningitis is complicated by cerebral vasculitis (p. 495), dural sinus thrombosis (p. 224), cerebral or subdural abscess (p. 503) or encephalitis (p. 498). Seizures are unusual in adults but more common in children. In severe cases raised intracranial pressure and coma develop. Papilloedema is rare and suggests a cerebral abscess or hydrocephalus.

Traps for the unwary:

- Elderly patients may present merely with a pyrexia of unknown origin, confusion and drowsiness.
- Neonates and infants may not have meningism but present with fever, apathy, vomiting, anorexia, seizures, drowsiness and occasionally a bulging anterior fontanelle.
- Meningism sometimes disappears in coma.

Differential diagnosis

Usually the clinical diagnosis is not difficult, although other disorders may sometimes masquerade as 'meningitis'.
- subarachnoid haemorrhage (p. 228) has a sudden onset but can be confused with bacterial meningitis in a comatose patient with no available history
- acute painful neck conditions, e.g. prolapsed cervical disc (p. 326)
- cerebral abscess and subdural empyema (p. 503)
- migraine (p. 137)

- acute tonsillitis, parotitis, cervical lymphadenitis and pneumonia may cause neck pain in children but seldom meningism
- pituitary apoplexy (p. 273)

Investigations

These aim to confirm the clinical diagnosis and identify the microbial cause of the meningitis, to find out where the infection has come from, and to decide quickly on the appropriate specific treatment. The CSF must be examined immediately. However, if there are focal neurological signs and/or evidence of raised intracranial pressure (e.g. coma, papilloedema, p. 256), a CT scan is needed to exclude cerebral abscess or subdural empyema (carotid angiography if scanning is not available) *before* doing a lumbar puncture; 'blind' antibiotics (p. 496) should be started at once while the appropriate imaging is being organized.

CSF

- *Pressure* is raised in severe meningitis.
- *Appearance* is cloudy or turbid in bacterial meningitis but usually clear in viral meningitis. In tuberculous meningitis (p. 512), it may be clear or turbid.
- *White cell count* is raised. In bacterial meningitis it is almost always more than 1000/ml with a predominance (greater than 50% of total white cells) or polymorphonuclear neutrophils. However, in infants and in very severe infections the total count can be much lower or even normal and if anti-biotics have been given it can be lymphocytic (*Note*: listeria meningitis, p. 511, usually is lymphocytic). In viral, tuberculous and fungal meningitis the lymphocyte count is increased, seldom greater then 1000/ml, but in the first few days there may be neutrophil predominance. An eosinophilic CSF can be found in helminthic infections (p. 537), drug allergies and the hyper-eosinophilic syndrome (p. 459).
- *Protein content* is usually modestly raised (about 1 g/l) but in chronic infection, particularly tuberculous or fungal, it may be very high (greater then 10 g/l) and the CSF clots.
- *Glucose* must be measured in the CSF *and* the blood simultaneously. In normals, the CSF/blood ratio is greater than 0.5. In bacterial meningitis this ratio is very low or zero, in viral infections it is normal and in tuberculous and fungal infections it is usually low but can be normal. A low ratio is also found in malignant meningitis (p. 277), sarcoidosis (p. 472), subarachnoid haemorrhage (p. 230) and cerebral malaria (p. 534).
- *Microscopy* of the centrifuged deposit and then Gram staining is vital even if the fluid is lymphocytic. Gram positive cocci are probably pneumococci, Gram negative cocci meningococci, and Gram negative rods haemophilus. If there is no obvious bacterial infection, then a Ziehl–Neelsen stain or ultra-violet microscopy for acid fast bacilli, and Indian ink staining for cryptococci,

are necessary, often on several samples if the diagnosis of tuberculous or fungal meningitis is a clinical possibility.

• *Culture* for aerobic and anaerobic bacteria and, unless bacterial or viral meningitis is certain, for TB and fungi as well. Special media are needed for mycoplasma. Antibiotic sensitivities must be carried out. Usually viral culture is unsuccessful.

• *Countercurrent immunoelectrophoresis* or latex agglutination of the CSF (and serum) to detect specific bacterial antigens is a quick method to diagnose pneumococcal, meningococcal and haemophilus meningitis and is particularly helpful if previous antibiotic treatment has reduced the chances of staining or growing the organism. Cryptococcal antigen must be looked for in appropriate cases.

• *Lactate* levels tend to be high in bacterial meningitis but are not particularly helpful in diagnosis.

If the CSF is contaminated by blood from a traumatic tap, the number of introduced white blood cells (WBC) can be calculated from the formula:

$$\frac{\text{WBC in peripheral blood}}{\text{RBC in peripheral blood}} \times \text{RBC CSF}$$

Then, the true CSF WBC count can be estimated as the number observed minus the number introduced. However, this formula tends to *over-estimate* the true CSF WBC count. A *definite* excess WBC count in the CSF is highly likely if the ratio of observed CSF WBC to calculated number of WBC introduced is greater than 10.

An alternative is to repeat the CSF after a few hours, provided it is clinically acceptable to wait for this length of time.

Other necessary investigations

• Full blood count and ESR. A neutrophil leucocytosis and raised ESR are typical of bacterial infections but not invariable. Severe viral infections can cause similar changes.

• Blood cultures are essential in all cases since bacteria are often easier to isolate from the blood than CSF.

• Syphilis serology in lymphocytic meningitis.

• HIV serum antibody in at-risk individuals.

• Other viral antibodies in acute and convalescent blood samples and the CSF in difficult infections. Which viral antibodies to screen for depends on the local pattern of infection and the isolation of any viruses from body fluids (see below). Some non-viral infections may also be diagnosed serologically, e.g. brucellosis (p. 510), legionella (p. 510), leptospirosis (p. 517), borrelia (p. 517), toxoplasmosis (p. 536).

• Culture (bacterial and viral) from throat swab, stool, septic sites and biopsy material.

- Skin tests for tuberculosis but they are not always positive in tuberculous meningitis (p. 512).
- Chest X-ray may be abnormal in tuberculosis (p. 512), legionella (p. 510), pneumococcal (p. 507) and mycoplasma (p. 521) infection.
- Skull and paranasal sinus X-rays in bacterial meningitis may show chronic infection or fracture.
- CT scan if focal neurological signs, raised intracranial pressure or if intracranial complications develop (see below).

Note:
- Effective and frequent liaison with microbiologists is essential.
- Do not hesitate to repeat the lumbar puncture in cases which clearly are clinically serious and in which no organism has been isolated.
- In seriously ill patients take all possible cultures before starting 'blind' antibiotics (see p. 496). It may not be possible to culture the CSF first if a CT has to be organized to exclude an intracranial abscess (p. 503).
- If the CSF opening pressure, cell count and protein are *all* normal, then further microscopy and culture to exclude infectious meningitis are unnecessary except in the immunocompromised and children.

Complications

- Hydrocephalus (p. 259), acutely or subacutely, as a result of inflammatory exudate obstructing the flow of CSF or delayed to cause 'normal' pressure hydrocephalus (p. 262) but not in viral meningitis.
- Cranial nerve palsies due to basal inflammatory meningitis can complicate bacterial, tuberculous, fungal and syphilitic infections; diplopia, sensorineural deafness, vertigo, facial palsy and blindness.
- Cerebral vasculitis causing focal infarction, seizures and cognitive impairment is due to inflammation spreading from the meninges to the cerebral arteries and veins.
- Cerebral abscess and subdural empyema (p. 503) in bacterial meningitis.
- Asymptomatic subdural effusions may develop in neonates and infants; sometimes they cause raised intracranial pressure.
- Direct microbial invasion of the brain or spinal cord leading to encephalitis or myelitis respectively.
- Bacterial endocarditis.
- Electrolyte imbalance, particularly hyponatraemia.

Bacterial meningitis is still a serious disease with a case fatality of about 10% and is particularly severe in neonates, immunocompromised hosts and with pneumococcal infection. Survivors are usually normal but some are left with blindness, deafness, seizures or mental handicap. Most patients with viral meningitis recover completely except after polio (p. 522) or unless there is complicating encephalitis.

Recurrent meningitis is unusual and can be caused by:

• CSF leak as a result of skull fracture, neurosurgery or spinal dysraphism (p. 329) with a midline cranial or spinal dermal sinus, particularly in the lumbosacral and cervical regions

• untreated middle ear and paranasal sinus suppuration

• immunocompromised host (p. 490)

• Mollaret's meningitis (p. 491)

• craniopharyngioma (p. 274) or cholesteatoma (p. 274) causing chemical meningitis (p. 491)

• sarcoidosis (p. 472)

• collagen vascular disorders (p. 444)

• Vogt–Koyanagi–Harada syndrome (uveitis, alopecia, white hair, vitiligo and meningoencephalitis)

Treatment of bacterial meningitis

Bacterial infections should be treated at once with the antibiotics most likely to be effective (see under the individual infections) and the choice refined when the antibiotic sensitivities of the particular infecting organism are known. Antibiotics should be given intravenously in boluses, unless otherwise stated, until the patient has been afebrile for some days (for further details see under individual infections).

If bacterial meningitis is a likely diagnosis clinically and on the CSF results, and if an organism cannot be stained in the CSF, then 'blind' antibiotic treatment must be started immediately. Which antibiotics to use under these circumstances depends on the local pattern of infection and resistance. In the UK recommendations are as follows:

Adults (meningococcal, p. 506, or pneumococcal infection, p. 507, likely; haemophilus, p. 506, very unlikely):
    i.v. benzylpenicillin, 150 mg/kg/day in 4-hourly boluses. Do *not* give intrathecally. If allergic to penicillin, then give i.v. chloramphenicol, 3 g daily in 8-hourly boluses.

Children under about 5 years (haemophilus, p. 506, likely and usually insensitive to penicillin):
    i.v. chloramphenicol, 75 mg/kg/day in 8-hourly boluses (the i.m. route can be painful, the oral route is satisfactory if swallowing possible). Particular care and monitoring of serum concentrations in children.

Neonates (*E. coli*, p. 509, *Strep. agalactiae*, p. 508, or listeria likely, p. 511):
    i.v. ampicillin, 200 mg/kg/day in 3 or 4 divided doses plus i.v. gentamicin 6 mg/kg/day in 3 or 4 divided doses, or an 'extended spectrum' cephalosporin such as cefotaxime instead of the gentamicin: i.v. 150–200 mg/kg/day in 3 or 4 divided doses.

Note:

• Adjust choice and dose of antibiotic when sensitivity of organism is known and in the light of serum concentrations if very high doses over long periods of time are necessary (particularly important for chloramphenicol in children and also gentamicin).

• Do not use intrathecal antibiotics.

• Only use corticosteroids if the patient is critically ill, if there is any sign of acute adrenal failure (see meningococcal meningitis, p. 506) and perhaps if there is raised intracranial pressure. In children i.v. dexamethasone 0.15 mg/kg every 6 hours for 4 days seems to reduce the risk of deafness complicating severe bacterial infections.

• Repeating the CSF examination is unnecessary if the patient is doing well.

• Persistent fever may be due to wrong diagnosis, inadequate dose of antibiotics, drug reaction, local collection of pus, subdural effusion, bacterial endocarditis, a resistant organism or thrombophlebitis at intravenous injection sites. Therefore, review the diagnosis and antibiotics.

• Treat headache with appropriate analgesics, if necessary intramuscular. It is a common cause of a restless patient.

• Treat seizures on their merits with the usual drugs (p. 82).

• Ensure adequate hydration, feeding, etc., with particular avoidance of hyponatraemia.

• Treat contacts (see meningococcal, p. 506, and haemophilus, p. 506, infections).

• Report notifiable infections (see p. 540).

Subacute and chronic meningitis and/or encephalitis

This may arise from an inadequately treated bacterial meningitis or as a consequence of chronic bacterial infection after head injury, intracranial surgery and the use of intracranial shunts. However, if it arises *de novo*, there are various possibilities:

• infections:
  bacterial
    brucellosis (p. 510)
    listeria (p. 511)
    tuberculosis (p. 512)
    syphilis (p. 515)
    leptospirosis (p. 517)
    borrelia (p. 517)
    actinomycosis (p. 512)
    nocardia (p. 512)
    Whipple's disease (p. 463)
  viral
    AIDS (p. 526)

fungal
  cryptococcus, others very rare in UK (p. 533)
  toxoplasmosis (p. 536)
  cysticercosis (p. 538)
- collagen vascular disorders:
  systemic vasculitis (p. 477)
  systemic lupus erythematosus (p. 444)
  Sjögren's syndrome (p. 449)
  Behçet's syndrome (p. 449)
  isolated granulomatous angiitis of the nervous system (p. 450)
- sarcoidosis (p. 472)
- malignant meningitis (p. 277)
- lymphoma (p. 275) and malignant angioendotheliosis (p. 276)
- chemical meningitis (p. 491)
- steroid responsive chronic meningitis (see below)

Patients present with an indolent illness, malaise, headache, meningism, possibly fever, loss of weight, with or without focal neurological features, papilloedema and cranial nerve palsies depending on the cause. If the usual investigations for meningitis (p. 493) are unhelpful, it is important to:
- re-examine the CSF on several occasions. Microscopy, culture, malignant cells, cryptococcal antigen and other antigens and antibodies as appropriate from the list of causes above. Usually lymphocytes predominate, occasionally neutrophils. If there is any suspicion of lymphoma, then the CSF lymphocytes should be typed
- repeat blood serology for brucellosis, borrelia, leptospirosis, AIDS, fungal antibodies
- test for antinuclear factor, DNA binding, etc.
- CT scan for focal collection of pus or possibly parameningeal infection such as intracranial (or spinal) subdural empyema
- search for general clues by abdominal examination and ultrasound (liver secondaries, etc.), pelvic examination (infection) and a chest X-ray (TB)
- biopsy with microscopy *and* culture of extraneural sites (e.g. lymph nodes, liver) if there is clinical involvement, and occasionally brain and meninges

If there is no defined cause, and if the patient is sick, then 'blind' antituberculous therapy is reasonable (p. 514). If there is still no clinical response and fungi are ruled out, then corticosteroids may cure some patients who appear to have a steroid-responsive chronic meningitis which may relapse when treatment is withdrawn.

Encephalitis

Encephalitis means 'inflammation of the brain' but is normally taken to imply acute *viral* infection of the brain. Almost always there is some meningeal inflammation or infection as well (i.e. meningitis). It is hard, if not impossible, to distinguish encephalitis from acute post-infectious encephalomyelitis (p. 502). 'Cerebritis' refers to diffuse *bacterial* infection of the brain which may complicate bacterial meningitis and cerebral abscess.

Encephalitis is rare. Usually no viral cause can be identified, although many viruses can produce the condition. In the UK herpes simplex (p. 523) is the most common virus identified, but causes no more than 100 cases per annum. In many countries arthropod-borne viruses (p. 526) are more often the cause. Other viral causes are listed in Table 18.1 and are described later.

Clinical features

There is usually a prodrome of malaise, fever and myalgia. Within a day or

Table 18.1 Organisms which cause infections of the nervous system and their usual sites of predilection.

	A	B	C	D	E	F	G	H	I	J
BACTERIA										
Meningococcus (p. 506)	++	−	−	−	−	−	−	−	−	−
Haemophilus (p. 506)	++	−	−	−	−	−	−	−	−	−
Strep. pyogenes (p. 507)	+	−	−	−	+	−	−	−	−	−
Pneumococcus* (p. 507)	++	−	+	+	−	−	−	−	−	−
Strep. milleri (p. 508)	+	−	++	++	−	−	−	−	−	−
Strep. agalactiae (p. 508)	+	−	−	−	−	−	−	−	−	−
Strep. suis (p. 508)	+	−	−	−	−	−	−	−	−	−
Staph. aureus (p. 508)	+	−	+	+	+	−	−	−	−	+
Staph. epidermidis (p. 508)	+	−	−	−	−	−	−	−	−	−
Salmonella (p. 509)	+	−	+	−	−	−	−	−	−	−
E. coli (p. 509)	+	−	−	−	−	−	−	−	−	−
Proteus (p. 509)	+	−	+	+	−	−	−	−	−	−
Pseudomonas* (p. 509)	+	−	−	−	−	−	−	−	−	−
Brucella (p. 510)	+	+	−	−	+	+	+	−	−	−
Legionella (p. 510)	−	+	−	−	−	−	−	−	+	−
Listeria* (p. 511)	+	+	+	−	−	−	−	−	−	−
Campylobacter (p. 511)	+	+	−	−	−	−	−	−	+	−
B. anthracis (p. 511)	+	−	−	−	−	−	−	−	−	−
Actinomyces (p. 512)	+	−	+	−	−	−	−	−	−	−
Nocardia* (p. 512)	+	−	+	−	−	−	−	−	−	−
M. tuberculosis (p. 512)	++	−	+	−	+	−	−	−	−	−
M. leprae (p. 514)	−	−	−	−	−	−	++	−	−	−
T. pallidum (p. 515)	+	+	−	−	−	+	−	−	−	−
Leptospira (p. 517)	+	−	−	−	−	−	−	−	−	−
Borrelia (p. 517)	+	+	−	−	−	+	++	−	−	−
Clostridium tetani (p. 518)	−	−	−	−	−	−	−	+	−	−
Clostridium botulinum (p. 520)	−	−	−	−	−	−	−	+	−	−
C. diphtheriae (p. 520)	−	−	−	−	−	−	−	+	−	−
RICKETTSIA (p. 521)	−	+	−	−	−	−	−	−	−	−
MYCOPLASMA (p. 521)	+	+	−	−	−	+	−	−	+	−

Table 18.1 continued

	A	B	C	D	E	F	G	H	I	J
VIRUSES										
Enteroviruses (p. 522)	++	+	−	−	−	+	−	−	−	+
Herpes simplex (p. 523)	+	++	−	−	−	+	+	−	−	−
Varicella-zoster (p. 523)	−	+	−	−	−	+	++	−	+	−
Epstein−Barr virus (p. 524)	+	+	−	−	−	+	−	−	+	−
Cytomegalovirus* (p. 525)	−	+	−	−	−	−	−	−	+	−
Mumps (p. 525)	+	+	−	−	−	−	−	−	−	−
Measles (p. 525)	−	+	−	−	−	−	−	−	−	−
Rubella (p. 526)	−	+	−	−	−	+	−	−	+	−
Influenza (p. 526)	−	+	−	−	−	−	−	−	+	+
Lymphocytic choriomeningitis (p. 526)	+	+	−	−	−	−	−	−	−	−
Arthropod-borne viruses (p. 526)	−	+	−	−	−	−	−	−	−	−
HIV (p. 526)	+	++	−	−	−	+	+	−	−	+
HTLV-1 (p. 529)	−	−	−	−	−	+	−	−	−	−
Rabies (p. 529)	−	+	−	−	−	+	+	−	−	−
Papovavirus (p. 530)	−	+	−	−	−	−	−	−	−	−
FUNGI										
Cryptococcus* (p. 533)	+	+	+	−	−	−	−	−	−	−
Candida* (p. 533)	+	+	+	−	−	+	−	−	−	−
Mucormycosis* (p. 533)	+	+	−	−	−	−	−	−	−	−
Histoplasma* (p. 534)	+	−	+	−	−	−	−	−	−	−
Aspergillus* (p. 534)	+	−	+	−	−	−	−	−	−	−
Coccidioides (p. 534)	+	−	−	−	−	−	−	−	−	−
PROTOZOA										
Malaria (p. 534)	−	+	−	−	−	−	−	−	+	−
Toxoplasma* (p. 536)	−	+	+	−	−	−	−	−	−	−
Trypanosoma (p. 536)	−	+	−	−	−	−	−	−	−	−
Blastocystis (p. 537)	+	−	+	−	−	+	−	−	−	−
HELMINTHS										
Toxocara (p. 537)	−	+	−	−	−	−	−	−	−	−
Trichinosis (p. 537)	−	+	−	−	−	+	−	−	−	+
Gnathostomiasis (p. 537)	+	+	−	−	−	+	+	−	−	−
Angiostrongyliasis (p. 538)	+	+	−	−	−	−	−	−	−	−
Cysticercosis (p. 538)	+	+	+	−	+	−	−	−	−	+
Hydatid (p. 539)	−	−	+	−	−	−	−	−	−	−
Schistosomiasis (p. 539)	−	+	+	−	+	+	−	−	−	−
AMOEBA										
Entamoeba histolytica (p. 540)	−	−	+	−	−	−	−	−	−	−
Naegleria fowleri (p. 540)	+	+	−	−	−	−	−	−	−	−

* Particularly likely in immunocompromised patients.

(++) most common site of infection; (+) frequent site of infection; (−) very unusual or never occurs.

A = meningitis; B = encephalitis; C = cerebral abscess; D = subdural empyema; E = spinal epidural abscess; F = myelitis; G = peripheral nerve/root; H = neurotoxin; I = Guillain−Barré syndrome; J = muscle.

two, headache, drowsiness and focal or generalized seizures occur. The patient becomes confused, combative and then lapses into coma, often with raised intracranial pressure. Sometimes there is evidence of myelitis as well (p. 332). Obvious focal neurological signs are not common, although in herpes encephalitis there may be particular involvement of the temporal lobes with aphasia detectable in the pre-coma stage. Sometimes there is meningism. The reflexes are usually brisk with bilateral extensor plantar responses. Clinical differentiation of the various viral causes is impossible unless there are clearcut pathognomonic features (e.g. the characteristic rash of herpes zoster, p. 523, or measles, p. 525, the hydrophobia of rabies, p. 529).

Diagnosis

The clinical features of encephalitis are distinctive but must be distinguished from other intracranial disorders, particularly those that require specific treatment:
- tuberculous meningitis (p. 512)
- bacterial meningitis (p. 491)
- fungal meningitis (p. 532)
- intracranial abscess (p. 503)
- cerebral malaria (p. 534)
- metabolic and toxic encephalopathies (p. 124)
- intracranial venous thrombosis (p. 224)
- acute fulminating multiple sclerosis (p. 346)

The general investigations are identical to those for meningitis (p. 493). The confirmation of the diagnosis of encephalitis and the exclusion of other disorders depends mostly on the following:
- *The CSF* usually contains a modest number of lymphocytes (50–200 per ml) and a slight rise in protein content (up to about 1 g/l) with a normal or slightly reduced CSF/blood glucose ratio. Occasionally it is normal or contains only a few neutrophils or red blood cells. These findings are similar in tuberculous meningitis (p. 512), fungal meningitis (p. 532) and intracranial abscess (p. 503). Virus is seldom cultured but specific antibodies may be raised in the CSF.
- The *EEG* shows bilateral slow wave activity, but this is not specific and can be found in any generalized encephalopathy. Repetitive, generalized and stereotyped sharp and slow wave discharges (periodic complexes) are often seen at some stage in herpes simplex encephalitis (p. 523); similar changes occur in subacute sclerosing panencephalitis (p. 525) and Creutzfeldt–Jakob disease (p. 531), but the clinical context is very different.
- *CT scan* is useful to rule out an intracranial abscess and other structural disorders. In encephalitis it is normal or shows brain swelling that is diffuse and/or focal (e.g. in the temporal lobes in herpes simplex encephalitis, p. 523). Haemorrhage and contrast enhancement may occur.

● *Brain biopsy* is rarely required. It is indicated when there is a serious but otherwise unproven possibility of a treatable disorder such as tuberculous meningitis (p. 512) or isolated granulomatous angiitis of the nervous system (p. 450). Herpes simplex virus may be detected by fluorescent antibody staining, electron microscopy and viral culture.

Treatment

Apart from general supportive measures there is no specific treatment except for herpes simplex encephalitis (p. 523): i.v. acyclovir 10 mg/kg infusion over one hour and repeated 8-hourly for about 10 days. The infusion can be made up in saline or dextrose saline, but 250 mg of acyclovir must be diluted in at least 50 ml of infusion fluid. It is important to maintain good hydration with particular caution in uraemic patients. Adverse effects are mild and reversible: renal failure, rash, lymphopenia, thrombocytopenia, nausea, headache, phlebitis.

Since there is no quick and reliable way of distinguishing herpes simplex encephalitis from other, usually less severe, forms of encephalitis without resorting to brain biopsy, and since acyclovir is safe, it is reasonable to use this treatment early in all definite and serious cases of encephalitis. The viral cause can sometimes be categorized serologically in retrospect, but this requires early and convalescent sera *plus* CSF, so that not only a rising titre to viral antibody can be detected but also a raised ratio of CSF/blood antibody, indicating intrathecal antibody production (provided the blood–brain barrier is intact, which can be shown by measuring the CSF/blood albumin ratio).

Corticosteroids should not be given routinely but only as a last resort in critically ill patients.

Most patients with encephalitis completely recover in a matter of days or weeks. However, herpes simplex encephalitis is particularly severe, with a 50% case fatality and severe memory impairment, aphasia and behavioural problems in survivors.

Acute post-infectious encephalomyelitis

This is also referred to as acute allergic or acute disseminated encephalomyelitis and acute haemorrhagic leucoencephalitis. Acute 'encephalitis', 'myelitis', or a combination of both, may be due not only to viral invasion of the brain and spinal cord but to a presumed immune response to a viral infection outside the nervous system; post-viral optic neuritis (p. 173) has a similar cause. There is perivenous inflammation and demyelination of the white matter.

Clinically, and from the CSF and EEG, one cannot usually differentiate encephalitis from post-infectious encephalomyelitis, although the latter tends to occur towards the end or a few days after the precipitating acute viral infection, e.g. measles (p. 525), rubella (p. 526), chicken pox (p. 523), Epstein–Barr virus (p. 524), influenza (p. 526), mumps (p. 525), non-specific influenza-like syndrome. The same disorder may follow vaccination (vaccinia, rabies). Sometimes there is no recognizable preceding illness.

In severe cases corticosteroids are given (prednisolone, 20 mg 4 times daily). Many cases recover spontaneously without a definite diagnosis being made.

Intracranial abscess (both cerebral and subdural)

A cerebral abscess is a localized collection of pus within the brain, usually supratentorial. Around its periphery, and also before the abscess cavity forms, there is diffuse bacterial infection and inflammation, so-called 'cerebritis'. Subdural empyema is a thin layer of pus spread over one or other side of the surface of the brain and eventually both sides, between the dura and the arachnoid membranes, frequently spreading into the parafalcine region between the cerebral hemispheres. Often there are several bacterial strains in a single abscess and sometimes nothing is grown or even seen on Gram stain. Anaerobic as well as aerobic cultures are important. Usual organisms are: *Streptococcus milleri* (p. 508), *Pneumococcus* (p. 507), *Bacteroides*, coliforms, *Staphylococcus aureus* (p. 508), very rarely a fungus (p. 532) or amoeba (p. 540).

Local spread of infection may cause a single intracerebral abscess, or subdural empyema; haematogenous spread usually leads to multiple intra-cerebral abscesses. The causes include:

- local infection:
  suppurative middle ear, paranasal sinus or dental disease
  bacterial meningitis (p. 491)
  orbital cellulitis
  CSF leak (head injury, neurosurgery, spinal dysraphism, p. 329, etc.)
  penetrating head injury or neurosurgical procedure
- haematogenous:
  septicaemia
  right to left intracardiac shunt
  pulmonary arteriovenous malformation (p. 234)
  suppuration in the chest (bronchiectasis, abscess, empyema)
  bacterial endocarditis

Clinical features

These are of a subacute progressive space-occupying lesion (raised intra-cranial pressure, p. 256, focal signs, seizures) usually in the context of malaise, a cause for the abscess (see above), and often, but not always, systemic evidence of bacterial infection (fever, blood leucocytosis, raised ESR) and possibly meningism.

Neurological deterioration is due to mass effect with transtentorial herniation, hydrocephalus, rupture of the abscess into the ventricles, cortical venous and dural sinus thrombophlebitis and cerebral arterial inflammation with subsequent infarction.

Subdural empyema is more likely than intracerebral abscess to cause severe headache (often unilateral), focal seizures, 3rd and 6th cranial nerve palsies, and severe disturbance of the underlying cerebral hemisphere. It is rare in the posterior fossa but when present there are focal cerebellar signs, meningism and the features of raised intracranial pressure.

Diagnosis

A high degree of clinical suspicion is important in the context of a patient who may at first sight appear to have bacterial meningitis (p. 491), tuberculous meningitis (p. 512), encephalitis (p. 498) or an intracranial 'tumour' (p. 267). The following investigations are likely to be particularly helpful:

• *Chest X-ray* may show lung suppuration, a cardiac abnormality or pulmonary arteriovenous malformation (coin lesion).

• *Skull X-ray* may show chronic sinusitis, mastoiditis, osteomyelitis, fracture, midline shift of the pineal.

• *CT scan* shows an abscess as a mass lesion, usually of low density with surrounding oedema and ring enhancement after intravenous contrast. Subdural empyema on the other hand is often so thin that it is invisible; there may be a thin rim of contrast enhancement over the cerebral hemisphere, swelling of the underlying hemisphere and midline shift of the brain. A parafalcine collection of pus is typical and requires scans to the vertex to be seen.

• *Carotid angiography* is required if there are no CT scanning facilities and, even if there are, may still be required if a subdural empyema is suspected, to demonstrate the avascular gap between the skull and the underlying cerebral hemisphere, or in the parafalcine region.

• *Culture* of pus from abscess, blood, sinuses, sputum, etc., both aerobically and anaerobically.

• *Lumbar puncture is contraindicated.* If it is done inadvertently, then the CSF may be normal or show merely a mild cellular reaction with a raised protein and normal glucose, and no visible organisms or bacterial growth (i.e. similar to acute viral encephalitis, tuberculous or viral meningitis).

If, despite several normal CT scans with i.v. contrast, a subdural empyema is still strongly suspected, then exploratory burr holes may be necessary.

Treatment

Whether to undertake burr hole aspiration or a formal craniotomy with excision of the abscess is a technical neurosurgical decision, but some kind of drainage is almost always necessary. Sinus, ear, mastoid and orbital sup-puration must be treated on their own merits.

In the first instance the antibiotic regime should be:

- i.v. benzylpenicillin, 200 mg/kg/day in 4-hourly boluses (omit if allergic to penicillin) *plus*
- i.v. chloramphenicol, 75 mg/kg/day in children and 3 g daily in adults in 8-hourly doses *plus*
- i.v. metronidazole, 500 mg (infused over 1 hour) 6-hourly (7.5 mg/kg 6-hourly in children)

If staphylococcal infection is likely (post-neurosurgery, ventricular shunts, etc.), then instead of benzylpenicillin use:

- i.v. fusidic acid, 500 mg over 6 hours 8-hourly (particularly if there is osteomyelitis), or
- i.v. flucloxacillin, 1 g 4-hourly, in children 50 mg/kg/day.

Intravenous therapy must be continued until the patient is neurologically stable, if not actually recovered, when it may be possible to change to oral therapy for several weeks. The final choice of antibiotics, and the dose, depends on bacterial sensitivities and serum levels.

Case fatality is about 20% and the morbidity amongst survivors is high, particularly seizures.

Spinal epidural abscess

Pus or infected granulation tissue in the epidural space is a complication of septicaemia, adjacent vertebral osteomyelitis or a local surgical procedure. Any part of the spine can be affected. The usual organisms are *Staph. aureus* (p. 508) or streptococci (p. 507), occasionally *Brucella* (p. 510), *Salmonella* (p. 509) or a fungus (p. 531) (also see spinal TB, p. 513).

The illness is usually subacute with local and severe back pain, tender-ness, root pain and the development of spinal cord and/or root disturbance (p. 320) as a result of compression or vasculitis in the context of the systemic signs of a bacterial infection (fever, malaise, blood leucocytosis, etc.).

The differential diagnosis includes:

- acute prolapsed disc (p. 326)
- epidural haemorrhage (p. 320)
- transverse myelitis (p. 332)
- spinal cord infarction (p. 333)

Spinal X-ray may reveal the bone changes of osteomyelitis and myelo-graphy shows cord compression. The CSF is sterile or contains an excess of polymorph neutrophils, lymphocytes and protein.

Treatment is surgical decompression and drainage and high doses of antibiotics appropriate for the infecting microorganism.

Bacterial infections

Meningococcus

Neisseria meningitidis, the meningococcus, is a Gram negative diplococcus commonly carried in the throat of asymptomatic individuals and spread by droplets. In a small proportion of people it causes clinical disease, most commonly bacterial meningitis at any age which may be sporadic or there may be outbreaks in families, schools and army camps.

The clinical and CSF features are similar to those of any other form of bacterial meningitis (p. 491) but, in this context, a petechial or purpuric rash (skin, conjunctiva, palate) is almost diagnostic. Meningococcaemia is common and there may be infective or allergic complications such as arthritis, episcleritis, myocarditis, pericarditis, disseminated intravascular coagulation and cutaneous vasculitis. Acute adrenal haemorrhagic necrosis complicates severe cases and may cause endotoxic shock (Waterhouse–Friederichsen syndrome).

Treatment

Treatment is with benzylpenicillin, i.v. 150 mg/kg/day in 4-hourly boluses for about 7 days.

If the organism turns out to be sensitive, oral sulphonamides can be substituted: sulphadiazine 100 mg/kg/day in adults, 200 mg/kg/day in children in 6-hourly doses.

If allergic to penicillin, use i.v. or i.m. chloramphenicol, 3 g daily in 8-hourly boluses (children 75 mg/kg/day), changing to the oral route when feasible for a total of about 7 days.

Hypotensive crisis should be treated with circulatory support, dopamine, and perhaps i.v. hydrocortisone.

Contacts and index cases on hospital discharge should be given oral rifampicin for 2 days: 600 mg twice daily in adults, 10 mg/kg twice daily in children; 5 mg/kg twice daily if under 1 year. If the organism in the index case is sensitive, then adult contacts can be given sulphadiazine 1 g twice daily, and 500 mg twice daily in children for 2 days. Vaccination against some strains may be feasible and can be offered in addition to chemoprophylaxis to close contacts, and as an alternative to distant contacts.

Haemophilus influenzae

H. influenzae is a Gram negative bacillus frequently carried in the nasopharynx of normal children and adults. The encapsulated type b strain is the most common cause of bacterial meningitis in small children, very few cases occurring outside the range of 3 months to 4 years. The clinical and CSF features are similar to those of other types of bacterial meningitis (p. 491), but it can be difficult to see the organisms on Gram stains of the CSF. Septic arthritis and epiglottitis may complicate the meningitis.

Treatment

Treatment is with chloramphenicol, 3 g daily in 8-hourly doses i.v. or i.m., and then oral as soon as swallowing is possible for a total of about 10 days (75 mg/kg/day in children). The risk of marrow suppression has been greatly exaggerated. In the UK less than 2% of strains are resistant and should then be treated with cefotaxime.

Household and nursery contacts aged less than 5 should be carefully observed and perhaps treated with oral rifampicin (see under meningococcal infection above) for 4 days to reduce the 2% risk of a second case. Small outbreaks occasionally occur but true epidemics do not.

Streptococcal infection

Streptococci are Gram positive cocci and several species cause infections of the nervous system. There is nothing particularly specific about the neurological features of streptococcal infection and the bacteriological diagnosis is straightforward.

Strep. pyogenes (group A streptococci)

This is a common cause of suppuration in the paranasal sinuses and middle ear which in very rare cases spreads locally to cause meningitis at any age, including neonates. Meningitis is an occasional complication of streptococcal septicaemia. Myositis is rare (p. 436).

Strep. pneumoniae (pneumococcus)

This is carried in the nasopharynx from where it can spread by droplets to cause pneumonia, sinusitis and otitis media. It is a common cause of bacterial meningitis at any age, particularly over the age of 40 and as a complication of head injury. There is a high case fatality (about 30%) even with appropriate treatment. The meninges are invaded by local or septicaemic spread and complicating cerebral abscess or subdural empyema can arise. Not all cases have an obvious source of infection such as pneumonia and in the elderly there may merely be a rather indolent illness with fever and increasing confusion without much in the way of meningism. Severe infection tends to occur in splenectomized patients or in those with hypogammaglobulinaemia, complement deficiencies and sickle cell disease.

Strep. milleri

This causes suppurative dental and sinus infection in the middle-aged and elderly and then complicating subdural empyema (p. 503), cerebral abscess (p. 503), bacterial meningitis (p. 491) and septicaemia.

Strep. agalactiae (group B streptococci)

This is a cause of neonatal bacterial meningitis (p. 491) and septicaemia and rarely causes infection in adults.

Strep. suis (group R streptococci)

This causes bacterial meningitis (p. 491) in meat handlers and farmers. Deafness is a common complication.

Treatment

Treatment is with penicillin since almost all streptococci are highly sensitive: i.v. benzylpenicillin, 150 mg/kg/day in 4-hourly boluses for about 14 days. For pneumococcal and *Strep. agalactiae* infections, and for other streptococcal infections which involve more than just the meninges, the dose should be 200 mg/kg/day and continued for 2–3 weeks.

If patients are allergic to penicillin, then chloramphenicol is an alternative (p. 507).

Note: Antibiotic sensitivities must be checked since penicillin-resistant pneumococci are now appearing.

Staphylococcal infection

Staph. aureus

Staph. aureus, a Gram positive coccus, is a common cause of suppuration in many organs, wound infection and septicaemia. However, it rarely causes infection of the nervous system; it is an unusual cause of bacterial meningitis (p. 491), but a rather more frequent cause of cerebral abscess (p. 503), subdural empyema (p. 503), spinal epidural abscess (p. 505) and myositis (p. 436). These infections are caused by septicaemia or local spread (head injury, neurosurgical procedure, ventricular shunt, CSF fistula).

Staph. epidermidis

Staph. epidermidis (*albus*) is a more likely cause of intraventricular shunt infection which can usually be eradicated only by removing the shunt.

Treatment

Since most staphylococci are resistant to penicillin, treatment should start 'blind' with flucloxacillin and, if bone is involved, fusidic acid as well. When antibiotic sensitivities are known, the treatment can be tailored accordingly:

- flucloxacillin, i.v. 1 g 4-hourly (in children 50 mg/kg/day)
- fusidic acid, i.v. 500 mg over 6 hours, 8-hourly, followed by oral 500 mg 8-hourly

For patients allergic to penicillin, vancomycin should be used.

Usually 7 days of treatment are sufficient, but if there is bone involvement or serious intracranial infection then at least 4 weeks are necessary.

Enterobacteria

These are Gram negative bacilli inhabiting the gastrointestinal tract. They tend to cause neurological infections in neonates and the elderly.

Salmonella

Salmonella infection of the bowel may be complicated by septicaemia and then rarely by focal infection in almost any organ. Meningitis and cerebral abscess have been described and also an indolent vertebral osteomyelitis which can cause spinal cord/root compression (p. 505).

During typhoid fever, as well as delirium or coma, there may be psychotic features (mutism, catatonia, paranoia) and also cerebellar ataxia of the limbs and gait.

E. coli

E. coli is an occasional cause of meningitis, particularly in neonates and the elderly.

Proteus mirabilis

This is another cause of neonatal meningitis and sometimes intracranial abscess.

Pseudomonas pyocyanea

This causes an intractable meningitis but usually only in debilitated or immunocompromised patients, in neonates or as a complication of neurosurgical procedures.

Treatment

Treatment depends on the antibiotic sensitivities of the infecting organism and, while chloramphenicol (p. 507) is usually appropriate for *Salmonella*, Gram negative infections in neonates and debilitated adults may require i.v. gentamycin or cefotaxime.

Intrathecal administration of gentamicin, usually via an indwelling reservoir, can be used in severe infection to improve the local tissue level of antibiotic and reduce systemic toxicity, but is seldom very successful.

Brucellosis

Brucellosis is caused by a Gram negative coccobacillus and occurs in people in close contact with infected animals and carcasses (cows, goats, sheep, camels) or after drinking infected milk. There is an acute form with fever and malaise and a more indolent recurrent form with lethargy, headache, fever, myalgia, anorexia and weight loss. Neurological complications may be the presenting feature or part of the generalized acute or chronic illness:
- subacute meningoencephalitis (p. 498) with a lymphocytic CSF, raised protein and sometimes a low glucose
- acute or chronic bacterial meningitis (p. 491)
- cerebellar syndrome with or without cranial nerve involvement
- acute or subacute myelitis (p. 332)
- spinal epidural abscess (p. 505)
- subacute proximal motor polyradiculopathy and/or peripheral neuropathy with raised CSF protein and lymphocytes (cf. Guillain–Barré syndrome, p. 398, borrelia, p. 517, HIV, p. 526)

The organism is difficult to culture from blood and CSF and the diagnosis is usually made serologically.

Treatment is a combination of tetracycline, 500 mg 4 times daily, oral, for 6 weeks, plus streptomycin, 1 g daily i.m. for 3 weeks, or doxycycline, 200 mg oral once daily, plus rifampicin, 900 mg oral once daily for at least 6 weeks, is probably more effective.

Legionnaire's disease

This is an acute febrile illness characterized by pneumonia, myalgia and diarrhoea. It is caused by a Gram negative bacillus. Neurological features are common but unexplained, since no neuropathological changes seem to account for them:
- Diffuse encephalopathy which in the acute phase is reversible; drowsiness, confusion, hallucinations, headache.
- Cerebellar ataxia acutely but it can persist. Dysarthria and truncal ataxia are more prominent than limb ataxia.

- Acute rise in muscle CK but no clinical correlate.
- Guillain–Barré syndrome (p. 398).

The CSF is usually normal and the diagnosis made serologically or occasionally by isolation of the organism from the sputum.

Treatment is erythromycin, 1 g 6-hourly i.v. for 3 weeks and/or rifampicin, 300 mg twice daily oral.

Listeria monocytogenes

This is a short Gram positive bacillus with a worldwide distribution. It tends to cause disease in neonates, pregnant women, elderly, debilitated and immunocompromised hosts but many patients are normal. Neurological involvement is severe and may be in the context of only the non-specific features of an acute febrile illness:

- Acute purulent meningitis (p. 491), with a typical CSF for bacterial meningitis, but there may be more lymphocytes than neutrophils.
- Encephalitis (p. 498), with similar clinical and CSF features to viral encephalitis. However, focal features are common, particularly brainstem signs.
- Abscess (p. 503) in the cerebrum, brainstem or spinal cord, often with a normal CSF.

The diagnosis depends on culturing the organism from the CSF or blood, usually requiring selective media.

Treatment is ampicillin, i.v. 300 mg/kg/day in 4 divided doses, depending on sensitivity, which varies from strain to strain, until a week or two after fever subsides.

Campylobacter

This a Gram negative flagellated bacterium. It is a common cause of acute enterocolitis, occasionally with a high fever, delirium and even generalized convulsions. The illness may be followed by the Guillain–Barré syndrome (p. 398). The diagnosis is made serologically since the organism has usually been cleared from the stool before the onset of neurological symptoms. It is a very rare cause of meningitis and encephalitis.

Anthrax

Bacillus anthracis is a spore-bearing Gram positive bacillus. It is transmitted to man from animals and tends to occur in people handling raw animal products (carcasses, hides, wool, hair, bone).

The disease is usually cutaneous or pulmonary but occasionally bacterial meningitis occurs either alone or with obvious disease elsewhere. The CSF is blood-stained which is distinctly unusual in any other bacterial meningitis.

Actinomycosis

Actinomyces israelii is a filamentous branching Gram positive bacterium which is a normal commensal in the oropharynx. It may cause subacute granulomatous lesions in several sites (cervico-facial, thoracic, abdominal, pelvic) and is a rare cause of cerebral abscess and meningitis. It is sensitive to penicillin.

Nocardiasis

Nocardia is a similar organism to *A. israelii* and tends to cause opportunistic infection. Pulmonary infections are the most common but sometimes there is haematogenous spread to cause cerebral abscess and chronic meningitis. The treatment is a sulphonamide or minocycline.

Tuberculosis

Human, and occasionally bovine, tuberculosis is unusual in Western societies, although it is still common in developing countries. In the UK, disease affecting the nervous system is now seen mainly in immigrants, the indigent, immunosuppressed hosts and after gastrectomy. It occurs at any age.

It takes three main forms which may coexist: tuberculous meningitis (below) and less often intracerebral tuberculoma (p. 513) and spinal tuberculosis (p. 513). They are secondary infections and can be part of miliary TB, but quite often no other evidence of TB is found except perhaps for inactive calcified lesions on the chest X-ray.

TUBERCULOUS MENINGITIS

This is a serious illness. It is more indolent and subacute than pyogenic bacterial meningitis and presents with headache, meningism, lassitude, low grade fever, irritability and drowsiness. It is particularly likely to be complicated by cranial nerve palsies, hydrocephalus and cerebral vasculitis causing seizures, cerebral infarction, coma and spinal cord infarction. Choroidal tubercles are uncommon. Even after effective treatment the patients may be left seriously neurologically disabled.

Diagnosis

- The white blood cell count and ESR are normal or raised.
- The skin test for tuberculosis is not always positive.
- The chest X-ray may show a primary focus or miliary change, but is often normal.
- CT scan often shows hydrocephalus and meningeal enhancement with

i.v. contrast. Also, any complicating infarction and tuberculomas may be seen (see below). The scan can be normal. However, a normal scan after i.v. enhancement in a drowsy patient more or less rules out tuberculous meningitis.

• The CSF is the most crucial diagnostic test (p. 493). If the clinical picture and CSF findings are suggestive but no acid fast bacilli can be stained, the CSF examination should be repeated, if necessary several times. Even then acid fast bacilli may not be seen and treatment has to be started 'blind' before there is a definite bacterial diagnosis on culture. The CSF should be cultured but this takes time and is not always conclusive.

• Microscopy and culture of other body fluids for tubercle bacilli, e.g. sputum, early morning urine, gastric aspirates.

• Enquire about TB in contacts.

The main differential diagnoses are:
• encephalitis (p. 498)
• bacterial meningitis (p. 491)
• fungal meningitis (p. 532)
• malignant meningitis (p. 277)
• sarcoidosis (p. 472)
• cerebral abscess (p. 503)
• subdural empyema (p. 503)

TUBERCULOMA

This can present as an intracranial space-occupying lesion with some combination of focal signs, seizures and raised intracranial pressure. Fever, weight loss and other features of systemic infection are usually absent. The CT scan shows one or more lesions of any density which may enhance with contrast, uniformly or as a ring; there may be surrounding oedema and occasionally some calcification. Diagnosis by biopsy is required, unless there is obvious active tuberculosis elsewhere, to exclude other causes of cerebral abscess or neoplastic conditions. In high prevalence areas antituberculous treatment is given and biopsy only undertaken if there is no clinical and CT response in a matter of weeks.

SPINAL TB

Spinal TB occurs as a result of localized spinal meningitis (Pott's disease of the spine) with vertebral body collapse and destruction of the adjacent discs. It may cause root and/or cord compression (p. 320), arteritis and infarction of the spinal cord (p. 333), spinal arachnoiditis (p. 335) and very rarely a spinal cord tuberculoma.

Treatment

Initially a combination of three antibiotics should be used:
- rifampicin:
  600 mg daily as a single oral dose, 20 mg/kg/day in children. Adverse effects: fever, rash, hepatitis, nausea, vomiting, diarrhoea, thrombocytopenia. An early but transient rise in liver enzymes is common. Soft contact lenses may discolour and saliva and urine turn orange-red.
- pyrazinamide:
  30 mg/kg as a daily oral dose. Adverse effects: flushing, fever, nausea, vomiting, urticaria, arthralgia, hepatitis, hyperuricaemia.
- isoniazid:
  400 mg daily as a single oral dose, 10 mg/kg/day in children. Adverse effects: nausea, vomiting, rash, arthralgia, peripheral neuropathy, confusional and psychotic states, seizures, hepatitis, pellagra (p. 471).
- pyridoxine:
  Should always be given with isoniazid to prevent the peripheral neuropathy, 20 mg daily, oral.

  If rifampicin causes intolerable adverse effects, then streptomycin can be substituted: 1 g daily i.m.; 20–40 mg/kg/day in children. If renal impairment occurs, the dose must be reduced and in most patients' serum levels should be monitored in any case. Adverse effects include rash, vertigo, tinnitus, deafness, ataxia, nephrotoxicity, and exacerbation of myasthenia gravis.

  Ethambutol is sometimes used instead of pyrazinamide: 25 mg/kg/day for the first month, then 15 mg/kg/day as a single oral dose. Adverse effects include blurred vision, optic atrophy, peripheral neuropathy, hepatitis. Avoid in uraemia and in children.

  After 2 months, if the mycobacterium is found to be sensitive to all three antibiotics *in vitro*, rifampicin and isoniazid (and pyridoxine) should be continued together for about another 7 months.

Note:
- The dose of streptomycin must be lowered in renal failure.
- Corticosteroids do not have any routine use.
- Contacts must be screened for TB.
- Surgery may be required to relieve hydrocephalus and to remove a tuberculoma causing raised intracranial pressure.
- Tuberculoma may appear or, if present already, transiently increase in size at the start of medical treatment even when the clinical picture is improving.

Leprosy

Leprosy is a chronic inflammatory disease caused by *Mycobacterium leprae* with particular involvement of the skin and peripheral nerves. The diagnosis should be considered in anyone from an endemic area who has hypopigmented, anaesthetic and anhidrotic skin lesions; thickened cutaneous and peripheral nerves with motor and/or sensory loss in their distributions; a widespread but often patchy peripheral neuropathy, with loss of cutaneous but normal positional sensation and a tendency to spare warm areas (groins, perineum, axillae, hairy scalp). In lepromatous cases there are extensive skin lesions with thickening, plaques and nodules; destruction of the nasal cartilage and bone; ulceration and loss of fingers and toes due to painless and repeated trauma. Weakness of the facial muscles, orbicularis oculi and frontalis muscles is common. The tendon reflexes are preserved and there is no autonomic involvement. Acute exacerbations ('reactions') of the dermal and neural lesions may occur during treatment.

The diagnosis is confirmed by skin biopsy and finding acid fast bacilli in all except the milder cases and, if necessary, by nerve biospy. *Note*: other causes of thickened nerves (p. 393).

Treatment is with a combination of dapsone, rifampicin and clofazimine.

Syphilis

Clinically evident infection of the nervous system with *Treponema pallidum* is now rare. However, because it is rare and takes many different forms, it is easy to forget. Since it is treatable, it is reasonable to ask for syphilis blood serology in most, if not all, patients with organic disease of the central nervous system if there is no other definite diagnosis.

There is considerable overlap between the main clinical syndromes:

Meningovascular syphilis may occur from the time of the secondary syphilis rash to 10 years after the primary infection. It is due to granulomatous syphilitic infiltration and vasculitis around the brainstem, spinal cord and spinal roots. The features include:
- acute, subacute and chronic meningitis (p. 491)
- acute and subacute cranial nerve palsies
- optic neuritis (p. 343), optic atrophy and choroidoretinitis
- Argyll Robertson pupils (p. 177)
- seizures
- stroke, transient ischaemic attacks and mental confusion
- acute and subacute deafness (unilateral at first)
- acute and subacute spinal cord and/or root syndromes (transverse myelitis, p. 332, spinal cord infarction, p. 333, compression, p. 320)
- hydrocephalus (p. 259)
  There is usually no fever.

Tabes dorsalis develops 20 years or so after the primary infection. There is neuronal loss in the posterior columns and dorsal root entry zones of the spinal cord. The features include:
- gait ataxia due to loss of joint position sense in the lower limbs

- hypotonia and loss of deep tendon reflexes in the legs and also perhaps the arms, sometimes with extensor plantar responses
- lightning pains in the legs and back
- loss of deep pain sensation in the legs
- patchy loss of superficial pain sensation on the face and limbs
- Charcot joints in the lower limbs (p. 00)
- trophic foot ulcers
- impotence
- urinary and faecal retention/incontinence and dysuria
- Argyll Robertson pupils (p. 00)
- postural hypotension (p. 00)
- sensorineural deafness
- optic atrophy (p. 00)
- ptosis
- abdominal pains and vomiting

General paresis of the insane (GPI) is due to widespread spirochaetal invasion of the brain and chronic meningovascular syphilis. It appears about 20 years after the primary infection and the clinical features include:
- dementia, delusional syndromes
- Argyll Robertson pupils (p. 177)
- seizures
- tremor

Diagnosis

In almost all cases blood serology is positive if both non-specific antibody (Wassermann reaction, WR, or now the venereal disease research laboratory slide test, VDRL) and specific antibody (*Treponema pallidum* haemagglutination test, TPHA, fluorescent treponemal antibody test, FTA, or treponema pallidum immobilization test, TPI) tests are carried out.

The CSF must be examined if:
- the clinical picture is very suggestive but the blood serology is negative
- there is positive blood serology and a compatible clinical picture

In *active* disease the CSF contains excess lymphocytes and a moderate increase in protein; if these are normal, the patient's disease is 'burnt out' or the diagnosis of syphilis is wrong. The specific serology is usually positive in the CSF; occasionally the VDRL is negative. The glucose is normal. Oligoclonal bands are common.

It is unnecessary to examine the CSF if the blood serological titres are low, the patient has had effective treatment for syphilis in the past, or the clinical picture is incompatible or clearly due to a non-syphilitic cause.

Note: Syphilis cannot be serologically differentiated from yaws, a spirochaetal disease which is endemic in the Caribbean.

Treatment

Treatment for active disease (i.e. with raised protein and/or lymphocytes in the CSF) is i.m. procaine penicillin, 600 mg daily for 21 days. If allergic to penicillin, erythromycin, 500 mg oral 6-hourly for 30 days. Probably a more effective alternative, but which has the disadvantage of hospital admission, is i.v. benzylpenicillin, 600 mg daily for 10 days.

For one day before and 3 days after beginning treatment give oral prednisolone, 40 mg daily, to avoid the Herxheimer reaction.

The CSF must be re-examined at 3 months, 6 months, 12 months and 24 months. If the raised cell count persists, then treatment should be repeated until it is normal. The protein level may not normalize for a year or so after successful treatment. The blood and CSF serology often remains positive for life, although the VDRL titres should fall.

Meningovascular syphilis can be cured and GPI and tabes dorsalis arrested, although fixed neurological deficits will likely remain along with any lightning pains. The latter may be helped by carbamazepine (p. 90).

Note: If in doubt whether the disease is active, then treat just in case it is.

Leptospirosis

Leptospirosis is caused by a spirochaete acquired by contact with infected animals (particularly rats and cattle) or with water contaminated by their urine. At-risk groups include farm workers, sewermen, miners and freshwater sportsmen.

It is a biphasic illness. The septicaemic phase lasts about a week with fever, headache, myalgia, conjunctivitis, rash, abdominal pain, renal failure and, in severe cases, jaundice and liver failure. In the second week an aseptic meningitis develops with uveitis, rash and recurrent fever. The CSF contains excess polymorph neutrophils or lymphocytes, but is otherwise normal. In the first phase the organism can be isolated from blood and urine, but later the diagnosis depends on serological tests.

Treatment is i.v. benzylpenicillin, 150 mg/kg/day in 6-hourly boluses for about 7 days.

Borrelia burgdorferi (Lyme disease or Bannwarth's syndrome)

The ixodes tick, which infests deer and small mammals, carries the spirochaete *B. burgdorferi* which is transmitted to man by a bite. Within a few days an erythematous papule appears which turns into an expanding annular lesion with a partially clearing centre (erythema chronicum migrans), sometimes with multiple secondary skin lesions and often accompanied by general malaise, headache and lymphadenopathy.

Sometimes a more indolent and debilitating illness follows or occurs *de novo* with increasing headache, neck stiffness, fever, fatigue, myalgia, arthralgia and cardiac arrhythmias. This may be followed some weeks later by recurrent arthritis and/or, in some patients, neurological complications including:

- 7th cranial nerve palsy, unilateral or bilateral (cf. Bell's palsy, p. 191), and occasionally other cranial nerve palsies
- polyradiculopathy with severe root pain, sensory and motor loss (cf. Guillain–Barré syndrome, p. 398)
- mononeuritis multiplex (p. 370)
- neuralgic amyotrophy (p. 368)
- subacute or chronic meningitis (p. 491)
- transverse myelitis (p. 332)
- subacute or chronic but usually rather mild encephalitis (p. 498)
- myositis

The neurological complications are mostly subacute, accompanied by fatigue rather than by any of the earlier features which have usually resolved by then, and usually recover spontaneously in weeks or months. In some patients there is no preceding skin lesion, not very much systemic upset, and no remembered insect bite.

Diagnosis

The disease usually appears in the summer in endemic areas: in the USA where it is known as Lyme disease, in Europe where it is called Bannwarth's syndrome, and in Australia. The peripheral blood white count is normal or lymphopenic and the ESR may be raised. If there are neurological complications, the CSF is lymphocytic with a raised protein but normal glucose, and a raised IgG/albumin ratio with oligoclonal bands; it can occasionally be normal. Isolation of the spirochaete from the blood, CSF and skin is difficult. Serological tests can be misleading; a raised serum IgG does not necessarily indicate active infection and the serum IgM may no longer be raised at the stage of neurological complications. CSF serology may be more helpful.

The differential diagnosis of the neurological complications includes viral encephalitis (p. 498), Bell's palsy (p. 191), chronic meningitis (p. 497) and the Guillain–Barré syndrome (p. 398), but in the latter there is no CSF pleocytosis.

Treatment

Benzylpenicillin, i.v. 200 mg/kg/day in 6-hourly doses for 14 days, or oral tetracycline, 500 mg 4 times daily for 30 days.

Tetanus

Clostridium tetani, a Gram positive bacillus, may contaminate deep and necrotic wounds and secrete a neurotoxin to cause tetanus. In some patients the wound is trivial or there is even no history of wounding. The disease is now rare in Western countries.

Clinical features

Within days or weeks of the injury there is, over a few days, the onset of stiffness, pain and rigidity in voluntary muscles — usually first the jaw, face and abdomen followed by neck, pharynx, back and sometimes limbs. The disease may be mild and progress no further. However, involuntary spasms of the affected muscles, which are painful and frightening, may develop. The rigidity and spasms cause:
- difficulty opening the jaw (trismus)
- facial stiffness and grimacing (risus sardonicus)
- dysphagia for food, liquids and even saliva
- neck and back hyperextension, occasionally causing vertebral body fracture
- respiratory failure due to laryngeal spasm, respiratory muscle spasm and inhalation pneumonia

Spasms are precipitated by startle, cough, touch and a full bladder. Laryngeal spasm can be precipitated by swallowing or the passage of a nasogastric tube.

Other features include:
- hyperreflexia
- little or no fever
- ophthalmoplegia and facial weakness are rare
- in severe cases, sympathetic overactivity and lability (labile blood pressure and heart rate, cardiac arrhythmias, sweating, fever, salivation, gastric stasis)

The disease progresses over about a week, stabilizes for another week, and then recovers over several weeks. It is of very variable severity with an overall case fatality of about 10%.

Diagnosis

This is entirely clinical with differentiation from:
- acute drug induced dystonia (p. 302)
- hysteria
- rabies (p. 529)
- other causes of trismus (infection in pterygomandibular space, facial or jaw trauma, psychogenic, drug-induced dystonia, strychnine poisoning)

The CSF is normal (cf. rabies).

Management

- Excise and debride any wound.
- Benzylpenicillin, i.v. 100 mg/kg/day in 6-hourly doses for one week.

- Human antitetanus immunoglobulin, i.m. at multiple sites because large volume, 100 units/kg, followed by routine immunization with toxoid.
- Good nursing in quiet surroundings.
- Sedation with oral or i.v. diazepam.
- Tracheostomy if rigidity or spasms interfere with swallowing or breathing.
- Paralysis and ventilation if spasms become severe.
- Nutrition and fluid balance maintained with i.v. line, or nasogastric tube if the spasms are not severe; if they are, the patient must be intubated and ventilated. Mild cases can be fed orally.
- Beta-blockade or combined alpha and beta-blockade as necessary for labile blood pressure and heart rate.
- Low dose heparin to prevent deep vein thrombosis (5000 units subcutaneously twice daily).

Botulism

Ingestion of food contaminated with *Clostridium botulinum* may, if the organism has released its neurotoxin, produce botulism which varies in severity from a mild self-limiting illness to severe weakness and death within hours. In infants the toxin can be produced by bacteria colonizing the gut. The neurotoxin blocks cholinergic transmission in motor and autonomic nerves. Botulism is extremely rare in the UK, tending to occur in outbreaks in relation to contaminated food.

Symptoms arise within hours or days of ingestion, with dry mouth and eyes, blurred vision, diplopia, imbalance, nausea, vomiting, dysphagia and dysarthria. At this stage there is lower motor neurone weakness of muscles innervated by the cranial nerves and unreactive pupils. The flaccid weakness then spreads to the limbs, trunk and respiratory muscles and is of the lower motor neurone type. Other autonomic features include constipation, urinary retention and hypotension. There is no fever, there are very rarely any sensory features and consciousness is normal. The CSF is normal.

The differential diagnosis is:
- myasthenia gravis (Chapter 15)
- Guillain–Barré syndrome (p. 398)
- atropine and organophosphorus poisoning (p. 548)
- diphtheria (below)
- polio (p. 522)
- porphyria (p. 398)

The diagnosis can be supported by EMG and confirmed by finding toxin in the serum, faeces or stomach contents by innoculation into mice; also, by isolating the organism from the suspect food or its container.

Diphtheria

Diphtheria is now almost extinct in the UK but is still common in some developing countries. The acute febrile and toxic illness, particularly if involving the nasopharynx, is sometimes complicated a few weeks later by progressive lower motor neurone paralysis; palatal weakness is common and may be followed by weakness of the extraocular, pharyngeal, laryngeal, respiratory and limb muscles. This is due to a neurotoxin secreted by the bacillus which causes a demyelinating peripheral neuropathy, predominantly motor.

Antitoxin and penicillin are probably ineffective once paralysis is present. Good nursing and respiratory care may allow survival until natural recovery occurs.

Cat scratch disease

This is probably due to a bacterial infection and may occasionally be complicated by encephalitis, transverse myelitis, radiculitis and cerebral arteritis. The diagnosis depends on the history of cat scratch, characteristic lymph node histology (epitrochlear usually involved) and an antigen skin test.

Rickettsial diseases

Rickettsiae are obligate intracellular parasites, not true bacteria. The reservoir is in mammals (particularly rodents) and the vectors are arthropods (ticks, lice, etc.). Disease in man includes rocky mountain spotted fever, Q-fever and epidemic murine and scrub typhus. Encephalitis is an occasional complication due to direct infection, vasculitis or both. Treatment is chloramphenicol or a tetracycline.

Mycoplasma pneumoniae

This is a micro-organism without a cell wall, but free living like bacteria, which causes upper respiratory tract symptoms and a rather protracted pneumonic and febrile illness. Occasionally this can be complicated by various self-limiting neurological disorders which do not appear to be due to direct infection of the nervous system:

- meningitis (p. 491)
- encephalitis (p. 498)
- cranial nerve palsy
- transverse myelitis (p. 332)
- acute cerebellar syndrome
- Guillain–Barré syndrome (p. 398)

Sometimes there is no obvious pneumonic component. The CSF is either normal or shows a lymphocytic response. The diagnosis is serological and about 50% have cold agglutinins in the blood.

Treatment is tetracycline or erythromycin.

Viral infections

Mild degrees of neck stiffness, drowsiness and even confusion with diffuse slowing of the EEG are common in a wide range of acute febrile illnesses caused by viral infection. This probably represents a mild form of meningitis or even encephalitis and, if the CSF is examined, there may be a mild excess of lymphocytes and protein. However, it is only when neurological features become more obvious that the diagnosis of meningitis or encephalitis becomes relevant or even entertained (e.g. severe headache, neck stiffness, coma, seizures). Certain viruses are more likely than others to cause neurological problems and these are described individually.

Enteroviruses

These are widespread and commonly cause a non-specific febrile respiratory illness, particularly in the summer, and affect children more often than adults. Sometimes there is a maculopapular or other type of rash. Coxsackie, echo and polio infection may be complicated by meningitis (p. 491) and rarely by encephalitis (p. 498), transverse myelitis (p. 332) and acute cerebellar ataxia. Generalized or focal myositis (Bornholm disease, p. 437) is a characteristic complication, usually of Coxsackie.

Paralytic polio is now a rare complication of any enteroviral meningitic illness but it is most severe and most likely with polio virus infection. Over a few days, usually just after the early meningitic phase, a flaccid paralysis develops with loss of the tendon reflexes, often with fasciculations. It is due to viral infection of the spinal anterior horn cells and/or the motor nuclei of the brainstem. The severity and distribution of weakness vary and it is usually asymmetrical. Limb, respiratory, facial and bulbar muscles can all be affected. Back and limb pains are common. Transient urinary retention may occur.

Most patients recover in a few weeks, some are left with mild lower motor neurone paralysis and a few remain severely paralysed. Occasionally very slow deterioration of motor function occurs in survivors after many years of stable weakness and disability; more common late complications are progressive scoliosis, alveolar hypoventilation and chest infections causing respiratory failure leading to fatigue, morning headache, excessive day-time sleepiness and generalized weakness which can be relieved by respiratory support, particularly at night. Pressure palsies (p. 369) and spondylosis (p. 327) are other complications.

Occasionally paralytic polio develops in individuals, or their contacts, who have been given live polio vaccine; the risk is less than 1 case per million doses of vaccine.

The main differential diagnosis is the Guillain–Barré syndrome (p. 398), but polio usually causes fever and a lymphocytic CSF.

Herpes viruses

Herpes viruses all share a tendency to cause primary infection followed by a period of latency and then recrudescence, particularly in immunocompromised hosts.

Herpes simplex type 1 infection

This infection (the main cause of herpetic cold sores) can cause a severe necrotizing encephalitis at any age, probably by direct viral invasion of the brain. Clinically it cannot be reliably distinguished from other viral causes of encephalitis (p. 498). Acyclovir is the specific treatment (p. 502).

Herpes simplex type 2 infection

This is the main cause of anogenital herpes, which can occasionally be complicated by meningitis (p. 491), transverse myelitis (p. 332) and lumbosacral radiculitis (p. 368). The last of these may cause urinary retention, constipation, impotence and dermatomal sensory disturbance over the perineum. Encephalitis is very unusual except in neonates and the immunocompromised. Recovery is spontaneous.

Chicken pox (varicella-zoster virus)

This is occasionally complicated by encephalitis (p. 498), post-infectious encephalomyelitis (p. 502), involuntary movements, acute cerebellar ataxia, bilateral optic neuritis (p. 343) and the Guillain–Barré syndrome (p. 398). The diagnosis is obvious from the typical rash.

Herpes zoster

Herpes zoster is due to a recrudescence of the varicella virus which has remained latent in sensory nerve root ganglia after an episode of chicken pox. Usually zoster appears in otherwise normal people, but sometimes there is an underlying lymphoma, AIDS or other cause of immunosuppression. Neurological complications are easily diagnosable if there has been a typical vesicular rash either at the time or within the previous few weeks, or if vesicles can be found by an assiduous search (NB palate, external auditory meatus, behind the ear). The diagnosis is confirmed by a rise in the titre of antibodies in the serum and/or culture of vesicular fluid. Just occasionally there is pain but no rash, making the clinical diagnosis particularly difficult.

    The neurological complications are as follows:
- Sensory radiculopathy is common. There is pain for a few days before, during and sometimes after the rash, usually in much the same place. Dermatomal cutaneous sensory loss and dysaesthesia are common (usually in

the distribution of the rash) and may persist. The first division of the tri-geminal nerve and the thoracic roots are the most often involved.

- Motor radiculopathy is usually more or less in the radicular distribution corresponding to the rash. Flaccid weakness of variable severity develops over a matter of a few days and may affect the limbs, face (sometimes with loss of taste), diaphragm (phrenic nerve involvement), extraocular muscles, palate and other cranial nerves very rarely. Recovery takes weeks but some-times the weakness persists.
- Encephalitis (p. 498), acute post-infectious encephalomyelitis (p. 502) and transverse myelitis (p. 332) are all rare. Some patients with encephalitis have a widespread vasculitis identical to isolated granulomatous angiitis of the nervous system (p. 450).
- Guillain–Barré syndrome is rare (p. 398).
- Sacral radiculopathy may cause urinary retention, constipation, impo-tence and perineal pain and loss of sensation. The rash is usually over the sacral dermatomes (buttocks, anal canal, scrotum).
- Intracranial subintimal fibromuscular proliferative vasculopathy may cause ischaemic or much less often haemorrhagic stroke(s) usually a few weeks after the onset of ophthalmic zoster, and usually within the ipsilateral middle cerebral artery distribution.

If there is neurological involvement, the CSF usually has a modest excess of lymphocytes and protein.

Treatment: i.v. acyclovir (p. 502), only for neurologically serious or im-munocompromised cases since recovery is usually spontaneous and the drug has no major effect on post-herpetic neuralgia. If given orally, the dose must be 800 mg 5 times daily.

Epstein–Barr (EB) virus

This is the most common cause of the glandular fever syndrome or infectious mononucleosis. Neurological complications occur in perhaps 1%, usually during the acute illness, sometimes as a presenting feature, and rarely in isolation without 'glandular' features:

- acute viral meningitis (p. 491)
- acute encephalitis which is often mild and manifest by generalized seizures and CSF lymphocytosis (p. 498)
- acute cerebellar syndrome with limb and truncal ataxia, dysarthria and inconstant nystagmus
- Guillain–Barré syndrome (p. 398)
- isolated cranial nerve palsies, particularly the 7th
- transverse myelitis (p. 332)
- optic neuritis (p. 173)

Usually the neurological complications recover. The diagnosis is made from the associated glandular fever, atypical blood lymphocytes, a positive monospot or Paul–Bunnell test, a rising titre of EB virus antibodies and positive IgM antibody.

Cytomegalovirus (CMV)

This is usually acquired subclinically but sometimes causes a glandular fever-like syndrome. Infection with CMV may be followed by the Guillain–Barré syndrome (p. 398) and it occasionally causes an encephalitis (p. 498). Immunocompromised hosts are particularly vulnerable to CMV infections of all kinds. In AIDS (p. 526) there is a subacute progressive encephalopathy, which is sometimes caused by CMV, with a modest increase in CSF cells and protein. The CT scan is normal or shows atrophy. AIDS patients may also develop a subacute cauda equina syndrome, often painful, due to CMV radiculitis.

Congenitally acquired CMV damages the fetus and neurological features include mental retardation, microcephaly, seizures, deafness, hydrocephalus, choroidoretinitis and optic atrophy.

Diagnosis of CMV infection is made serologically but can be difficult since significant antibody titres are commonly found in asymptomatic individuals and CMV may be reactivated by other infections, so causing a raised IgM antibody.

Mumps

This virus may cause:
- acute meningitis, clinically no different from any other viral meningitis (p. 491); often there is no accompanying parotitis
- encephalitis (p. 498), sometimes with polio-like paralytic features and an acute cerebellar syndrome
- acute post-infectious encephalomyelitis (p. 502)

Measles

This may affect the nervous system in four main ways:
- Acute encephalitis (p. 498), sometimes manifested only by drowsiness and generalized seizures. It is mild and occurs during the acute exanthem. The brain is invaded by virus.
- Acute post-infectious encephalomyelitis (p. 502) is a more severe illness which is clinically indistinguishable from encephalitis except that it is said to start later in the exanthem.
- Subacute delayed measles inclusion body encephalitis develops months or years after measles. Often the patients are immunosuppressed. This is a progressive encephalopathic illness, often fatal.
- Subacute sclerosing panencephalitis is an extremely rare disease in children and adolescents caused by persistent measles infection of the brain. A

few years after measles, or in rare cases live measles vaccination, the patient gradually becomes demented and develops myoclonic jerks, spasticity and rigidity. Death occurs in about 2 years. In the CSF the total protein and cells are usually normal, but there are oligoclonal bands and a very high gamma globulin level. The CSF measles antibody titre is extremely high as it is in the blood. Characteristic periodic complexes (p. 54) appear on the EEG. Inosiplex is said to prolong survival by a year or two: oral, 100 mg/kg/day in 4-hourly doses.

Rubella

This is a particularly important cause of intra-uterine infection leading to the 'congenital rubella syndrome' which includes neurological features such as deafness, microcephaly and mental retardation. Occasionally acquired rubella may be complicated by:
- encephalitis, probably of the post-infectious type (p. 502)
- transverse myelitis (p. 332)
- Guillain–Barré syndrome (p. 398)
- a very rare progressive chronic encephalitis in children appearing some years after rubella or the 'congenital rubella syndrome'. Serum and CSF rubella antibodies are raised, with a markedly raised CSF IgG and oligoclonal bands

Influenza

In rare cases this is complicated by encephalitis (p. 498), post-infectious encephalomyelitis (p. 502), the Guillain–Barré syndrome (p. 398) and myositis (p. 436).

Lymphocytic choriomeningitis

This is a rare cause of meningoencephalitis with fever and myalgia. Human infections are secondary to contact with an infected (usually symptomatic) rodent, e.g. mouse, hamster, gerbil. The diagnosis is made serologically.

Arthropod-borne viruses

Numerous viruses transmitted mostly by mosquitoes and ticks cause encephalitis within the context of an acute febrile illness. None occur in the UK but patients may arrive by air already infected. Most of the warmer parts of the world have endemic areas and in central Europe the viral transmission is usually via ticks.

Acquired immune deficiency syndrome (AIDS)

This is caused by infection with the human immunodeficiency virus (HIV) and, in the UK, is at present largely confined to homosexual and bisexual men, with a few cases in intravenous drug abusers, recipients of infected blood, heterosexual contacts of infected patients and babies born to infected mothers. Neurological complications of AIDS are common but their frequency and inter-relationships are still being worked out.

Direct viral infection of the nervous system may cause:
* acute meningoencephalitis soon after infection and preceding or co-inciding with seroconversion. Clinically it is similar to any other viral encephalitis (p. 498) or meningitis (p. 491) and neurological recovery occurs in a few weeks although the underlying HIV infection remains
* subacute polyneuritis at the time of seroconversion. Although the clinical picture is similar to that of the Guillain–Barré syndrome (p. 398), the CSF contains lymphocytes. Usually the patient recovers
* AIDS dementia complex is the most common neurological feature of the full blown AIDS syndrome, with insidious onset of dementia, usually some years after infection and seroconversion. Focal cognitive defects are unusual (aphasia, apraxia, etc.); apathy, poor concentration and memory, and depression are more characteristic, with increasing clumsiness and ataxia. The CSF shows an excess of lymphocytes; excess IgG and oligoclonal bands are present and HIV can be grown. CT shows rapidly progressive cortical atrophy with ventricular dilatation
* chronic meningitis (p. 497) may cause persisting headache, cranial nerve palsies and a lymphocytic CSF usually in the pre-AIDS stage. This may remit
* chronic spinal cord syndrome (vacuolar myelopathy) often accompanies the AIDS dementia complex and chronic peripheral neuropathies. The white matter is involved, leading to paraplegia, ataxia and incontinence of urine
* chronic distal sensorimotor and autonomic neuropathy, mononeuropathies and mononeuritis multiplex, are frequent in full blown AIDS; the CSF may contain excess lymphocytes but does have a high IgG level and oligoclonal bands
* polymyositis can precede or accompany AIDS. *Note*: zidovudine may cause an inflammatory myopathy

Opportunistic infections of the nervous system in AIDS:
* toxoplasmosis (p. 536), with encephalitis and granulomas, is the most common
* herpes zoster is also common (p. 523)
* cytomegalovirus encephalitis, retinitis and painful radiculitis (p. 525)
* cryptococcal meningitis (p. 533)
* tuberculosis and other mycobacterial infections are unusual (p. 512)
* herpes simplex encephalitis, radiculitis, myelitis (p. 523)
* progressive multifocal leucoencephalopathy (p. 530)
* candida is rare (p. 533)

These opportunistic infections are common in AIDS and more than one may be present at any one time. They can be difficult to distinguish from the direct neurological effects of HIV but this is important since some are treatable.

Cerebrovascular complications are unusual:
• intracranial haemorrhage due to thrombocytopenia
• cerebral infarction due to marantic endocarditis (p. 477), herpes zoster vasculopathy (p. 524)

CNS malignancies may occur:
• primary CNS lymphoma (p. 275)
• systemic lymphoma with CNS involvement
• Kaposi's sarcoma (very rare)

Also the patient may be affected by the other complications of AIDS (e.g. pneumocystis pneumonia), drugs used to treat AIDS, poor nutrition, alcoholism, drug abuse and the emotional reaction to having the disease.

Diagnosis

Usually the patient with neurological symptoms is known to be HIV positive, or to have full blown AIDS, but the diagnosis of AIDS should be considered in *any* 'neurological' patient who is at risk (see at risk groups above) and it can be strongly argued that HIV antibody testing should be as routine as syphilis serology in all 'neurological' patients without some other definite diagnosis.

In HIV positive patients with spinal cord, peripheral nerve or muscle syndromes there are usually no directly treatable possibilities because they are largely due to direct HIV infection. However, it is still important to make the diagnosis of the site of the lesion and then, if reasonable, to exclude non-AIDS causes for the neurological syndrome, e.g. spinal cord compression, etc. Examination of the CSF may reveal infection or malignancy. If there are intracranial symptoms (dementia, headache, seizures, focal signs, cranial nerve palsies, etc.), then the first step is an enhanced CT scan. Enhancing focal lesions may be due to:
• toxoplasmosis (usually multiple) (p. 536)
• lymphoma (usually single) (p. 275)
• tuberculoma (multiple or single) (p. 513)

Atrophy on CT scan may indicate AIDS dementia complex but does not exclude other complications, and focal white matter hypodensity may indicate progressive multifocal leucoencephalopathy (p. 530). Whether the CT scan is normal or abnormal, provided it is safe to do so (p. 43), the CSF should be cultured and examined for excess cells and protein which can be minimal even when there is meningitis; opportunistic infections should be excluded by appropriate CSF and blood serology. Coincidental syphilis (p. 515) must be excluded.

Note: Cranial nerve palsies may be due not only to direct HIV infection but to fungal and TB meningitis, and lymphoma.

Treatment

The course of AIDS may be retarded by zidovudine (AZT) which is well absorbed orally with good CSF penetration; 3.5 mg/kg 4-hourly given indefinitely if anaemia and neutropenia are not limiting. Adverse effects include headache, nausea, vomiting, myalgia, insomnia, bluish nail pigmentation, marrow suppression, macrocytosis, anxiety, confusion, tremulousness, seizures and an inflammatory myopathy.

In neurological AIDS the main aim is to treat the treatable complications, which often has to be done empirically without confirmation of the exact diagnosis of any opportunistic infection. Moreover, there may be several simultaneous neurological complications, making exact diagnosis extremely difficult; the diagnosis of one complication certainly does not exclude others, so all treatable possibilities must be looked for. Also, most infections are not curable but merely containable for a while. Naturally the usual diagnostic procedures appropriate for possible infections and malignancies are necessary. The normal strategy is that, if there is a possibility of toxoplasmosis (one or more enhancing lesion on CT), to treat it 'blind' (p. 536) and only to resort to biopsy if there is no clinical or CT improvement in about 4 weeks.

Human T cell leukaemia/lymphoma retrovirus type I (HTLV-I)

This is associated with a chronic progressive paraparesis and sphincter involvement but little sensory disturbance. The disorder is seen mainly in people who have lived in tropical countries for some years and in Japan. Excess IgG antibodies are found both in serum and CSF and there are oligoclonal bands in the latter. It is said to be the most common cause of spastic paraplegia in developing countries (cf. tropical 'myeloneuropathies', p. 338)

Rabies

This cannot be caught in the UK but is endemic in most other countries. It is a zoonosis and infects a wide variety of mammals, being transmitted to man by a bite and infected saliva (most often from a dog, cat or bat which is usually rabid itself).

The incubation period is weeks or months. The onset is non-specific with malaise, fever, myalgia and headache. Within a day or two there is often paraesthesia or pain in the region of the bite and most patients enter into the form known as 'furious' rabies while a few develop 'dumb', or paralytic, rabies.

In 'furious' rabies the patient becomes excitable and anxious, complains of chest tightness and pains and may be febrile. Spasms of the neck, pharyngeal, laryngeal and respiratory muscles then appear, but the patient remains lucid. Hydrophobia does not always occur; it is due to laryngeal and pharyngeal spasm which strikes terror into the patient while attempting to drink, or even at the sight of water. Spasms may also be precipitated by draughts of air on the skin. Stupor, coma, seizures, renal failure and cardiac arrhythmias cause death in a matter of days.

In 'dumb' rabies the clinical picture is similar to the Guillain–Barré syndrome, fasciculation is seen, and in a matter of days the patient becomes paraplegic, unconscious or develops 'furious' rabies.

In both forms the CSF is normal or shows the changes of viral meningitis (p. 493). There is no reliable diagnostic test, although it may be possible to demonstrate rabies antigen in skin biopsies or in brain biopsy material if appropriate. It may be helpful to confirm the diagnosis of rabies in the infecting animal by brain histology and antigen detection, and by intracerebral inoculation of mice. Treatment is ineffective.

Progressive multifocal leucoencephalopathy (PML)

PML is a rare disease of immunocompromised adults. A papovavirus (usually JC) invades the brain to cause patchy demyelination throughout the white matter.

The clinical course is progressive, leading to death in about 6 months. Usually the cerebral hemispheres are involved asymmetrically and sometimes the brainstem and cerebellum. There is progressive hemiparesis, dysphasia, other focal neurological features and dementia. Seizures are rare.

Diagnosis

The CT scan shows small low density non-enhancing areas in the cerebral white matter and these enlarge and coalesce. The scan is often far less abnormal than anticipated from the clinical features, and on occasion it is normal. The CSF is usually normal, but JC viral antibody titres can be high. The definitive diagnosis is made by brain biopsy followed by viral culture, immunofluorescence to detect viral antigen and electron microscopy.

Treatment

Treatment is ineffective, although cytarabine is often tried. Occasional spontaneous remissions are said to occur.

'Slow virus' infections

Creutzfeldt–Jakob disease

This is an extremely rare (0.1/100 000 population/annum), untreatable and fatal disease which can be transmitted experimentally from man to primates and rodents, and from man to man by neurosurgical instruments, corneal grafts and human pituitary growth hormone. The pathology is characteristic, with spongiform change in the grey matter of the brain and spinal cord. The infectious agent has not been identified but it is resistant to normal methods of destroying micro-organisms.

Most patients are middle-aged or elderly and present subacutely. The onset is vague, with apathy, forgetfulness, depression and confusion. Obvious dementia follows, often with visual distortion and hallucinations, cortical blindness, cerebellar ataxia, aphasia and weakness. Myoclonus appears and finally the patient becomes mute, rigid and decorticate. Death occurs within weeks or months from onset. About 10% of cases are chronic, death not occurring for several years; wasting and muscle fasciculations are prominent, myoclonus is rare, and in these cases transmission to animals has failed.

The diagnosis is made clinically and at some stage in the course the EEG shows periodic complexes (p. 54). Confirmation is neuropathological. The CT scan and CSF are normal apart from a slightly raised protein in some cases.

Differential diagnosis includes:
- Alzheimer's disease with myoclonus, but the course is much more prolonged (p. 160)
- motor neurone disease, but no dementia (Chapter 13)
- corpus callosum glioma, but the CT scan is diagnostic

It is sensible to nurse patients similarly to others with 'normal' infectious diseases and to use disposable pins and lumbar puncture needles for all patients with a rapidly progressive dementia.

Kuru

Cases occur only in New Guinea and are probably transmitted by cannibalism. It can be transmitted experimentally to primates. Cerebellar ataxia develops over a few months and the patients die in about a year. The neuropathology is similar to that of Creutzfeldt–Jakob disease.

Fungal and yeast infections

Fungal and yeast infections are becoming more common since they most often occur in immunocompromised hosts, particularly patients taking corticosteroids and cytotoxic drugs, seriously ill patients receiving multiple antibiotics or parenteral nutrition, and in intravenous drug abusers. Patients of any age can be affected. In the UK the most common infections are cryptococcosis, candidiasis and mucormycosis.

Fungal infections produce various combinations of:
- meningitis, which is usually subacute or chronic (p. 497), with a marked tendency to be complicated by hydrocephalus and cranial nerve palsies. Lymphocytes predominate in the CSF, the glucose is normal or low, and the protein is normal or mildly raised. Sometimes there are neutrophils in the CSF
- granulomatous encephalitis (p. 498)
- abscess or granuloma acting as an intracranial space occupying lesion (p. 503) or causing spinal cord compression (p. 505)
- cerebral vasculitis, causing ischaemic or haemorrhagic strokes
- fever, raised ESR and blood leucocytosis are often absent
  The main differential diagnoses are:
- tuberculous meningitis (p. 512)
- malignant meningitis (p. 277)
- cord compression syndromes (p. 320)
- intracranial space occupying lesion (p. 266)
- sarcoidosis (p. 472)

Diagnosis

Diagnosis is made by:
- biopsy of a granuloma with microscopy and culture
- CSF examination, although both microscopy and culture can be surprisingly normal and the examination may need to be repeated several times
- blood serology and culture
- antigen detection for cryptococcosis in CSF and blood is particularly useful (p. 533)

Treatment

Amphotericin is the most effective treatment for systemic fungal disease but mortality and morbidity remain high; 5 mg i.v. test dose, then i.v. 0.25 mg/kg/day as an infusion (in 500 ml 5% dextrose over 4 hours). If tolerated, the dosage can be increased over a matter of some days to 1 mg/kg/day. In severe disease, or if there is renal toxicity, this drug can be given intrathecally via an indwelling reservoir.

Adverse effects include phlebitis, renal failure, hypokalaemia, nausea, vomiting, diarrhoea, abdominal pain, muscle pain, tinnitus, fever, hypotension and anaphylaxis.

For cryptococcosis and candidiasis a lower and less nephrotoxic dose of amphotericin (0.3 mg/kg/day) may be combined with oral flucytosine in a dose of 150 mg/kg/day divided and given 6-hourly, but in a lower dose if there is renal impairment. The adverse effects include marrow depression, nausea, vomiting, diarrhoea and rash. In AIDS, the combination is probably no more effective than amphotericin alone.

Treatment is required for at least 6 weeks and relapse is common. Naturally any underlying disease should be treated if possible and surgical debridement may be necessary (e.g. for mucormycosis, below). In AIDS some degree of chronic maintenance therapy is necessary.

Cryptococcosis (torulosis)

This is the most common cause of fungal meningitis in the UK but it is still a very rare disease. Many patients also have evidence of pulmonary involvement and most are immunocompromised. Case fatality is about 50%.

There is an acute, subacute or chronic meningoencephalitis, often with cranial nerve palsies, papilloedema, blindness, seizures and hydrocephalus. It can be surprisingly indolent with an apparently active CSF for months or even years. Intracerebral granulomas occasionally occur and present as isolated mass lesions. The diagnosis can be difficult and should be pursued in several ways:
- antigen detection in CSF and blood is the most sensitive
- CSF and blood culture
- microscopy of CSF using Indian ink to stain the organisms, which can be mistaken for red blood cells
- antibody detection in CSF and blood

Note: In AIDS the CSF protein and cell count can be normal.

Candidiasis

This causes meningitis, intracranial abscesses and granulomas, and sometimes spinal cord compression. There may also be a cerebral vasculitis. Patients are usually immunocompromised, drug abusers or are having long-term intravenous treatment. There is often candidal infection elsewhere (urine, endocarditis, etc.).

Since candidal infection is so frequent on the skin and at drip sites, the culture of candida in the CSF may be mistakenly ignored. Serological diagnosis in blood and CSF can be helpful.

Mucormycosis (zygomycete fungi)

This is usually a complication of diabetes mellitus and sometimes occurs in immunocompromised hosts. The invasive infection starts in the nose and spreads to the paranasal sinuses, orbits and through the cribriform plate and orbital apex to the brain, where it may cause a cerebral vasculitis with secondary venous and arterial thrombosis. Intracranial granulomas from haematogenous spread are unusual. Patients seldom survive.

Facial swelling, orbital cellulitis and pain, proptosis, extraocular muscle weakness, blindness, cranial nerve palsies, dark nasal discharge and headache are all common. The diagnosis is made from microscopy and culture of lesion scrapings or biopsy material and perhaps serologically. It must be distinguished from bacterial cavernous sinus thrombosis (p. 188).

Histoplasmosis

This becomes a disseminated infection in immunocompromised hosts and may cause meningitis, cerebral abscess and miliary granulomas. There is usually a primary lung focus.

Aspergillosis

This infects the brain by direct spread from the upper respiratory tract, via the blood from a primary lung focus or by intravenous contamination in drug abusers. Usually the infection is disseminated and the host immunocompromised. Neurological features include:
● multiple brain abscesses and granulomas, often with vasculitis and secondary thrombosis and haemorrhage; spinal cord compression is unusual
● meningitis is unusual

Coccidioidomycosis

This can affect healthy or immunocompromised hosts and causes disseminated infections and a chronic granulomatous meningitis. It is found in arid parts of America.

Protozoal infections

Cerebral malaria

Cerebral malaria is the most serious form of malaria and is caused by protozoal infection with *Plasmodium falciparum*. The incubation period is about 2 weeks after the mosquito bite and the illness begins acutely with fever, rigors, headache and malaise. Within hours or days the patient becomes confused and, in severe infections, lapses into coma. Seizures and bilateral extensor plantar responses may be present but there are no focal neurological features.

The differential diagnosis is:

- viral encephalitis (p. 498)
- tuberculous (p. 512) or bacterial meningitis (p. 491)
- other causes of coma (p. 122)

Complications include acute renal failure, intravascular haemolysis, haemoglobinuria, disseminated intravascular coagulation, metabolic acidosis, hypoglycaemia, hyponatraemia, pulmonary oedema, shock and bacterial infection. The case fatality is about 20% but survivors do not appear to have any neurological deficit and relapses do not occur.

Diagnosis

This is made by examination of thin and thick blood films for parasites within the red blood cells. This should be repeated several times if the diagnosis is clinically likely, particularly in patients who are, or were within the previous 3 weeks, in an endemic area (or who have had a blood transfusion). Sometimes there are *no* parasites in the peripheral blood, but in such cases they can usually be found in bone marrow smears or fluid squeezed from intradermal punctures. The white blood cell count is normal or low.

In endemic areas parasitaemia does not necessarily exclude an alternative diagnosis (e.g. bacterial meningitis) and in a febrile unconscious patient lumbar puncture is mandatory; the CSF may shows a slightly raised protein, a low glucose, and a high lactate level, but there are usually no more than about 10 white cells per mm^3.

Treatment

Quinine dihydrochloride 16.7 mg as base/kg in 500 ml dextrose saline i.v. over 4 hours, then 8.4 mg/kg i.v. over 2 hours 8-hourly, with a change to the oral route when practical for a total of 7 days (i.m. dosing is satisfactory if i.v. is impractical).

Adverse effects include abdominal pain, nausea, vomiting, diarrhoea, deafness, tinnitus, dizziness, headache, blurred vision, skin rash, cardiac arrhythmias, hypotension; haemolysis, confusion and marrow suppression are rare. Hypoglycaemia may complicate i.v. doses, particularly in pregnancy. The dose should be lowered in renal failure.

Quinidine is as effective as quinine, has the same adverse effects and can be used for severe cases if parenteral quinine is unavailable. The dosage of quinidine gluconate is 15 mg of base/kg in 250 ml of normal saline infused slowly, then 7.5 mg/kg i.v. 8-hourly with a change to the oral route, when practical, as quinidine sulphate, for a total of 7 days.

Chloroquine can only be used in an area where parasites are known to be sensitive: i.v. infusion of 10 mg/kg over 8 hours, followed by three 8-hourly infusions of 5 mg/kg, and then oral 2.5 mg/kg twice daily for 3 days (if i.v. not feasible, it can be given i.m.).

Adverse effects include: dizziness, nausea, vomiting, blurred vision, pruritus, hypotension.

Note:
- exchange blood transfusion may be used for heavy parasitaemia
- it is important to monitor any hypoglycaemia and correct with dextrose
- prophylactic anticonvulsants are reasonable, particularly in severe cases
- the ECG should be monitored because of the risk of cardiac arrhythmias

Toxoplasmosis

Subclinical infection with the protozoan *Toxoplasma gondii* is common and only occasionally do lymphadenopathy and a 'glandular fever' like syndrome occur. This is almost always self-limiting and rarely complicated by encephalitis or the Guillain–Barré syndrome. However, in immunocompromised hosts, particularly AIDS (p. 526), a devastating and usually fatal encephalopathic illness can occur with or without the glandular syndrome. The presentation is acute or subacute and may be a generalized encephalopathy with seizures and coma or focal because of one or more space occupying granulomatous lesions.

Diagnosis

The CT scan can be normal but usually shows one or more non-specific low density and usually ring-enhancing lesions. If there is no obvious alternative explanation (metastasis or abscess) and the patient is immunocompromised or at risk of AIDS, then brain biopsy may be needed to make the definitive diagnosis showing cysts and organisms and eventually the organism can be isolated after inoculation into mice. Histology shows necrotizing granulomatous encephalitis. Serological tests in blood and CSF are not entirely reliable, particularly in immunocompromised hosts. The CSF is normal or shows a very non-specific increase in white cells and protein and the organisms are seldom seen or isolated from it.

Treatment

Treatment is a combination of oral pyrimethamine, 50 mg 3 times daily for 5 days, followed by 20 mg daily for 4 weeks, plus sulphadiazine, 6 g daily in 3 divided doses, supplemented by folinic acid to reduce the risk of thrombocytopenia and leucopenia. In AIDS, it is usual to continue the lower dose of pyrimethamine indefinitely and to halve the dose of sulphadiazine.

African trypanosomiasis (sleeping sickness)

The trypanosomes are transmitted to man by a tsetse fly bite. A few weeks later a nodular lesion appears at the site along with fever, malaise and lymphadenopathy lasting some months. Months or years later the meningo-encephalitic illness starts, with personality change, headache and disturbance of the normal sleep rhythm. Chorea, athetosis and seizures may appear followed by cachexia, stupor and death. The diagnosis is by CSF examination which shows a modest rise in lymphocytes and protein, trypanosomes in 50% and usually a high IgM level.

Blastomycosis

This usually affects healthy individuals. Meningitis, intracranial or spinal abscess and granuloma are associated with lung and skin involvement.

Helminthic infections

Nematode worms

Infection of man with some nematodes can cause neurological damage. The diagnosis is usually suspected because of a high blood eosinophil count, other cases in an outbreak and a history of exposure to the likely intermediate host.

Toxocara

The common dog round worm, *Toxocara canis*, may occasionally infect humans (usually infants and children in unhygienic conditions) to cause rash, fever, cough, eosinophilia, hepatosplenomegaly, pulmonary infiltrates and ophthalmitis. Occasionally seizures occur due to brain involvement. The diagnosis is made serologically or by biopsy of infected tissue.

Trichinosis

This is contracted by eating undercooked pork or horse meat. It is found worldwide. There may be parasitation of muscle, particularly the diaphragm, with pain and raised muscle enzymes along with fever, urticarial rash, diarrhoea, facial oedema and eosinophilia. Encephalitis and myelitis are rare.

Gnathostomiasis

This is transmitted by infested and undercooked fresh water fish, duck and chicken in South East Asia. Cutaneous migratory swellings are variable and, if they occur, the worm can be recovered from them. As the worm migrates into the nervous system, it causes meningitis, severe radicular pain and myelitis. Encephalitis, cranial nerve palsies and subarachnoid haemorrhage are less common. The CSF is eosinophilic and lymphocytic with a normal or low glucose and a raised protein.

Angiostrongyliasis

This may be contracted from eating snails, freshwater molluscs, crustacea and fish in Asia and the Pacific basin. It causes an eosinophilic meningitis with severe headache, nausea and vomiting. Encephalopathy and cranial nerve lesions are uncommon. The CSF is similar to that for gnathostomiasis (p. 537) and larvae may occasionally be seen.

Cestode worms

Cysticercosis

This is caused by the larval form of the pork tapeworm, *Taenia solium*, invading the body tissues and encysting, particularly in the brain. It is rare in temperate countries. Infested patients are often asymptomatic or only become symptomatic after many years. The disease may be active and aggressive but more often is indolent with little more than seizures. The clinical features include:
● subacute or chronic meningoencephalitis due to an inflammatory reaction around cysts in the brain, spinal cord, ventricles and in the subarachnoid space. This type of active disease causes seizures, hydrocephalus, raised intracranial pressure, cranial nerve palsies and sometimes vasculitic strokes. The prognosis is poor
● hydrocephalus caused by meningitis, cysts obstructing CSF flow or more insidiously by chronic arachnoiditis (p. 259)
● progressive cerebral mass lesion presenting as a 'tumour' (p. 266)
● chronic seizures, often without any history of active disease, but there can be cerebral lesion(s) on CT
● spinal cord compression (p. 320) and arachnoiditis (p. 335)
● acute myositis is uncommon
● subcutaneous nodules due to cysts are uncommon

Diagnosis. This is difficult and depends on the clinical picture along with:
● CT scan; single or more often multiple (up to 5 cm diameter) low density areas which may enhance with contrast and be surrounded by oedema. Calcification can occur but is seldom enough to be shown on skull X-ray
● CSF may show a non-specific increase in lymphocytes, neutrophils (occasionally eosinophils) and protein
● X-ray of thigh muscles may show calcified cysts but only in chronic or inactive disease
● serology is unreliable
● biopsy of brain or subcutaneous nodules may be required for a definitive diagnosis

Treatment. For active disease: praziquantel 50 mg/kg/day, oral, divided in 3 doses, for 21 days. A drug-induced inflammatory reaction may occur with increased headache, drowsiness and seizures, with increasing cells in the CSF, but usually this resolves. Adverse effects include indigestion, nausea, diarrhoea, fever and pruritus.

Symptomatic hydrocephalus may require relief, and surgical removal of solitary lesions is sometimes necessary.

Hydatid disease

This disease is caused by the echinococcus or dog tapeworm which is widespread in most countries. Clinical disease is rare. Ingestion of the eggs leads to cysts in the liver and lung but rarely in the brain and spinal cord. A cyst is often several centimetres across, may calcify, and presents like any other slowly progressive space occupying lesion. On CT scan there is a spherical low density area with a sharp border and no surrounding oedema or contrast enhancement. Multiloculated budding cysts are a less common variant.

Serological tests are helpful but not entirely reliable. The treatment is surgical removal. Albendazole is a promising new chemotherapeutic agent.

Schistosomiasis (bilharzia)

This is caused by chronic trematode worm infection in Asia, Africa, the Caribbean and South America. The freshwater snail is the intermediate host. Neurological involvement is rare but when it occurs it is serious and consists of a granulomatous inflammatory reaction to large collections of eggs. This causes:
- spinal cord/root compression by granuloma (particularly in the lumbosacral region) (p. 320)
- transverse myelitis/intramedullary granuloma (particularly in the conus medullaris) (p. 322)
- meningoencephalitis (p. 498)
- space occupying intracranial granulomas with seizures, raised intracranial pressure, etc. (p. 266)

In asymptomatic individuals in endemic areas it is common to find ova in the faeces, positive blood serology and a blood eosinophilia, so the only proof of invasive disease is by finding ova in neurological biopsy material. The CSF is not helpful since it is only non-specifically lymphocytic and does not contain ova. Treatment with praziquantel (see above) may have to be given on circumstantial evidence when biopsy is not feasible.

Amoebic infections

Amoebic CNS infection is rare.

Entamoeba histolytica

This is the cause of amoebic dysentery. It may cause an amoebic liver abscess and spread via the bloodstream to produce a cerebral abscess.

Naegleria fowleri

This is a free living amoeba found in the soil and warm fresh water, particularly spa springs. It probably enters the nasal mucosa and spreads from there to cause an acute necrotizing meningoencephalitis which is fatal. The differential diagnosis is bacterial meningitis and the CSF findings are similar (p. 493). Amoebae can be found in fresh wet specimens of centrifuged CSF. The treatment is amphotericin (p. 532).

Notifiable diseases

The following infectious diseases are compulsorily notifiable in England and Wales:

Anthrax
Cholera
Diphtheria
Dysentery (amoebic and bacillary)
Encephalitis
Food poisoning
Leprosy
Leptospirosis
Malaria
Measles
Meningitis
Meningococcal septicaemia
    (without meningitis)
Mumps
Ophthalmia neonatorum

Paratyphoid fever
Plague
Polio
Relapsing fever
Rubella
Scarlet fever
Smallpox
Tetanus
Tuberculosis
Typhoid fever
Typhus fever
Viral haemorrhagic fever
Viral hepatitis
Whooping cough
Yellow fever

19 Toxins and the nervous system

Numerous toxins affect the nervous system, often along with other systems, as a result of deliberate or accidental exposure, acutely or chronically. Many are of only historical or forensic interest but some still cause problems frequently enough to be clinically important:

- alcohols and glycols (p. 542)
- organic solvents (p. 546)
- metals (p. 547)
- organophosphorus compounds (p. 548)
- carbon monoxide (p. 549)
- miscellaneous chemicals (p. 549)
- subacute myelo-optico-neuropathy (SMON) (p. 550)
- drug abuse (p. 551)
- animal venoms and toxins (p. 551)
- plants (p. 552)

Note: More than one toxin may be involved, which can make the clinical picture confusing and less than 'pure'.

Individual susceptibility varies widely, making interpretation of the concentration of chemicals in blood, urine, hair, etc. difficult.

Contamination of the apparent toxin with another chemical may be as responsible as, or more responsible than, what is written on the label of any container in terms of clinical effects.

Alcohols and glycols

Ethanol

Excessive alcohol consumption causes various neurological syndromes, often in combination:

- acute intoxication (p. 543)
- withdrawal symptoms (p. 543)
- seizures (p. 543)
- Wernicke–Korsakoff syndrome (p. 468)
- head injury (p. 544)
- dementia (p. 544)
- central pontine myelinolysis (p. 465)
- Marchiafava–Bignami disease (p. 544)
- stroke (p. 544)
- peripheral neuropathy (p. 544)
- myopathy (p. 544)
- cerebellar degeneration and atrophy (p. 545)
- tobacco–alcohol amblyopia (p. 545)

- neurological complications of liver failure (p. 467)
- neurological complications of hypoglycaemia (p. 108)

One standard unit of alcohol (about 10 g) ≡ half pint beer *or* 1 tot of spirits *or* 1 glass of sherry *or* 1 glass of wine. The upper limit for relatively safe regular drinking is about 6 units per day in men and 3 units per day in women. However, there is wide individual variation in tolerance to both the acute and chronic neurological effects of alcohol. In chronic alcoholics it is unclear how much of the neurological damage is a consequence of malnutrition; probably it is mostly due to the direct toxic effects of alcohol.

Acute intoxication

This causes disinhibition, impaired judgement, nausea and vomiting, leading on to combativeness, cerebellar ataxia, dysarthria, nystagmus, confusion, drowsiness and eventually coma. Often the patient is amnesic for much of the period of intoxication. Paroxysmal atrial fibrillation may cause stroke (p. 544). Falls may cause head and other injuries. Headache and insomnia are common after a binge.

Note: In patients smelling of alcohol, coma may *also* be due to, or exacerbated by, associated head injury, subdural haematoma (p. 235), hypoglycaemia (p. 108), liver failure (p. 467), hyponatraemia (p. 464), seizures (see below) and drug abuse. Alcohol is an unlikely cause of coma if the blood level is less than 200 mg/dl (44 mmol/l).

Withdrawal symptoms

These are unpredictable and variable. Early morning tremor of the limbs and head, agitation, anxiety, clumsiness and hyperreflexia are early signs of chronic alcoholism and are relieved by taking another drink. Visual and auditory hallucinations are more serious manifestations of withdrawal and full-blown delirium tremens may occur a day or two after withdrawal: agitation, sweating, tachycardia, resting and action tremor, confusion, disorientation, fear, delusions, hallucinations (usually visual and often of animals on or around the bed) and tonic-clonic seizures.

Seizures

One or more tonic-clonic seizures are common in chronic alcoholics and may be due to alcohol itself, withdrawal from alcohol, hypoglycaemia (p. 108), hyponatraemia (p. 464), head injury or drug abuse. Anticonvulsants are not particularly effective, especially if the patient continues to drink and compliance is erratic.

Head injury

Head injury is common as a result of fights, falls (see below) and seizures.

Dementia

Dementia is a sad and common culmination of chronic alcoholism and is a result of some combination of direct alcoholic brain damage, nutritional deficiency, head injuries, stroke and liver failure. Cortical atrophy is seen on CT. Delusions, paranoia and antisocial behaviour are all too common.

Marchiafava–Bignami disease

This is an unusual consequence of chronic alcoholism with demyelination of the corpus callosum, usually diagnosed only at postmortem. It is associated with alcoholic dementia.

Stroke

Stroke, both haemorrhagic and ischaemic, is more common than expected in chronic alcoholics and after binge drinking. Possible causes include:
- chronic hypertension due to excessive alcohol consumption (p. 213)
- atrial fibrillation in acute intoxication, or as a result of alcoholic cardio-myopathy, with intra-atrial thrombus and embolization
- cardiomyopathy with intraventricular thrombus followed by embolization
- neck injury with dissection of carotid or vertebral arteries (p. 214)

Peripheral neuropathy

Peripheral neuropathy with axonal degeneration is due to both chronic alco-holic damage and nutritional deficiency, particularly of vitamin B_1 (p. 468). It can be subacute or chronic. Burning pains, dysaesthesia and skin tenderness are common features in the feet and legs, less so in the hands. Eventually distal weakness occurs, along with autonomic features sometimes.

Note: disulfiram (or Antabuse) causes peripheral neuropathy.

Myopathy

This is usually chronic, progressive, painless and proximal. An acute form occurs in chronic alcoholics after binge drinking; there is muscle pain, swelling and tenderness perhaps with rhabdomyolysis (p. 432).

Cerebellar degeneration and atrophy

This is a result of chronic alcoholism. There is slowly progressive ataxia of gait, imbalance, and ataxia of the legs more than of the arms. Dysarthria and nystagmus are unusual. It is one cause of unexpected falls in alcoholics, others being:

- acute intoxication
- seizures
- hypoglycaemia
- postural sense loss due to peripheral neuropathy
- postural hypotension due to autonomic neuropathy

Tobacco–alcohol amblyopia

This is occasionally seen in chronic alcoholics who smoke heavily. The optic nerves and chiasm degenerate, leading to subacute bilateral impairment of vision with central-caecal scotomata.

Treatment

Treatment of neurological complications of alcoholism is largely symptomatic along with a good diet with vitamin supplementation (particularly with B_1), social rehabilitation and attempting to stop the patient drinking.

Methanol

Methanol is found in solvents, antifreeze and adulterated wine. Inhalation, ingestion or absorption through the skin may cause merely a mild confusional state and drowsiness. However, some hours after a high dose patients develop nausea, vomiting, abdominal pain, headache, dizziness, ataxia, confusion and coma. Often there is a severe metabolic acidosis, hyperglycaemia and raised plasma amylase. The optic nerves are particularly affected, with bilateral reduced acuity, perhaps with papilloedema. Usually there is no recovery of vision. CT may show hypodensity in the basal ganglia.

Isopropyl alcohol

This is found in sterilizing agents, disinfectants and cleaning solutions. It is oxidized by the liver to acetone. The acute neurological effects are similar to those of alcohol but, in addition, there is a smell of acetone on the breath. Haematemesis, acute renal tubular necrosis and haemolytic anaemia may occur.

Ethylene glycol

This is the main constituent of antifreeze and has been used to adulterate wine. Ingestion causes similar symptoms to alcohol intoxication but there is no smell on the breath. It leads to metabolic acidosis, renal failure, partial and generalized seizures, optic neuropathy with papilloedema, extraocular muscle palsies, nystagmus and coma.

Organic solvents

Organic solvents are used in numerous industrial processes and are found in common household items (glue, paint stripper, paint, lighter fuel, etc.). Acute intoxication most commonly occurs deliberately ('glue' sniffing, usually of toluene-based glues and paint strippers) and sometimes in industrial accidents. Chronic intoxication may occur in regular 'glue' sniffers and possibly in workers frequently exposed to low levels of solvents in confined spaces (industrial workers, painters and decorators).

Acute intoxication (e.g. with toluene, xylene, styrene, n-hexane, carbon tetrachloride, carbon disulphide, chloroform, trichloroethylene, methyl bromide, methyl chloride) at first causes euphoria and headache; then nausea, vomiting, visual hallucinations, confusion, dysarthria, ataxia; and eventually seizures, delirium and coma. Also asphyxia can occur because of inhalation of vomit, rebreathing in a plastic bag and solvent-induced cardiac arrhythmias.

Chronic exposure (to the same solvents as above) can cause:
• chronic encephalopathy: irritability, apathy, headache, tiredness, confusion, dementia and cortical atrophy on CT
• cerebellar degeneration causing predominantly gait and leg ataxia
• pyramidal signs but usually no weakness
• optic atrophy and blindness
• deafness

Exposure to n-hexane, methyl butyl ketone, carbon disulphide and possibly toluene causes a peripheral neuropathy. Also carbon disulphide can cause a parkinsonian syndrome and trichloroethylene a cranial neuropathy (particularly bilateral facial numbness).

Diagnosis

Diagnosis of acute toxicity is by measurement of solvent in blood and urine. Often there is metabolic acidosis.

Note: 'Glue' sniffers may also be abusing other chemicals likely to affect the nervous system, e.g. alcohol, amphetamines.

Metals

Environmental contamination is now rare in the UK. Exposure to metals is usually accidental. The effects can be rather variable depending on whether exposure is acute or chronic, and whether more than one toxin is involved.

Lead

Inorganic lead poisoning causes a predominantly motor peripheral neuropathy, anaemia, colic, constipation and a blue line on the gums. It used to occur in painters and lead battery workers. Children exposed to inorganic lead may develop an encephalopathy with irritability, ataxia, confusion, seizures and coma. Symptoms are unlikely unless the blood level is above 60 µg/100 ml; blood levels are a reflection of *current* rather than past exposure.

Organic lead

Organic lead (tetraethyl lead in petrol) exposure occurs in men cleaning petrol storage tanks. It causes nightmares, insomnia, agitation, hallucinations and psychosis.

Mercury

Inorganic mercury poisoning causes insomnia, anxiety, depression, rest tremor, excess salivation, gingivitis, hallucinations and psychosis.

Organic mercury exposure (e.g. methyl mercury discharged into water and entering fish, or contaminating grain from fungicides) causes paraesthesia and numbness around the mouth, face and extremities; ataxia with cerebellar signs; constriction of the visual fields; memory impairment; pyramidal signs and weakness; fasciculation; blindness and deafness.

Arsenic

This is contained in insecticides and weed killers. Ingestion causes immediate vomiting and diarrhoea, followed, 1–3 weeks later, by a distal sensorimotor neuropathy; dense white bands in the nails; desquamation of the skin on the hands and feet; hyperkeratosis of the palms and soles; raindrop pigmentation over the abdomen.

Organic tin

This causes raised intracranial pressure, paraplegia, sensory neuropathy, confusion, deafness, tonic-clonic seizures and cerebellar dysfunction.

Thallium

Thallium is a constituent of rat poison and other pesticides. Ingestion causes vomiting and diarrhoea followed a few days later by a subacute and profound peripheral neuropathy clinically similar to the Guillain–Barré syndrome (p. 398), involuntary movements and alopecia.

Manganese poisoning

This occurs in miners. In causes insomnia, irritability and emotional lability followed by parkinsonism and pyramidal signs.

Bismuth intoxication

Bismuth intoxication (usually from treatment with its salt) causes irritability, insomnia, anxiety, depression and tremulousness followed by confusion, memory impairment, myoclonus, tonic-clonic seizures, dysarthria and ataxia of gait.

Gold

Gold, used to treat rheumatoid arthritis, can cause a peripheral neuropathy with myokymia and fasciculation.

Platinum

Platinum, in cisplatin, can cause tinnitus, deafness and a sensory peripheral neuropathy with Lhermitte's symptom.

Aluminium (see dialysis dementia, p. 467)

Organophosphorus compounds

These are used as pesticides, plasticizers and in nerve gas. Exposure may be by suicidal intent or accidental in agricultural and other workers. The chemicals are inhaled, or absorbed through the skin. They inhibit acetyl cholinesterase in autonomic ganglia, parasympathetic nerve endings and at neuromuscular junctions. This causes a cholinergic crisis: salivation, sweating, small pupils, colic, vomiting, diarrhoea, headache and weakness leading to muscle fasciculation, urine incontinence, seizures, confusion, coma, bronchoconstriction, respiratory depression and death. Different compounds tend to cause rather different combinations of symptoms. Patients usually recover with symptomatic support and specific antidotes.

A few days after recovery, some patients develop proximal limb, neck flexor, respiratory, and cranial nerve innervated muscle weakness with depressed reflexes and normal sensation. A few weeks after recovery other patients develop a distal sensorimotor neuropathy.

Note: Triorthocresylphosphate (TCP), widely used in lubricating oils, may contaminate edible oils and cause a subacute sensorimotor neuropathy.

Carbon monoxide

Carbon monoxide (CO) gas sources are car exhaust fumes, household gas where natural gas is not used, fumes from incomplete combustion of fossil fuels, particularly in poorly ventilated heating systems, and by metabolic conversion of methylene chloride (found in paint strippers). The clinical picture depends on the rate and amount of exposure and is due to binding of CO to haemoglobin and consequent tissue hypoxia.

Massive and sudden exposure causes confusion, seizures, coma and death. Survivors may have, or may develop in a few days, a parkinsonian syndrome, memory impairment, gait ataxia, urine incontinence and sometimes involuntary movements. CT shows low density in the globus pallidus, ventricular enlargement and cortical atrophy. Recovery may or may not occur.

Chronic low level exposure causes irritability, fatigue, headache, nausea and mild mental confusion.

Diagnosis is made by being alert enough to the possibility of exposure to measure the blood carboxyhaemoglobin level (less than 10% is not symptomatic) in patients with symptoms from chronic headache to coma.

Miscellaneous chemicals

Acrylamide

Workers may be exposed during synthesis of the polymer and develop a peripheral sensorimotor neuropathy and cerebellar ataxia.

Cyanide

Cyanide is found in rat poisons, fertilizers, plants (p. 553) and smoke from polyurethane foams. It is widely used in industrial processes. Poisoning is usually a result of suicide or homicide and causes palpitations, chest constriction, shortness of breath, pulmonary oedema, headache, dizziness, vertigo, ataxia, seizures, metabolic acidosis and coma. The breath may smell of almonds.

Chronic exposure can cause tobacco–alcohol amblyopia (p. 545) and cassava poisoning (p. 553).

Ethylene oxide

This is a gas used in sterilizers. Acute toxicity causes headache, confusion and coma. Long-term overexposure can cause a peripheral sensorimotor neuropathy.

Methyl bromide gas

This is used as a fumigating agent. Acute exposure is followed a few hours later by headache, dizziness, nausea, vomiting, abdominal pain, malaise, blurred vision and breathlessness leading on to ataxia, paraesthesia, hallucinations, seizures and coma. Chronic exposure can cause a peripheral sensorimotor neuropathy.

Nitrous oxide

If chronically abused, which is a hazard for dentists, this can cause a chronic peripheral neuropathy and spinal cord syndrome similar to subacute combined degeneration of the spinal cord (p. 470). Possibly this is due to interference with vitamin B_{12} metabolism.

Pyridylmethyl nitrophenyl urea (PNU)

PNU is used as a rat poison. Within hours of accidental or deliberate ingestion it causes diabetes mellitus and widespread neurological damage; peripheral and autonomic neuropathy, and sometimes encephalopathy with drowsiness and memory impairment.

Subacute myelo-optico-neuropathy (SMON)

Prolonged and high doses of clioquinol (Enterovioform) can cause the subacute onset of a neurological syndrome (often preceded by abdominal symptoms such as diarrhoea, constipation and pain), but more or less only in the Japanese. It has almost completely disappeared now that the drug is far less widely available. The onset is with burning and tingling in the feet which spreads up the legs over a few days, weakness of the legs with pyramidal signs, and sometimes impaired visual acuity bilaterally due to degeneration of the optic nerves, chiasm and tracts. Neurones in the spinal cord and peripheral nerves degenerate. The tongue is often discoloured green. The CSF is normal.

It tended to appear in young adults and, if recovery occurred, it took months or years.

Note: A few hours after a single large dose of clioquinol a confusional state and global amnesia occur lasting for several days.

Drug abuse

Since abused drugs are taken for their CNS affects, it is hardly surprising that they can all cause confusion, hallucinations, psychosis, seizures, drowsiness and coma. Intravenous injection may cause septicaemia with secondary brain abscess; endocarditis with embolism to the brain or mycotic aneurysm rupture; myelopathy; and HIV infection (p. 526).

Specific effects of drugs

Amphetamines

Amphetamines and other sympathomimetic drugs such as ephedrine, methylphenidate, phenylpropanolamine cause:
- insomnia
- headache
- tremor and hyperreflexia
- stroke due to intracranial haemorrhage (and perhaps cerebral infarction)
- rhabdomyolysis

Barbiturates

- cerebellar ataxia, nystagmus, dysarthria

Cocaine/Crack

- intracranial haemorrhage due to hypertension or vasculitis
- cerebral infarction
- hyperpyrexia
- rhabdomyolysis

Heroin

- cerebral infarction (? due to vasculitis)
- rhabdomyolysis

Animal venoms and toxins

Snake bites

Snake bites and injection of venom cause a variety of neurological (and other) effects, systemic and local:

- paralysis due to blocked neuromuscular transmission, e.g. cobra, krait, coral snake
- rhabdomyolysis, e.g. sea snake, terrestrial Australasian snakes
- intracranial haemorrhage, e.g. Russell's viper

Fish stings

These are rarely more than painful. However, the venom of rays, scorpion fish and stone fish can cause nausea, vomiting, diarrhoea, sweating, hypersalivation, cardiac arrhythmias, seizures and coma.

Marine animals

Marine animal ingestion may be a cause of botulism (p. 520) or methyl mercury poisoning (p. 547). Toxins in seafood can cause 'pelagic paralysis'; paraesthesia and numbness of the face and limbs, ataxia and flaccid paralysis. These toxins are found at certain times in ciguatera fish, puffer fish and shell fish.

Insect stings

These occasionally cause direct neurological complications such as muscle spasm, seizures and paralysis (scorpions and a few spiders). Anaphylactic shock is far more common and occasionally leads to cerebral anoxia.

Plants

Atropine-like effects

These effects include blurred vision, dilated pupils, dry mouth, hot and dry skin, retention of urine, constipation, tachycardia, fever, headache, confusion, delirium, hallucinations, seizures, coma.
- deadly nightshade (*Atropa*)
- henbane (*Hyoscyamus*)
- jessamine (*Cestrum*)
- thornapple (*Datura*)

Nicotine-like effects

These effects include nausea, vomiting, salivation, headache, thirst, confusion, hallucinations, seizures.
- hemlock (*Conium*)
- laburnum
- lobelia
- tobacco (*Nicotiana*)

Convulsants

Convulsants are also found in:
- arbor vitae (*Thuja*)
- cowbane (*Cicuta*)
- cypress (*Cupressus*)
- juniper (*Juniperus*)
- strychnos
- tansy (*Tanacetum*)
- water dropwort (*Oenanthe*)

Hallucinogens

These are found in:
- hemp (*Cannabis*)
- morning glory (*Ipomoea* and *Rivea*)
- nutmeg (*Myristica*)
- periwinkle (*Vinca*)
- peyote (*Lophophora*)

Cyanogens

Cyanogens are found in:
- cassava (see below)
- seed kernels of almond, apricot, cherry and peach

Cassava

The roots are consumed in large quantities throughout the tropics, usually without ill effect even though they contain cyanide. However, during famine or drought it seems that the plant can cause chronic cyanide poisoning as a result of more being eaten, an increase in cyanide content of the plant, or a change in methods of preparation. This can cause a painful peripheral neuropathy, sensory ataxia, optic atrophy and pyramidal signs. It tends to occur in epidemics and the onset is acute or subacute.

Strychnine poisoning

This is usually deliberate. It causes heightened awareness, muscle spasms (particularly of the face, neck and back), so mimicking tetanus (p. 518).

Mushrooms and toadstools

These may contain a variety of pharmacologically active substances:

- muscarine, causing nausea, salivation, colic, lacrimation, visual blurring, weakness
- hallucinogens such as ibotenic acid, muscimol, psilocin, psilocybin

Appendix 1: Neurological disorders and driving in the UK

The holders of a driving licence are obliged by law to inform the Driver and Vehicle Licensing Centre (DVLC), Medical Advisory Branch, Oldway Centre, Orchard Street, Swansea SA1 1TU, if they have any disability likely to make them, now or in the future, a danger when driving, and to do so as soon as they become aware of it unless it is expected to last less than 3 months (e.g. fractures). This rule is clearly stated on the driving licence and doctors should remind patients of it and that failure to notify the DVLC may compromise the validity of their motor insurance. Even if the disability is temporary, it may still be serious enough to bar driving until recovery. Standards are higher for holders of heavy goods vehicle (HGV) and public service vehicle (PSV) licences and for other professional drivers (police, chauffeurs, etc.) than for those with ordinary driving licences.

Intermittent neurological disability (e.g. epilepsy, p. 66, TIA, p. 219, narcolepsy syndrome, p. 114) is much harder to assess than chronic physical or cognitive disability (e.g. stroke, Chapter 8, dementia, Chapter 6, Parkinson's disease, p. 280, head injury, established multiple sclerosis, Chapter 12), when a driving assessment can be used to decide whether a patient is competent to drive.

In uncertain cases the DVLC is extremely helpful either in response to the patients, or their doctors, who should not reveal the patients' names without their permission. The DVLC has an important role in protecting the doctor–patient relationship when it takes the blame for withdrawing a driving licence. Patients have the right of appeal if their licence is withdrawn.

Note: For private motorists, a greater than 20% risk of a sudden and disabling event (e.g. loss of consciousness) in a year is regarded as unacceptable. For HGV and PSV licence holders the figure is about 2%.

Epilepsy (Chapter 2)

Patients with seizures are forbidden to hold an ordinary driving licence unless they have been free of any type of seizure, from whatever cause, for at least 2 years. If, however, the seizures occur *only* while asleep, then a licence is allowed, even if the seizures are continuing and there have been awake attacks more than 3 years previously, *provided* the sleep-associated seizures have been occurring for at least the last 3 years. In any case, the patient's driving should not be regarded as a danger to the public. These regulations apply whether or not the patient is taking anticonvulsants. Patients should not drive if they are intoxicated with anticonvulsants.

Even after a single first seizure (while awake or asleep) it is obligatory for the patient to inform the DVLC; they should not drive for 12 months, but longer if there is a significant intracranial cause for the seizures which is likely to progress (e.g. a tumour), or clearcut seizure activity (spike and wave) on the EEG. However, it is not obligatory for the doctor to look for a tumour after a single seizure (by doing a CT scan, for example) or to carry out an EEG.

When withdrawing anticonvulsants, patients with a licence are under no legal obligation to inform the DVLC or their insurance company, or to stop driving, but it is sensible to drive as little as possible until a few months after anticonvulsants have been stopped, when the risk of any recurrence is less than during the withdrawal period. If a recurrence does arise, the patient must inform the DVLC, even if anticonvulsants are resumed, and may not always have his/her licence revoked for a full 2 years without another seizure; patients should be made aware of this possibility before withdrawal of anticonvulsants.

Some patients have seizures provoked by stimuli which can be recognized and avoided in the future, e.g. myelography, anoxia, tricyclic antidepressants, etc. Under these circumstances the advice of the DVLC should be sought and usually the driving licence will not be withdrawn if the provoking factor can be avoided.

Patients who have a continuing and relevant disability (i.e. more than one seizure) are *obliged* to inform the DVLC and are wise to inform their car insurers as well. Doctors must tell the patients this, but certainly not tell the DVLC without the patients' consent, unless in their judgement they believe the public interest overrules their duty of maintaining the patients' confidence. It is sensible to make a record in the notes of exactly what driving advice is given to patients. Some patients, and neurologists, are surprised at the generous way the DVLC often interprets the regulations, sometimes more generously than many neurologists.

Patients who have had *any* seizures under *any* circumstances over the age of 5 are barred from holding either a heavy goods vehicle or a public service vehicle licence.

The risk of having a seizure at the wheel is determined not just by the probability of a seizure but also by the time spent driving. In cases of doubt, when driving is not illegal but unwise, this risk can be reduced by driving as little as possible.

Note: Patients with an episode(s) of sudden disabling giddiness, faintness or loss of consciousness should be advised to inform the DVLC and not to drive until the cause is found, after which the normal rules for seizures, pacemakers, etc. usually apply. If no explanation is found, they will probably be barred from driving for a year after the last attack. These rules obviously do not apply to disorders such as postural giddiness and micturition syncope which do not occur at the wheel.

Patients at risk of seizures

Many intracranial disorders cause seizures in their acute phase (e.g. cerebral abscess, p. 503, encephalitis, p. 498, subarachnoid haemorrhage, p. 228, head injury, supratentorial neurosurgery, stroke, p. 246), and the 2-year rule usually applies provided there is no physical or mental bar to driving. It is difficult to give sensible advice to patients with these conditions who have *not* had a seizure but who are clearly at excess risk of having one. On the whole, patients should not drive for 12 months after:

- any supratentorial neurosurgical procedure
- intracranial abscess (p. 503)
- encephalitis (p. 498)
- head injury complicated by intracerebral haematoma, depressed skull fracture, dural tear or focal signs of cortical damage.
- subarachnoid haemorrhage due to aneurysm or artriovenous malformation (p. 228)

In general, patients with a malignant or inoperable intracranial tumour should not drive at all. If an isolated metastasis is removed from the brain, then driving may be allowed if the patient is seizure free for about 4 years.

Physical disability

Patients with a fixed physical disability (e.g. disabling stroke, spinal cord trauma, etc.) or even in the early stages of a progressive disability (e.g. from multiple sclerosis, Parkinson's disease, etc.) are often able to drive, particularly if the car is suitably adapted. They should inform the DVLC. Advice about car choice and adaptations, etc. can be obtained from the following:

Mobility Advice and Vehicle Information Service
Department of Transport
TRRL
Crowthorne
Berkshire RG11 6AU
Tel: 0344-770456

Disabled Drivers Association
Ashwellthorpe House
Ashwellthorpe
Norwich NR16 1EZ
Tel: 0508-41449

If there is any doubt about driving ability, the DVLC can arrange for the patient to have a free driving assessment. Standards for HGV and PSV licences are much more stringent than for ordinary licences.

Cognitive and mental impairment

Patients are not allowed to drive if they are confused, have serious memory impairment, visuospatial problems or severe mental subnormality such that they cannot live an independent life or guard themselves against serious exploitation. In uncertain cases a free driving assessment can be arranged by the DVLC.

Cerebrovascular disease (Chapter 8)

Patients with stroke or TIA should inform the DVLC. After a stroke driving is usually allowed within 3 months of onset (provided there is no physical disability which bars driving), as it is after a single TIA. After recurrent TIAs the bar is usually for 6 months but will probably depend on the character of the attacks (e.g. amaurosis fugax being less disabling from the point of view of driving than brainstem attacks with vertigo).

Vision

The statutory requirement is to read a clean number plate with figures 3½ inches high at 25 yards in good daylight, wearing glasses if necessary. There is no bar for *monocular* visual loss. Patients with a homonymous hemianopia or visual inattention should not drive; this rule is often relaxed if the field defect is in the upper quadrants only. Diplopia is a bar to driving except perhaps when one eye is occluded by a patch.

Excessive daytime sleepiness (Chapter 3)

There are no definite rules, but patients having day-time sleep attacks without warning should be advised not to drive, as should anyone who is excessively lethargic and sleepy during the day.

Appendix 2: Adverse effects of drugs on the nervous system

The function and sometimes structure of the central and peripheral nervous systems may be disturbed by many drugs used in routine clinical practice, and illicitly. Depending on their nature, these adverse effects are referred to in the appropriate chapters (e.g. on movement disorders, myopathies, etc.). Rather than expecting a comprehensive list of all the neurological adverse effects of innumerable drugs, the reader must refer to the index where a drug of interest can be looked up under its pharmacopoeial (non-proprietary or generic) title and the page numbers refer to all the places in the book where it is mentioned. Page numbers in bold refer to pages where the main indications are described.

Note: Adverse effects may be the result of not just the drug (excessive dosage, interaction with other drugs, idiosyncrasy) but also the patient (age, body size, genetic variation, etc.) and disease (renal failure, gastrectomy, myasthenia, etc.).

If a neurological adverse effect is suspected, usually because it has been described before and coincides in time with the drug being started or increased in dosage, then the drug should be stopped if possible or at least reduced in dosage. If the putative adverse effect resolves, then, if it is safe to do so, rechallenge with the drug may be required for confirmation; rechallenge with placebo to disentangle a real from placebo adverse effect is seldom practical. Rechallenge is unnecessary if the drug is not indicated at all (e.g. prochlorperazine for prevention of vertigo) or if an alternative is available and unlikely to cause the same adverse effect. Adverse effects are occasionally permanent even after drug withdrawal.

Reducing the risk of adverse effects

- use drugs only when really indicated
- keep indication for repeat prescriptions under review
- use the minimum number of drugs necessary
- before starting a drug, check what else the patient is taking, including self-medications, and consider interactions
- avoid fixed-dose combinations if possible
- before starting a drug, check the patient's previous experience of it
- use drugs with which one is familiar
- start with a small dose and slowly increase as necessary unless the clinical situation demands urgent full dose treatment
- keep the dosage regimen as simple as possible (i.e. once daily)
- give clear instructions, if necessary in writing, to the patient and, if appropriate, to relative or carer

- for any one drug try to use only one size of tablet
- ask the patient to discard drugs which are no longer required
- ensure clear communication between general practitioner and hospital, if appropriate by using a shared care card
- if patients cannot be seen by the same doctor on each hospital visit, then consider discharging the patient back to the general practitioner where continuity of care should be better

Useful address

Committee on Safety of Medicines
Freepost
London SW8 5BR
Tel: 071-720-2188

24 hour Freephone service for advice and information: Dial 100 and ask for 'CSM Freephone'.

Appendix 3: Useful addresses

Action for Research in Multiple Sclerosis
(ARMS)
4A Chapel Hill
Stansted
Essex CM24 8AG
Tel: 0279-815553

Alzheimer's Disease Society
158/160 Balham High Road
London SW12 9BN
Tel: 081-675-6557

Ann's Neurological Trust Society (ANTS)
Jocelyn Lodge
Keythorpe
Tugby
Leicester LE7 9XJ
Tel: 053-756-244

Association for Spina Bifida &
Hydrocephalus
ASBAH House
42 Park Road
Peterborough
Cambs PE1 2UQ
Tel: 0733-555-988

Association to Combat Huntington's
Chorea
108 Battersey High Street
London SW11 3HP
Tel: 071-223-7000

British Association of Myasthenics
Keynes House
Central Office
77 Nottingham Road
Derby DE1 3QS
Tel: 0332-290219

British Epilepsy Association
Anstey House
40 Hanover Square
Leeds LS3 1BE
Tel: 0345-089599

British Migraine Association
178a High Road
Byfleet
Weybridge
Surrey KT14 7ED
Tel: 0932-352468

Chest, Heart and Stroke Association
CHSA House
Whitecross Street
London EC1Y 8JJ
Tel: 071-490-7999

Committee on Safety of Medicines
Freepost
London SW8 5BR
Tel: 071-720-2188

Disability Alliance
25 Denmark Street
London WC2H 8NJ
Tel: 071-240-0806

Disabled Drivers Association
Ashwellthorpe House
Ashwellthorpe
Norwich NR16 1EZ
Tel: 0508-41449

Disabled Living Foundation
Equipment Centre
380–384 Harrow Road
London W9 2HU
Tel: 071-289-6111

Driver and Vehicle Licensing Centre
(DVLC)
Medical Advisory Branch
Oldway Centre
Orchard Street
Swansea SA1 1TU
Tel: 0792-782-341

Dystonia Society
Omnibus Workspace
39–41 North Road
Islington
London N7 9DP
Tel: 071-700-4594

Equipment for the Disabled
Mary Marlborough Lodge
Nuffield Orthopaedic Centre
Headington
Oxford OX3 7LD
Tel: 0865-750103

Friedreich's Ataxia Group
Copse Edge
Thursley Road
Elstead
Godalming
Surrey GU8 6DJ
Tel: 0252-702864

Guillain–Barré Support Group
'Foxley'
Holdingham
Sleaford
Lincs NG34 8NR
Tel: 0529-304615

LINK, The Neurofibromatosis Association
Surrey House, Office No. B09
34 Eden Street
Kingston-Upon-Thames
Surrey KT1 1ER
Tel: 081-547-1636

Medic-Alert Foundation
17 Bridge Wharf
156 Caledonian Road
London N1 9UU
Tel: 071-833-3034

The Migraine Trust
45 Great Ormond Street
London WC1N 3HD
Tel: 071-278-2676

Mobility Advice and Vehicle Information
    Service
Department of Transport
TRRL
Crowthorne
Berkshire
RG11 6AU
Tel: 0344-770456

Motor Neurone Disease Association
PO Box 246
Northampton MN1 2PR
Tel: 0604-22269/250505

The Multiple Sclerosis Society
25 Effie Road
London SW6 1EE
Tel: 071-736-6267/8

Muscular Dystrophy Association
Nattrass House
35 Macaulay Road
London SW4 0QP
Tel: 071-720-8055

National Society for Epilepsy
Chalfont Centre for Epilepsy
Chalfont St. Peter
Gerrards Cross
Bucks SL9 0RJ
Tel: 02407-3991

Parkinson's Disease Society
36 Portland Place
London W1N 3DG
Tel: 071-255-2432

Spastics Society
12 Park Crescent
London W1N 4EQ
Tel: 071-636-5020

Spinal Injuries Association
Yeoman House
76 St. James's Lane
London N10 3DF
Tel: 081-444-2121

SPOD
(Sexual & Personal Relationships of the
    Disabled)
286 Camden Road
London N7 0BJ
Tel: 071-607-8851

Tuberous Sclerosis Association of Great
    Britain
Little Bansley Farm
Milton Road
Catshill
Bromsgrove
Worcestershire B61 0NQ
Tel: 0527-71898

UK Association of Narcolepsy
South Hall
High Street
Farningham
Kent DA4 0DE
Tel: 0322-863195

Index

Page numbers in italic refer to tables and/or figures. Page numbers in bold refer to the main indications of drugs.